SAFETY AND HEALTH HANDBOOK FOR CYTOTOXIC DRUGS

SAMUEL J. MURFF

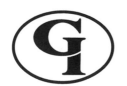

GOVERNMENT INSTITUTES
An imprint of The Scarecrow Press, Inc.
Lanham • Toronto • Plymouth, UK
2012

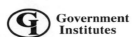 **Government Institutes**

Published by Government Institutes
An imprint of The Scarecrow Press, Inc.
A wholly owned subsidary of The Rowman & Littlefield Publishing Group, Inc.
4501 Forbes Boulevard, Suite 200, Lanham, Maryland 20706
www.rowman.com

10 Thornbury Road, Plymouth PL6 7PP, United Kingdom

British Library Cataloguing in Publication Information Available

Library of Congress Cataloging-in-Publication Data
Murff, Samuel J.
  Safety and health handbook for cytotoxic drugs / Samuel J. Murff.
     p. cm.
  Includes bibliographical references and index.
  ISBN 978-1-60590-704-8 (cloth : alk. paper)—ISBN 978-1-60590-705-5 (ebook)
  1. Antineoplastic agents—Safety measures—Handbooks, manuals, etc. 2. Drugs—Administration—Safety measures—Handbooks, manuals, etc. I. Title.
  RS431.A64M87 2012
  615.7'98—dc23   2011044657

♾™ The paper used in this publication meets the minimum requirements of American National Standard for Information Sciences—Permanence of Paper for Printed Library Materials, ANSI/NISO Z39.48-1992.

Printed in the United States of America

CONTENTS

Disclaimer

This publication is generated to distribute health, safety, and environmental data. To the best of our knowledge, the information contained herein is accurate. However, neither the author nor the publisher assumes any liability whatsoever for the accuracy or completeness of the information contained herein. Final determination of suitability of any material is the sole responsibility of the user. All materials may present unknown hazards and should be used with caution. Although certain hazards are described herein, we cannot guarantee that these are the only hazards that exist.

Furthermore, it is not a specification sheet and none of the displayed data should be construed as a specification. Information contained in the publication was obtained from sources which we believe are reliable, and we believe that the information is complete and accurate. However, the information is provided without any warranty, express or implied, regarding its correctness. Some of the information presented and conclusions drawn are from sources other than direct test data of the substance. The conditions or methods of handling, storage, medical monitoring, use, and disposal of the product are beyond our control and may also be beyond our knowledge. It is the user's responsibility to determine the suitability of any material for a specific purpose and to adopt such safety precautions as may be necessary.

Preface

You may be wondering how the concept of this manuscript handbook developed. Here is the story behind this manuscript.

Historically, most workers take hazard communications for granted when working with hazardous chemicals. Healthcare workers who are involved in cytotoxic drug transportation, preparation, storage, administration, spill cleanup, and disposal are asked routinely to handle these extremely hazardous chemicals (drugs) used in chemotherapy. But the occupational toxicological health effects of these drugs are not fully understood. And many do not know what precautions to take to reduce or eliminate occupational exposures or have the means to verify, by air or environmental sampling or by bioassay, that employees are not being overexposed. Safety and health information has always lagged behind the actual introduction of cytotoxic drugs into the healthcare workplace. No other occupations in America are allowed to work with extremely hazardous chemicals without the minimum safety and health information being made available to workers. The minimum safe guards and a means to detect overexposure are in place. All that is needed is information.

Cytotoxic drug contamination traces have been found in various places in the workplace environment, such as on the outside packages of cytotoxic drugs and in healthcare worker's urine. Several research papers and journal articles have alluded to the fact that some cytotoxic drugs, if opened in the workplace without using an approved biological safety cabinet, would immediately show up in the healthcare worker's urine. There is debate about what concentration of cytotoxic drugs detected in urine is harmful. But in most countries, dosing someone with anything without their permission and without any medical benefit is unlawful.

My experience working with cytotoxic drug safety and health issues started in a teaching medical center and medical college in the early 1990s. I was trying to resolve cytotoxic drug safety and health issues concerning exposure assessments, the installation and maintenance of proper engineering controls, selection of personal protective equipment, lack of toxicological health information, handling of incidents of employee exposures and spill cleanup, and employees' unexplained illnesses. Many of these issues were never completely resolved while I was employed there because of the lack of technical information and availability of resources—in other words, system-related problems.

Likewise, several years ago while being deployed on active duty in support of Operation Iraqi Freedom; I was involved with designing and conducting a cytotoxic drug program audit of various military community hospitals and medical centers. These audits revealed that the same safety and health cytotoxic drug issues from the 1990s existed across all hospitals visited regardless of size, and were still not being addressed by healthcare institutions even though new sources of information were available, such as research papers, journals, and regulatory documents.

During one of these audits, a nursing supervisor, who had just been through an employee cytotoxic drug exposure and spill incident that was handled improperly (from spill response and cleanup, occupational health consultation to employee hazard communications), made a suggestion. She said, "The nursing staff is willing to do the right thing, if they know the right thing to do. But do not expect them to be safety professionals because they are hired with the skill set to be expert care givers, not safety professionals."

Over the next several years the concept for this manuscript was developed and the manuscript was written using the most current technical information from research papers, journals, material safety data sheets, pharmaceutical product information, regulatory guidelines, proposed guidelines, and feedback from healthcare professionals to create a comprehensive reference that will resolve nearly all the systemic safety and health issues related to cytotoxic drugs.

This handbook is dedicated to all the hardworking healthcare professionals that I have enjoyed working with over the past thirty years that continued to provide exceptional healthcare services under adverse working conditions. This handbook is my first step in making the healthcare workplace a healthier one. Additional technical references covering program development, sampling strategies, sampling mythology, and environmental issues related to cytotoxic drugs worldwide will be forthcoming.

INTRODUCTION 1

Introduction to the Safety and Health Handbook for Cytotoxic Drugs

1.1. Introduction

Information provided in this handbook is intended only as a technical resource (refer to the disclaimer located at the beginning of the handbook). The user should first review the manufacturer's Material Safety Data Sheet (MSDS) before using other sources of information. The users should make their own investigations to determine the suitability of the information for their particular purposes. This handbook covers cytotoxic drugs and associated drugs used with chemotherapy. Furthermore, cytotoxic-antineoplastic drugs are only one segment of the classification "hazardous drugs" as defined by the Occupational Safety and Health Administration (OSHA). This handbook is just one reference of a set of three references designed to provide comprehensive references concerning every aspect of cytotoxic drugs from safety, health, and environmental aspects.

There is limited but increasing scientific evidence that personnel involved in the preparation and administration of parenteral cytotoxic-antineoplastic drugs may be at some risk due to potential mutegenicity, teratogenicity, and/or carcinogenicity of these agents. The toxicological properties of some cytotoxic drugs have been neither fully investigated, nor examined as it pertains to occupational exposure of workers. Often, there are no known safe established occupational exposure levels (OEL) to cytotoxic drugs. Based on the foregoing declaration, prudent safe work practices must be designed to reduce human exposure to the lowest level practicable, engineering controls, and personal protective equipment must be utilized to reduce potential exposure and environmental contamination levels to as low as reasonably achievable (ALARA). (Refer to 3.9, Rationale for Adopting the Environmental Sentinel Contamination Action Level [ESCAL] Concept.)

The Environmental Sentinel Contamination Action Level (ESCAL) is an analyte used routinely that has an analytical method and is the lowest feasible detection concentration of a drug based on the established analytic practical quantitation limit (PQL). A PQL is normally three to ten times the method detection limit (MDL) and is considered the lowest concentration that can be accurately measured, as opposed to just detected. If a PQL is not available for the specific method, use the level of detection (LOD) or the level of quantification (LOQ) until a PQL is established.

Sections 3.16, 3.17, and 3.18 contain internal and consensus occupational exposure limits/levels for cytotoxic drugs. Information contained in these sections can be reviewed and environmental sentinel contamination action levels may be chosen.

The Comprehensive Cytotoxic Drugs Table reviewed drugs based on individual aspect of exposure not in combination with other drugs (chemicals, substances, etc). Only the cytotoxic portion of a mixture was reviewed and listed in this table. Sections 2.2 and 2.3 contain registered trademark information.

The definition of "Target Organs/Systems" is defined a little differently than conventional definitions. Target Organs/Systems refers to not only chronic affects but also acute effects to organs and system. In some cases the clinical/therapeutic effects on organs and systems were listed under this heading (Target Organs/Systems).

1.2. Personnel Decontamination

Contamination of protective equipment or clothing, or direct skin or eye contact should be treated by:

> Immediately removing the contaminated clothing (gloves, gown, shoes, etc.). Place contaminated clothing into a closed container designed for chemotherapy (cytotoxic) drugs;
>
> Follow the general first aid guidance unless specific medical information is available from the chemical/drug MSDS or from other technical references (e.g., *Safety and Health Handbook for Cytotoxic Drugs*, section 2.0, Cytotoxic Drug Table);
>
> Employee and supervisor (if possible) should report to the emergency room with accident/incident paperwork and the Material Safety Data Sheets (MSDS) for the specific cytotoxic-antineoplastic drug(s) involved; if no MSDS is available or the required information is not on the MSDS then use the cytotoxic drug table found in Section 2.0 of this handbook.

1.3. Small Spills Cleanup

Small spills are less than 5 ml.

(*Note*: If no specific spill cleanup procedure is listed in attached cytotoxic table drug tables [refer to section 2.0], use general small spill cleanup procedures below.)

The 5-ml volume of material should be used to categorize spills as large or small. Spills of less than 5 ml or 5 gm outside an approved biological safety cabinet should be cleaned up immediately by trained personnel wearing appropriate PPE (e.g., gowns, shoe coverings, double cytotoxic gloves, and splash goggles/shield). An appropriate NIOSH-approved respirator (100 or better) should be used for either powder or liquid spills where airborne powder or aerosol is or has been generated. Please refer to section located below (or contact your local safety and health staff for assistance) for specific safety equipment and PPE requirements.

> Isolate the spill;
>
> Remove personnel and patients at risk of exposure to spill;
>
> Obtain MSDS for spilled substance(s), and check if soap and water are suitable for cleanup;
>
> Notify the safety manager or other designated points of contact (i.e., Industrial Hygiene, Occupational Health, etc.);
>
> Locate the chemotherapy/cytotoxic spill kit, which should be identified by a sign;
>
> Wearing appropriate PPE, use absorbent towels and pads included in the spill kit to absorb as much of the drug as possible. When available use specific spills response information provided in the MSDS or from other sources (e.g., this handbook);
>
> Place contaminated materials into plastic cytotoxic disposable bag obtained from spill kit;
>
> Place this bag inside labeled chemotherapy/cytotoxic waste bag obtained from spill kit;
>
> Use detergent and water, if applicable, otherwise use methods listed in attached Comprehensive Cytotoxic Drug Table (section 2.0) to wash surfacing in contact with cytotoxic drugs and place in labeled chemotherapy/cytotoxic waste bag;
>
> Use fresh detergent solution, if applicable, to clean equipment such as IV pumps, vital sign equipment, etc.;
>
> Place all cleaning and disposable PPE in the labeled chemotherapy/cytotoxic waste bag and seal bag with tie in kit;
>
> Place the bag inside the dedicated chemotherapy/cytotoxic container and keep secured until released for disposal as directed by your local procedure or policy.

1.4. Large Spills Cleanup

Large spills are greater than 5 ml.

(*Note*: If no specific spill cleanup procedure is listed in the cytotoxic drug tables [refer to section 2.0] for large spills, then use the general large spill cleanup procedures below.)

When a large spill occurs outside an approved biological safety cabinet (BSC), the affected area should be isolated and aerosol generation avoided. Most cytotoxic drugs are not volatile; however, this may not be true for all hazardous drugs.

Immediately remove personnel and patients from room;

All exposed or potentially exposed individuals should comply with personnel decontamination procedures (see above);

Secure area;

Turn off ventilation system; keep doors and windows closed if feasible;

Obtain MSDS for spilled substance(s); review manufacturers cleanup and neutralizing procedures, if information is provided on the MSDS;

Activate internal emergency response plan or notify appropriate emergency response organizations (fire department, safety manager, industrial hygiene, etc.);

Provide MSDS, deactivation/neutralizing solutions, and other relevant information (e.g., located in the Comprehensive Cytotoxic Drug Table located in section 2.0) to responders;

Monitoring should be performed (if available, retain in your facility) to verify decontamination is complete. Keep affected area closed until released by appropriate official. Documentation is retained in accordance with your local Hazardous Drugs Safety and Health plan.

1.5. Decontamination and Spill Cleanup in Biological Safety Cabinet (BSC)

All spills (large and small) occurring within a properly operating approved BSC dedicated to cytotoxic drugs should be dealt with as follows:

The cabinet should be cleaned according to the manufacture's instructions.

Some manufacturers have recommended weekly decontamination, as well as whenever spills occur, or when the cabinet requires moving, service, or certification.

Decontamination should consist of surface cleaning with water and detergent followed by thorough sensing. The use of detergent is recommended because there is no single accepted method of chemical deactivation/neutralization for all drugs involved. Quaternary ammonium cleaners should be avoided due to the possibility of vapor build-up in recirculated air. Ethyl alcohol (ethanol) or 70 percent isopropyl alcohol may be used with the cleaner if the contamination is soluble only in alcohol (refer to the MSDS and section 2.0 specific cytotoxic drug tables for chemical properties). Alcohol vapor build-up has also been a concern, so the use of alcohol should be avoided in BSCs where air is recirculated. Spray cleaners should also be avoided due to risk of spraying the HEPA filter. Ordinary decontamination procedures, which include fumigation with a germicidal agent, are inappropriate in a BSC for hazardous drugs (cytotoxic drugs) because such procedures do not remove or deactivate the drugs.

Removable work trays, if present, should be lifted in the BSC so the back and any sump below can be cleaned. During cleaning, the worker should wear PPE similar to that used for spills. Ideally, the sash should remain down during cleaning; however, a NIOSH-approved respirator appropriate for the hazard must be worn by the worker if the sash will be lifted during the process. The exhaust fan/blower should be left on. Cleaning should proceed from least to most contaminated areas. The drain spillage through area should be cleaned at least twice since it can become heavily contaminated. All materials from the decontamination process should be handled as HDs (hazardous drugs) and disposed of in accordance with federal, state, and local laws.

For additional information on barrier isolators, contact: CDC-NIOSH, OSHA

For additional information on barrier isolators manufacturers, contact your organization's safety and health personnel.

1.6. General First Aid Measures

(*Note*: If there are no specific first aid measures listed in the Comprehensive Cytotoxic Drug Table [refer to section 2.0], then use the general first aid measures below.)

Move victim to a safe area away from the spill. Always ensure that your safety is paramount—take prudent precautions to protect yourself and other personnel. Use substance specific technical/medical information from MSDS, SOPS, a regional poison center, and other reference materials, if readily accessible;

Call for medical/emergency assistance;

Give artificial respiration if not breathing;

Do not use mouth-to-mouth method if victim ingested or inhaled the substance/drug. Give artificial respiration with the aid of pocket-mask equipped with a one-way valve or other proper respiratory medical device;

Administer oxygen if breathing is difficult (if available and no ignition sources are present);

Remove and isolate contaminated clothing to include shoes;

In case of skin (dermal) contact with substance (drug), immediately flush skin with soap and cool running water for at least 20 minutes. Do not use solvents;

In case of eye contact with substance (drug), check for and remove any contact lenses, immediately flush eyes with plenty of water for at least 15 minutes, occasionally lifting the upper and lower lids;

In case of ingestion, wash out mouth with water provided person is conscious. Do not induce vomiting unless recommended by medical personnel or substance specific medical information, which may be found in section 2 of this handbook;

Keep victim warm and quiet; and keep victim under observation;

Effects of exposure (inhalation, ingestion, or skin contact) to substances may be delayed.

As needed, treat symptomatically if trained and qualified.

Ensure that medical personnel are aware of the substance(s) involved and take precautions to protect themselves.

1.7. Regional Emergency Contacts

Below are some of the regional emergency contacts that may be used in case of an emergency.

Occupational Safety and Health Administration (OSHA)

Additional information about exposure to hazardous drugs (cytotoxic drugs) is available online at www.osha.gov.

OSHA Regional and Area Offices

Region VI—AR, LA, NM, OK, TX
525 Griffin Street, Room 602, Dallas, TX 75202
(214) 767-4731 or (214) 767-4736 x224

Region VII—IA, KS, MO, NE
City Center Square, 1100 Main Street, Suite 800, Kansas City, MO 64105
(816) 426-5861

Region VIII—CO, MT, ND, SD, UT, WY
1999 Broadway, Suite 1690, Denver, CO 80202-5716
(303) 844-1600

Region IX—American Samoa, AZ, CA, HI, NV, Northern Mariana Islands
71 Stevenson Street, Room 420, San Francisco, CA 94105
(415) 975-4310

Region X—AK, ID, OR, WA
1111 Third Avenue, Suite 715, Seattle, WA 98101-3212
(206) 553-5930

OSHA Regional Offices
Region I—CT, ME, MA, NH, RI, VT
JFK Federal Building, Room E340, Boston, MA 02203
(617) 565-9860

Region II—NJ, NY, PR, VI
201 Varick Street, Room 670, New York, NY 10014
(212) 337-2378

Region III—DE, DC, MD, PA, VA, WV
The Curtis Center, 170 S. Independence Mall West, Suite 740 West, Philadelphia, PA 19106-3309
(215) 861-4900

Region IV—AL, FL, GA, KY, MS, NC, SC, TN
Atlanta Federal Center, 61 Forsyth Street, SW, Room 6T50, Atlanta, GA 30303
(404) 562-2300

Region V—IL, IN, MI, MN, OH, WI
230 South Dearborn Street, Room 3244, Chicago, IL 60604
(312) 353-2220

National Institute for Occupational Safety and Health (NIOSH)
Additional information about exposure to hazardous drugs is available at 1-800-35-NIOSH (1-800-356-4674); fax: 1-513-533-8573; e-mail: pubstaft@cdc.gov; website: www.cdc.gov/NIOSH.

1.8. Local Emergency Contacts
List your local emergency and safety contacts for quick reference in the space provided.

List of other local emergency contacts:

- Fire Department:

- Emergency Services:

- Safety and Health Personnel:

- Other:

1.9. Job Hazard Analysis/Job Safety Analysis (JHA/JSA)
A Job Hazard Analysis or Job Safety Analysis (JHA/JSA) process is the breaking down into its component parts of any method or procedure to determine the hazards connected with each key step and the requirements for performing it safely. Both the job hazard analysis and the job safety analysis will be considered interchangeable for the purpose of this publication. A JHA/JSA is required to determine what hazards are involved in the job/task being performed and to mitigate the identified hazards. One of the benefits that come out of this process is that this process will assist you in selecting the appropriate personal protective equipment and required engineering controls. Once this information is available, it should be formalized by placing this information on a Hazard Assessment Certification Form (refer to

section 3.8) and having it signed by the immediate supervisor or manager and briefed to employees. Another benefit is this information can be a valuable tool in training new employees and writing effective procedures.

The four basic stages in conducting a JHA/JSA are selecting the job/task to be analyzed, breaking the job/task down into a sequence of steps, identifying potential hazards, and determining preventive measures to overcome these hazards.

A job hazard analysis is an exercise in detective work. Your goal is to discover the following:

- What can go wrong?
- What are the consequences?
- How could it arise?
- What are other contributing factors?
- How likely is it that the hazard will occur?

A JHA/JSA form or chart (refer to section 3.6) can be developed to show the sequence of tasks, hazards, and preventive measures. Ideally, after you identify uncontrolled hazards, you will take steps to eliminate or reduce them to an acceptable risk level. Section 3.7 (PPE and Engineering Controls Listing for Cytotoxic Drugs) provide a quick reference list of personal protective equipment and engineering controls that are typically used in mitigating risks of handling, preparation, and administrating cytotoxic drugs (hazardous drugs). This listing should assist in completing the JHA and Hazard Certification forms (refer to sections 3.6 and 3.8) When hazards are mitigated to a lowest level risk possible than the task can be preformed safely using engineering control measures, personal protective equipment, administrative controls and/or substitution on a drug that is less hazardous to handle and administered.

Contact your organization's safety and health representatives or your regional Occupational Health and Safety Administrative office for assistance.

1.10. Selection Guidelines for Chemotherapy Gloves

Table 1.1 lists selection criterion and recommended guidelines necessary to select appropriate chemotherapy gloves.

A list of glove and personal protective equipment manufacturers is provided in section 3.5. Furthermore, manufacturer's breakthrough (permeation) times for certain gloves are depicted in section 3.4.

1.11. Recommended Respiratory Protection

Use respirators in accordance with OSHA (29 CFR 1910.134) and NOISH recommendations. Select particulate respirator filters in accordance with NIOSH (42 CFR 84). A respiratory protection program that meets OSHA's 29 CFR 1910.134 and ANSI Z88.2 requirements must be followed whenever workplace conditions warrant a respirator's use.

General information is provided in section 3.3 concerning respirator selection and use. Your local safety and health professional should assist you in the selection of appropriate respiratory protection based on existing or potential workplace hazards.

1.12. Specific Personal Protection Equipment (PPE) Requirements

Hazardous Drugs Operations Personal Protective Equipment Requirements

An unambiguous reference that contains information on the selection, use, and maintenance of personal protective equipment (PPE) required for hazardous drug operations/procedures are listed in USACHPPM TG 149, chapter 6, Personal Protective Equipment/OSHA Guidelines for Hazardous Drugs. This reference is available on the internet and was particularly designed for healthcare facilities. Additional information is available in sections 3.3 and 3.5.

Your local safety and health professional should assist you in the selection of appropriate PPE based on existing or potential workplace hazards.

Table 1.1. Recommended Chemotherapy Gloves Selection Guidelines*

Selection Criterion for Gloves	Oncology Nursing Society, 2nd edition, 1997	American Society of Health-System Pharmacists (ASHP) (1990)	Occupational Safety and Health Administration (OSHA)	Recommended Guidelines
Thickness and Miscellaneous Selection Criteria	Thickness, contact time, and latex sensitivity	Fingertip thickness, fit, length, tactile sensation, and latex sensitivity	Thickness more important than type of material	Use recommended specific gloves when provided on the MSDS by the drug manufacturer and/or data provided by the glove manufacturer based on the following selection criterion:
Ambidextrous or Hand-Specific	Not specified	Hand-specific (surgical) for better fit and tactile sensation, particularly in drug preparation area	Not specified	User specified
Thickness (at Fingertips)	0.007 inches or 0.178 mm (ASTM minimum 0.10 mm)	Not specified, but surgical glove is recommended (ASTM minimum 0.10 mm; thicker fingertips considered optimal)	Not specified; however, thickness of glove is more important than the type of material	User specified
Powder-Free	Yes	Yes; if powder-free is unavailable, then the outside of a powdered glove should be washed before use	Minimal or no powder preferred because powder may absorb any spilled hazardous material	No powder preferred because powder may absorb any spilled hazardous material/drug
Glove Material Recommendation	Latex or nitrile; PVC only as a double glove beneath latex glove, if necessary for latex allergy; subject to manufacturer test data	Latex	Latex, unless manufacturer specifically stipulates that some other glove provides better protection	Use chemotherapy gloves with specifications that meet or exceed breakthrough time, permeation rate, and degradation rating as specified by the manufacturer for specific chemotherapy drug(s) of interest Avoid latex because of allergy implications
Length	Long enough to be worn under and/or over the cuffs of a gown	Long enough to be worn under and/or over the cuffs of a gown	Long enough to be worn under and/or over the cuffs of a gown	Long enough to be worn under and/or over the cuffs of a gown
Specific Breakthrough Times for Specific Chemotherapy Drug	Not specified	Not specified	Not specified	Minimum: 60 minutes Optimal: more than 120 minutes
Permeation Rate	Not specified	Not specified	Not specified	Not specified
Degradation	Not specified	Not specified	Not specified	Select the highest glove rating for various chemotherapy drugs used in the workplace

(continued)

Table 1.1. (*Continued*)

Selection Criterion for Gloves	Oncology Nursing Society, 2nd edition, 1997	American Society of Health-System Pharmacists (ASHP) (1990)	Occupational Safety and Health Administration (OSHA)	Recommended Guidelines
Double Gloving	Yes, due to variability in permeation within and between glove lots	Yes, unless evidence shows that a single glove is sufficiently protective	Yes, due to variability in permeation within and between glove lots	Yes, due to variability in permeation within and between glove lots, and as a safety factor in case of the outer glove fails
Glove Change Frequency	Hourly or when damaged or contaminated	Hourly, between batches, or when damaged or contaminated	Hourly or when damaged or contaminated	At least hourly, between batches, when damaged or contaminated, or when glove manufacturer's testing specifications permit a longer period of use
Hand Wash Frequency	Before and after donning	Before and after donning	Before and after donning	Before and after donning

*Some of the selection criterion depicted for chemotherapy gloves may be used for selection of aprons and other chemotherapy drug resistant garments. The primary selection criterion for aprons and other garments should be the specific breakthrough times for specific chemotherapy drugs that are transported, prepared, handled, administered, and disposed of in the workplace.

1.13. General Cytotoxic Drugs Medical Surveillance Recommendations

Cytotoxic-Antineoplastic Drugs Medical Surveillance

In accordance with prudent industrial hygiene practices, Technical Guide 149, chapter 4, and other guidance documents, all employees working with cytotoxic drugs (CDs) (transporting, preparation, administrating, waste disposal, storage, cytotoxic drugs spill cleanup, and equipment maintenance or certification) will receive medical surveillance (before working with cytotoxic drugs, periodically and post cytotoxic drugs employment) through your local occupational health service. There are other occasions that medical surveillance may be necessary such as acute exposure to CDs and pregnancy/reproductive decisions.

Typically, medical surveillance consists of a pre-placement and transfer or termination examinations, and subsequently a periodic examination. Medical screening examination as part of a comprehensive surveillance program is one of several tools aimed at protecting workers who are exposed or potentially exposed to hazardous substances in the workplace. Medical surveillance programs are designed based on workplace hazards and are preventative in nature. Medical surveillance testing that looks for damage is *not* a substitute for controlling exposure through use of engineering and safe work practices.

Another medical surveillance requirement is to document workers acute exposures to hazardous materials, and to established and maintain an employee registry documenting who handle CDs. This register should be maintained. Furthermore, in all cases, employee should carefully fill out a specific medical history questionnaire for potential hazards found in their workplace. The primary source of information should be the manufacturer's Material Safety Data Sheet (MSDS) that sometimes contains essential information on suggested medical screening tests, health hazards engineering controls, and PPE selection and use. Listed below are some of the typical baseline tests:

Typical minimum baseline medical testing includes:

- Medical history questionnaire based on potential workplace hazards;
- Hematology;
- Complete blood count (HGB, HCT, WBW, MCV, MCH, MCHC);
- Differential white blood cell count;
- Urinalyses with microscopic or equivalent test.

Depending on potential workplace hazards and/or preexisting health problems, additional medical testing may be warranted.

Typical supplementary medical testing or medical examinations include:

- Pregnancy tests
- Reproductive tests
- Kidney function test
- Liver function test
- EKG and cardiovascular examination
- Examination of the eyes and vision
- Examination of eyes, ears, and nails
- Examination of skin periodically for abnormal growths
- Examination of the nervous system

All employees with potential exposure to hazardous substances to include cytotoxic drugs (CDs) must receive OSHA Hazard Communication training along with other specific safety and health training designated by your supervisor or safety officer. Contact your local safety and health professional for additional information and assistance.

Specific medical surveillance information is included in section 2.1 when provided by the manufacturer and other technical sources.

1.14. Recommended Engineering Controls—Biological Safety Cabinets and Barrier Isolators

In section 3.11 a detailed discussion of engineering controls is provided. Use of engineering controls can reduce or eliminate occupational exposure to cancer chemotherapy drugs in the workplace and are considered necessary to reduce exposures to as low as reasonable achievable (ALARA). This section discussion entails closed-system devices, locking systems, glovebags, needleless systems, special sharp containers, isolator barriers, and biological safety cabinets.

1.15. Unique Occupational Safety and Health Act Compliance Issues

It is not the purpose of this handbook to provide a comprehensive overview of Occupational Safety and Health Act compliance process but there are two unique areas that are of significant importance to the hazardous drugs program that they will be mentioned; the General Duty Clause and Material Safety Data Sheet (MSDS) containing specific personal protective equipment and engineering control requirements.

OSHA's General Duty Clause

The OSHA's General Duty Clause 29 U.S.C 654 5(a)1 states: "Each employer shall furnish to each of his employees employment and a place of employment which are free from recognized hazards that are causing or are likely to cause death or serious physical harm to his employees."

Furthermore, it states in 29 U.S.C 654 5(a)2: "Each employer shall comply with occupational safety and health standards promulgated under this act and 29 U.S.C 654 5(b). Each employee shall comply with occupational safety and health standards and all rules, regulations, and orders issued pursuant to this Act which are applicable to his own actions and conduct."

In other words, once the hazard in the workplace is known it must be abated even if not written in OSHA standards. This principle can also be traced back to labor and compensation laws; and the no fault compensation law if safety and health rules are followed.

MSDS Specific Requirements

As part of the Hazard Communication Standard, MSDSs, are required to be maintained on site, readily available to workers, and workers are trained accordingly to information contained on the MSDS provided by the manufacturer. Section 3.12 provides an introduction to applied toxicology that will enhance the use of MSDS information. Section 3.19 contains a table that summarizes hazards associated with antineoplatic drugs. This table is ideal for providing hazard communication training to employees. In sections 3.14 and 3.15 various hazard information systems (DOD, HMIS, and NFPA) are discussed. Furthermore, an MSDS discussion is provided in section 3.13 on how to read and understand MSDS. Only two sections will be discuss; the personal protection equipment (PPE) and engineering controls sections.

The MSDS PPE sections provide recommendations for personal protective equipment such as respiratory, eye protection, chemical gloves, and other safety equipment. Let's provide a hypothetical example to demonstrate a potential problem. A manufacturer stated on the MSDS that a self-contained breathing apparatus must be worn while preparing and administering the cytotoxic drug (Brand X). The standard of practice in most hospitals is to provide a P100 respirator to employees while preparing Brand X cytotoxic drug. An OSHA compliance officer arrives to perform an inspection of the worksite. The compliance officer asks for the MSDSs for all cytotoxic drugs. While observing the preparation and administering of cytotoxic drugs, the compliance officer notices that P100 respirators were used by employees and that all employees have been placed on the organization's respiratory protection program and medical surveillance was started. While reviewing the MSDS for Brand X cytotoxic drug, the compliance officer notices that the manufacturer requires a higher respiratory protection then that is being used by the hospital staff (P100). This situation could result in a compliance action being taken against the hospital because of the manufacturer's recommendation for specific respiratory protection was not implemented. Ideally, any disagreement with the manufacturer information contained within a MSDS should be addressed before OSHA compliance inspection, not during an inspection.

Another situation that has been happening in the recent past, whereby an OSHA compliance officer reviewed MSDSs for cytotoxic drugs being prepared and administered by the hospital staff. The manufacturer recommended a higher level of biological hood then was being used by the hospital. The compliance officer started compliance actions against the hospital for not making available the appropriate engineering controls to mitigate risks to an acceptable level. Ideally, a disagreement with the manufacturer information contained within an MSDS should be addressed before OSHA compliance inspection, not during an inspection.

Sections 3.20 and 3.21 will provide guidance in performing an assessment of areas that prepare, administer, handle, transport, and store hazardous drugs (cytotoxic drugs), while section 3.21 also provides information on nine cytotoxic drugs that are considered hazardous wastes in the United States.

A

ABATACEPT (*a-BAY-ta-sept*)
ORENCIA®1 (oh-REN-see-ah)

Abstract Chemical Service (CAS) Registry
Number: 332348-12-6
National Drug Code Number: 0003 2187 10

Health & Safety Hazards/US Department of Transportation (DOT)/US Environmental Protection Agency (EPA)—Sources
Not otherwise specified

Administration: ABATACEPT is for infusion into a vein.

First Aid Medical Information/ Occupational Exposure Limits
First Aid Measures to include: Use general first aid measures except for the following:

- Symptoms of an overdose
  Ingestion: Not otherwise specified
  Physician's note: Not otherwise specified
  Medical Information: Not otherwise specified
  Caution and Warning Statements: Not otherwise specified
  Routes of entry: Not otherwise specified
  Target Organs/Systems: Not otherwise specified
  Medical Conditions Generally Aggravated by Exposure: Not otherwise specified
  Specific Medical: Not otherwise specified
  Surveillance Information: Not otherwise specified
  Occupational Exposure Level/Limit (OEL) & Sampling Methods: Not otherwise specified
  Environmental Sentinel Contamination Action Level (ESCAL): Not otherwise specified

Supplemental Response Information
Extinguishing Media: Not otherwise specified. Use extinguishing agent which is the most appropriate to extinguish surrounding fire (carbon dioxide, foam, dry chemical or water fog as extinguishing media).
Solubility: ABATACEPT (ORENCIA®1) is reconstituted with sterile water (no other information is available).
Chemical Degradation/Neutralization Method: Not otherwise specified
> **Note**: If a specific degradation or neutralization method is not provided in this section and you do not have other specific information that will guide you on how to clean up the specific material spilled, then follow the general spill procedure found in the introduction section of this handbook.

Incompatibility: Not otherwise specified

ACLARUBICIN (Free Base) (ak-la-ru-bee-sin)
ACLACINOMYCIN®34

Chemical Abstract Service (CAS) Registry
Number: 57576-44-0
Registry of Toxic Effects of Chemical Substances
(RTECS): QI9279300
National Cancer Institute: NSC208734
$C_{42}H_{53}NO_{15}$

ACLARUBICIN HYDROCHLORIDE

Chemical Abstract Service (CAS) Registry
Number: 75443-99-1

Registry of Toxic Effects of Chemical Substances (RTECS): QI9283500

$C_{42}H_{54}ClNO_{15}$

$C_{42}-H_{53}-N-O_{15}$

$C_{42}-H_{53}-N-O_{15}\cdot CLH$

Health & Safety Hazards/US Department of Transportation (DOT)/US Environmental Protection Agency (EPA)—Sources

Mutagen—University of Maryland at College Park, Mutagen—Toxic Material Safety Data Sheet, Teratogen—University of Maryland at College Park, Reproductive Effector—Material Safety Data Sheet, Reproductive Effector—Toxic Material Safety Data Sheet, Toxic—Material Safety Data Sheet, Irritant—Material Safety Data Sheet, Permeator—Material Safety Data Sheet, Vesicant—Administration, National Fire Protection Association Hazard Rating Health (2) Flammability (0) Instability/Reactivity (1)—Material Safety Data Sheet, National Fire Protection Association Hazard Rating Health (3) Flammability (1) Instability/Reactivity (0)—Material Safety Data Sheet, Hazardous Materials Identification System (R) and/or US Department of Defense System Health (3★) with additional chronic hazard present Reactivity (1) Reactivity (0) Personal Protective Code (E) (Safety Glasses, Chemical Gloves, Dust Respirator)—Material Safety Data Sheet, Hazardous Materials Identification System (R) and/or US Department of Defense System Health (2) Fire Hazard (0) Reactivity (1) Personal Protective Code (None stated)—Material Safety Data Sheet, Hazardous Materials Identification System (R) and/or US Department of Defense System Health (2★) with additional chronic hazard present Fire Hazard (0) Reactivity (1)—Material Safety Data Sheet. UN 2811 Class 6.1.

ACLACINOMYCIN®34 is a yellow or orange solid.

ACLARUBICIN is an anthracycline antineoplastic antibiotic isolated from streptomyces galilaeus.

First Aid Medical Information/ Occupational Exposure Limits

First Aid Measures to include: Use general first aid measures.

Medical Information: Not otherwise specified

Caution and Warning Statements: Toxic by inhalation, in contact with skin and if swallowed.

ACLARUBICIN (ACLACINOMYCIN®34) is harmful if absorbed through skin or if swallowed. This drug is very hazardous in case of skin contact (permeator). Severe exposure can result in death. Ingestion may be fatal. It is a primary irritant and may be a reproductive effector. The toxicity of this drug has not been thoroughly investigated.

ACLARUBICIN is an oligosaccharide anthracycline antineoplastic antibiotic isolated from the bacterium streptomyces galilaeus. ACLARUBICIN intercalates into DNA and interacts with topoisomerases I and II, thereby inhibiting DNA replication, repair, RNA, and protein synthesis. ACLARUBICIN is antagonistic to other agents that inhibit topoisomerase II, such as ETOPOSIDE, TENIPOSIDE and AMSACRINE. This agent is less cardiotoxic than DOXORUBICIN and DAUNORUBICIN.

Caution: Females and males planning to have a child, pregnant women, and nursing mothers should exercise caution regarding potential occupational exposure to this cytotoxic drug. No information or not enough information exists or was provided concerning occupational exposure that may potentially occur while handling this drug and its affects on reproductive systems, the fetus, and/or if it is secreted along with breast milk, which may harm nursing infants. Staff members should consult with the occupational health physician monitoring workers' health in your facility to be apprised of potential hazards and should be advised to avoid becoming pregnant and/or breastfeeding or should be transferred in accordance with policy/procedures to other duties that do not involve preparation, handling, and administering this drug.

Therapeutic Levels: Safe use of ACLARUBICIN in pregnancy has not been established. There are no adequate and well-controlled studies in pregnant women. Women of childbearing age should be advised to avoid becoming pregnant if they are under treatment or the potential for occupational exposure.

Target Organs/Systems: Heart and gastrointestinal tract

Medical Conditions Generally Aggravated by Exposure:

- Repeated exposure to a highly toxic material may produce general deterioration of health by an accumulation in one or more human organs.
- Reproductive and pregnancy issues.

Specific Medical Surveillance Information: Reproductive and pregnancy counseling.

Medical surveillance should include a complete blood count and an EKG.

Occupational Exposure Level/Limit (OEL) & Sampling Methods: Not otherwise specified

Environmental Sentinel Contamination Action Level (ESCAL): Not otherwise specified

Supplemental Response Information

Extinguishing Media: Use extinguishing agent which is the most appropriate to extinguish surrounding fire (carbon dioxide, foam, dry chemical or water fog as extinguishing media).

Solubility: ACLARUBICIN (ACLACINOMY-CIN®34) is partly soluble to soluble in methanol, chloroform, and ethyl acetate. ACLARUBICIN HCL is soluble in ethanol and chloroform (pH = 6.2).

Chemical Degradation/Neutralization Method: The International Agency for Research on Cancer recommends treating spill surfaces with a 5.25% sodium hypochlorite (bleach) solution after absorbing liquids with inert absorbent pads or removing any powder present: allow solution to stand for up to one hour, and then thoroughly wash spilled surfaces with soap and water; sample to determine if surface contamination is still present (if sampling method is available). If drug is still present, repeat above steps; dispose of wastes in accordance with your local procedures, state, and federal regulations.

Incompatibility: ACLARUBICIN is incompatible with strong oxidizing agents.

ADRIAMYCIN (ay-dre-ah-MI-sin)
DOXORUBICIN (DOCKS-e-ROU-bi-sin) (For Free Base)

> Chemical Abstract Service (CAS) Registry
>   Number: 23214-92-8
> Registry of Toxic Effects of Chemical Substances
>   (RTECS): AV9800000
> National Cancer Institute: NSC123127
> $C_{27}H_{29}NO_{11}$

ADRIAMYCIN with hydrochloride

> Chemical Abstract Service (CAS) Registry
>   Number: 25316-40-9 (Mixture)
> Registry of Toxic Effects of Chemical Substances
>   (RTECS): QI9295900
> $C_{27}-H_{29}-NO_{11}.HCl$

Health & Safety Hazards/US Department of Transportation (DOT)/US Environmental Protection Agency (EPA)—Sources

Carcinogen G2A—International Agency For Research On Cancer, Carcinogen C2—US National Toxicology Program, Carcinogen—University of Maryland at College Park, Carcinogen—Material Safety Data Sheet, Possible-Carcinogen—Occupational Safety and Health Administration, Teratogen—University of Maryland at College Park, Teratogen—Material Safety Data Sheet, Embryotoxic—Material Safety Data Sheet, Reproductive Effector—Material Safety Data Sheet, Highly Toxic—Material Safety Data Sheet, Mutagen—Material Safety Data Sheet, Mutagen—University of Maryland at College Park, Lactation Immune Suppression & Concentrated In Human Milk—US Navy, Pregnancy Category (D)—Administration, Sensitizer—Material Safety Data Sheet, Cytotoxic—British Columbia Cancer Agency Canada, Vesicant—Material Safety Data Sheet, Carcinogen and Reproductive Effector Male—US California State Proposition 65, National Fire Protection Association Hazard Rating of Health (2) Flammability (1) Instability/Reactivity (0)—Material Safety Data Sheet, National Fire Protection Association Hazard Rating Health (2) Flammability (0) Instability/Reactivity (0)—Material Safety Data Sheet, National Fire Protection Association Hazard Rating Health (2) Flammability (0) Instability/Reactivity (1)—Material Safety Data Sheet, Hazardous Materials Identification System (R) and/or US Department of Defense System Health (2★) with additional chronic hazard present Fire Hazard (0) Reactivity (1) Personal Protection Code (-) (None stated)—Material Safety Data Sheet; Hazardous Materials Identification System (R) and/or US Department of Defense System Health (3) Fire Hazard (0) Reactivity (0) Personal Protective Code (X) (Ask Supervisor)—Material Safety Data Sheet.

DOXORUBICIN HYDROCHLORIDE is a red-orange, hydroscopic crystalline powder

DOXORUBICIN HCL is a red fluid (10 mg, 20 mg, 50 mg, and 200 mg).

(UV fluorescence at 465 nm, emitting orange-red light in the 580 nm range)

DOXORUBICIN: Breastfeeding is contraindicated; concentrated in human milk, with possible immune suppression, avoid breastfeeding.

First Aid Medical Information/ Occupational Exposure Limits

First Aid Measures to include: Use general first aid measures except for the following:

Ingestion: If victim is conscious and alert, rinse mouth and drink 2-4 cups of milk or water. Do not induce vomiting.

Physician's note: Treatment of acute overdosage consists of treatment of the severely myelosuppressed patient with hospitalization, antibiotics, platelet and granulocyte transfusions, and symptomatic treatment of mucositis. For ingestion, consider gastric lavage.

Medical Information: Not otherwise specified

Caution and Warning Statements:

DOXORUBICIN HCL (ADRIAMYCIN) may cause cancer, heritable genetic damage and may cause harm to the unborn child. Material may have myelo-suppression cardiotoxicity effects. Exposure may cause pigmentation of skin and may cause respiratory and digestive tract irritation. Contact with eyes may cause chemical conjunctivitis. Exposure may cause nausea, vomiting and diarrhea, delayed pulmonary edema, and allergic skin reaction. It is advisable to avoid exposure to ADRIAMYCIN during pregnancy. Overexposure may cause discoloration of urine. British Columbia Cancer Agency lists doxorubicin as a vesicant.

DOXORUBICIN HYDROCHLORIDE is a cytotoxic agent and hydrochloride a potential human carcinogen. All work practices must be designed to reduce human exposure to the lowest level. Registry of Toxic Effects of Chemical Substances (RTECS) lists DOXORUBICIN HYDROCHLORIDE as a suspected carcinogen and as a cardiovascular or blood toxicant.

Caution: Females and males planning to have a child, pregnant women, and nursing mothers should exercise caution regarding potential occupational exposure to this cytotoxic drug. No information or not enough information exists or was provided concerning occupational exposure that may potentially occur while handling this drug and its affects on reproductive systems, the fetus, and/or if it is secreted along with breast milk, which may harm nursing infants. Staff members should consult with the occupational health physician monitoring workers' health in your facility to be apprised of potential hazards and should be advised to avoid becoming pregnant and/or breastfeeding or should be transferred in accordance with policy/procedures to other duties that do not involve preparation, handling, and administering this drug.

Therapeutic Levels: Food and Drug Administration lists this drug as a Pregnancy Category (D). Safe Use of DOXORUBICIN in pregnancy has not been established. DOXORUBICIN is embryotoxic and teratogenic in rats; and embryotoxic and abortifacient in rabbits. There are no adequate and well-controlled studies in pregnant women.

Target Organs/Systems: Heart, kidneys, liver, blood, bone marrow, gastrointestinal tract, immune systems, nerves, male reproductive systems, skin, head, and possibly fetus

Medical Conditions Generally Aggravated by Exposure:

- Repeated exposure to a highly toxic material may produce general deterioration of health by an accumulation in one or many human organs.

- DOXIL (DOXORUBICIN HCL liposome injection) is contraindicated in patients who have a history of hypersensitivity reactions to a conventional formulation of DOXORUBICIN HCL or the components of DOXIL; heart problems, liver disorders, and muscular system disorders.
- Reproductive and pregnancy issues.

Specific Medical Surveillance Information: Reproductive and pregnancy counseling.

Medical surveillance should include a complete blood count, EKG, and examination of the nervous system.

Occupational Exposure Level/Limit (OEL) & Sampling Methods: Not otherwise specified

Environmental Sentinel Contamination Action Level (ESCAL): Air, Surface

Supplemental Response Information

Extinguishing Media: Use extinguishing agent which is the most appropriate to extinguish surrounding fire (carbon dioxide, foam, dry chemical or water fog as extinguishing media). (Do not use water jet.)

Solubility: ADRIAMYCIN is water soluble (10 mg/ml in water) (pH = 3 to 7.2) and is slightly soluble in methanol and aqueous alcohols. However, ADRIAMYCIN is insoluble in acetone, chloroform, and benzene.

Chemical Degradation/Neutralization Method: A manufacturer's Material Safety Data Sheet and the International Agency for Research On Cancer recommends treating spill surfaces with a 5.25% sodium hypochlorite (bleach) solution after absorbing liquids with inert absorbent pads or removing any powder present: allow solution to stand for up to one hour, and then thoroughly wash spilled surfaces with soap and water; sample to determine if surface contamination is still present (if sampling method is available). If drug is still present, repeat above steps; dispose of wastes in accordance with your local procedures, state, and federal regulations.

Incompatibility: ADRIAMYCIN (DOXORUBICIN) is incompatible with strong oxidizing agents.

ALDESLEUKIN (*al-des-LOO-kin*)
PROLEUKIN®2

Chemical Abstract Service (CAS) Registry Number: 110942-02-4
Registry of Toxic Effects of Chemical Substances (RTECS): NM9744500

L2-7001

$C_{690}-H_{1115}-N_{177}-O_{202}-S_6$

Health & Safety Hazards/US Department of Transportation (DOT)/US Environmental Protection Agency (EPA)—Sources

Cytotoxic—British Columbia Cancer Agency Canada, Nonvesicant—British Columbia Cancer Agency Canada, Pregnancy Category (C)—US Food and Drug Administration, Potent Mitogenic Agent—Material Safety Data Sheet, Hazardous Materials Identification System (R) and/or US Department of Defense System Health (1) Fire Hazard (1) Reactivity (0) Personal Protection Code (-) (None stated)—Material Safety Data Sheet, National Fire Protection Association Hazard Rating Health (1) Flammability (1) Instability/Reactivity (0)—Material Safety Data Sheet.

PROLEUKIN®2 powders used to make a fluid for injection.

First Aid Medical Information/ Occupational Exposure Limits

First Aid Measures to include: Use general first aid measures except for the following:

Ingestion: If ingestion of this product occurs, flush mouth with water and consult a physician. Induce vomiting only if professional medical attention is not available. Never induce vomiting with an unconscious person.

Physician's note: If symptoms occur, treat the symptoms, while alleviating the cause.

Medical Information: Not otherwise specified

Caution and Warning Statements:

Note: ALDESLEUKIN is one of the drugs that has little occupational hazards information. Therefore, therapeutic dose information was extrapolated below.

PROLEUKIN®2 is a potent mitogenic agent (capable of causing rapid and uncontrolled cell growth).

Caution: The toxicity of this drug has not been fully investigated, particularly with respect to occupational exposure. ALDESLEUKIN is one of the drugs that has little occupational hazard information available. Therefore, therapeutic dose information was extrapolated below to assist in determining occupational toxicity, and signs and symptoms of overexposure. Furthermore, it is prudent to minimize occupational exposure to ALDESLEUKIN. Some of the most common side effects from therapeutic protocol of ALDESLEUKIN are vomiting, loss of appetite, tiredness, weakness, general feeling of being unwell (malaise), headache, diarrhea, and dry skin.

Other possible side effects from therapeutic doses of ALDESLEUKIN are constipation, confusion, changes in mood, dizziness; changes in your vision, taste, or speech; muscle or bone aches, pains in the chest, abdomen, or back; weight gain, retaining water, and pain or redness at the site of injection; mouth blistering and fatigue. The potential for exposure is usually reduced in finished pharmaceutical form such as capsules and tablets; therefore, occupational exposure should be significantly lower than with therapeutic doses and severity of symptoms should be reduced. Exposure to ALDESLEUKIN may cause unusual bruising or bleeding, bleeding from the rectum, extreme sleepiness or tiredness, difficulty breathing, wheezing, yellowing of the skin or eyes, problems with urinating, itching or red rash, and fever chills or shaking. Avoid skin contact, eye contact, inhalation, and ingestion. Use appropriate prudent practices and administrative procedures to prevent opportunities for direct contact with the skin, eyes and/or to prevent inhalation.

Caution: Females and males planning to have a child, pregnant women, and nursing mothers should exercise caution regarding potential occupational exposure to this cytotoxic drug. No information or not enough information exists or was provided concerning occupational exposure that may potentially occur while handling this drug and its affects on reproductive systems, the fetus, and/or if it is secreted along with breast milk, which may harm nursing infants. Staff members should consult with the occupational health physician monitoring workers' health in your facility to be apprised of potential hazards and should be advised to avoid becoming pregnant and/or breastfeeding or should be transferred in accordance with policy/procedures to other duties that do not involve preparation, handling, and administering this drug.

Therapeutic Levels: The Food and Drug Administration lists this drug as a Pregnancy Category (C); (PROLEUKIN®2) has been shown to have embryo lethal effects in rats when given in doses at 27 to 36 times the human dose (scaled by body weight). Significant maternal toxicities were observed in pregnant rats administered (PROLEUKIN®2) by IV injection at doses 2.1 to 36 times higher than the human dose during critical period of organogenesis. No evidence of teratogenicity was observed other than that attributed to maternal toxicity. There are no adequate well-controlled studies of (PROLEUKIN®2) in pregnant women.

Target Organs/Systems: Heart, blood, fetus, and hematologic system

Medical Conditions Generally Aggravated by Exposure:

- Individuals who are sensitive to yeast should be especially careful when using (PROLEUKIN®2).
- Notify occupational health if you have had heart, lung, brain, kidney, liver, or autoimmune disease. Therapeutic dose exposure to ALDESLEUKIN has caused patients to be more sensitive to contrast dyes which are given to improve the pictures taken from x-rays or other scans. If planning to become pregnant contact your occupational health provider.
- Reproductive and pregnancy issues.

Specific Medical Surveillance Information: Reproductive and pregnancy counseling.

The most common side effect of ALDESLEUKIN is a decrease in the number of blood cells. A complete blood count with differentials may be used to monitor the blood.

Occupational Exposure Level/Limit (OEL) & Sampling Methods: Not otherwise specified

Environmental Sentinel Contamination Action Level (ESCAL): Not otherwise specified

Supplemental Response Information

Extinguishing Media: Use extinguishing agent which is the most appropriate to extinguish surrounding fire (carbon dioxide, foam, dry chemical or water fog as extinguishing media).

Solubility: ALDESLEUKIN is reconstituted with sterile water (water soluble); pH range from 7.2 to 7.8 (in reconstituted product).

Chemical Degradation/Neutralization Method:

A manufacturer's Material Safety Data Sheet recommends using alkaline soap/detergent and water to clean spill surfaces after absorbing liquids with inert absorbent pads or removing any powder present: repeat using soap and water at least three times; sample to determine if surface contamination is still present (if sampling method is available at your facility). If drug is still present, repeat above steps; dispose of wastes in accordance with your local procedures, state, and federal regulations.

Incompatibility: (PROLEUKIN®2) is not compatible with strong oxidizers.

ALEMTUZUMAB (*ay-lem-TOO-zuh-mab*) (CAMPATH®3) GENZYME CORP (BAYER SCHERING PHARMA)

Chemical Abstract Service (CAS) Registry Number: 216503-57-0 (Mixture)
$C_{6468}H_{10066}N_{1732}O_{2005}S_{40}$

Health & Safety Hazards/US Department of Transportation (DOT)/US Environmental Protection Agency (EPA)—Sources

Cytotoxic—British Columbia Cancer Agency Canada, Nonvesicant—British Columbia Cancer Agency Canada, Pregnancy Category (C)—US Food and Drug Administration, Reproductive Effector Male—Material Safety Data Sheet.

(CAMPATH®3) a solution for injection (10 mg/ml; 30 mg/ml).

First Aid Medical Information/ Occupational Exposure Limits

First Aid Measures to include: Use general first aid measures except for the following: Not otherwise specified

Medical Information: Not otherwise specified

Caution and Warning Statements:

Note: ALEMTUZUMAB is one of the drugs that has little occupational hazards information available. Therefore, therapeutic dose information was extrapolated below.

Caution: The toxicity of most cytotoxic drugs have not been fully investigated, particularly as it pertains to occupational exposure. ALEMTUZUMAB is one of the drugs that has little occupational hazards information available. Therefore, therapeutic dose information was extrapolated below to assist in determining occupational toxicity, and signs and symptoms of overexposure.

Furthermore, it is prudent to minimize occupational exposure to ALEMTUZUMAB. This material may cause heritable genetic damage. Exposure may cause fetal harm.

Symptoms of overdose (overexposure) are chest tightness, coughing, inability to urinate, shortness of breath, and troubled breathing. Avoid skin contact, eye contact, inhalation, and ingestion. Use appropriate prudent practices and administrative procedures to prevent opportunities for direct contact with the skin, eyes, and/or to prevent inhalation. Exposure may cause serious or fatal depression of the immune system and may cause low blood pressure, coldness, fever, shortness of breath, coughing, chills, rash, nausea, vomiting, fatigue, headache, and/or diarrhea.

Caution: Females and males planning to have a child, pregnant women, and nursing mothers should exercise caution regarding potential occupational exposure to this cytotoxic drug. No information or not enough information exists or was provided concerning occupational exposure that may potentially occur while handling this drug and its affects on reproductive systems, the fetus, and/or if it is secreted along with breast milk, which may harm nursing infants. Staff members should consult with the occupational health physician monitoring workers' health in your facility to be apprised of potential hazards and should be advised to avoid becoming pregnant and/or breastfeeding or should be transferred in accordance with policy/procedures to other duties that do not involve preparation, handling, and administering this drug.

Therapeutic Levels: The Food and Drug Administration lists this drug as a Pregnancy Category (C). Animal reproduction studies have not been conducted with (CAMPATH®3). It is not known whether (CAMPATH®3) can affect reproductive capacity or cause fetal harm when administered to a pregnant woman. However, human IgG is known to cross the placental barrier and therefore (CAMPATH®3) may cross the placental barrier and cause fetal B and T lymphocyte depletion. Nursing mothers, excretion of (CAMPATH®3) in human breast milk has not been studied. This material may cause heritable genetic damage. Exposure may cause fetal harm. Because many drugs including human IgG are excreted in human milk, breastfeeding should be discontinued during treatment and for at least three months following the last dose of (CAMPATH®3).

Target Organs/Systems: Bone marrow, blood, lymphatic system, immune, reproductive systems, and fetus

Medical Conditions Generally Aggravated by Exposure:

Note: ALEMTUZUMAB is one of the drugs that has little occupational hazards information available. Therefore, therapeutic dose information was extrapolated below.

- Notified occupational health if you have ever been treated with radiation or cancer medicines. Exposure to ALEMTUZUMAB may increase the effects of the exposure (ALEMTUZUMAB) on the blood.
- Other present or past medical problems that should be reported to occupational health are chickenpox (including recent exposure) or herpes zoster (shingles)—risk of severe disease affecting other parts of the body, heart disease—increased risk of low blood pressure, monitor blood pressure during therapy, bone marrow depression or infection—risk increased or worsening of infection by ALEMTUZUMAB, and immune deficiency condition—HIV infection may increase the risk of side effects of ALEMTUZUMAB.
- Reproductive and pregnancy issues.

Specific Medical Surveillance Information: Reproductive and pregnancy counseling.

Occupational Exposure Level/Limit (OEL) & Sampling Methods:

Environmental Sentinel Contamination Action Level (ESCAL): Not otherwise specified

Supplemental Response Information

Extinguishing Media: Use extinguishing agent which is the most appropriate to extinguish surrounding fire (carbon dioxide, foam, dry chemical or water fog as extinguishing media).

Solubility: (CAMPATH®3) is aqueous and completely miscible with water and has a pH range of 6.8–7.4.

Chemical Degradation/Neutralization Method:

Note: If a specific degradation or neutralization. Method is not provided in this section and you do not have other specific information that will guide you on how to clean up the specific material spilled, then follow the general spill procedure found in the introduction section of this handbook.

Incompatibility: Not otherwise specified

ALIMTA®4
PEMETREXED (PEM-e-TREX-ed)
ALIMTA®4

Chemical Abstract Service (CAS) Registry Number: 150399-23-8 (mixture 50% and 50% mannitol 69-65-8)
$C_{20}H_{19}N_5Na_2O_6 \cdot 7H_2O$

Health & Safety Hazards/US Department of Transportation (DOT)/US Environmental Protection Agency (EPA)—Sources

Mutagen—Material Safety Data Sheet, Irritant—Material Safety Data Sheet, Reproductive Effector—Material Safety Data Sheet, Antineoplastic Agent—Wikipedia.org, Pregnancy Category (D)—US Food and Drug Administration, National Fire Protection Association Hazard Rating Health (2) Flammability (1) Instability/Reactivity (0) with a special warning Reproductive—Material Safety Data Sheet, Lactation may be harmful to a nursing infant, breastfeeding is not recommended—US Navy.

A white to either light yellow or green-yellow lyophilized solid. Each 500-mg vial of (ALIMTA®4) contains PEMETREXED DISODIUM equivalent to 500 mg PEMETREXED and 500 mg of mannitol).

First Aid Medical Information/ Occupational Exposure Limits

First Aid Measures to include: Use general first aid measures except for the following:

Symptoms of an overdose: (ALIMTA®4) May include blood problems, sores in the mouth, rash, inflammation of mucous membranes, fatigue, fetal effects, reproductive, and diarrhea.

Ingestion: Do not induce vomiting. Call a physician or poison control center. If available, administer activated charcoal (6–8 heaping teaspoons) with 2–3 glasses of water. Do not give anything by mouth to an unconscious person. Immediately transport to a medical care facility and see a physician.

Physician's note: PEMETREXED DISODIUM—If overdose occurs, general supportive measures should be instituted as deemed necessary by the treating physician. Management of PEMETREXED overdose should include consideration of the use of leucovorin or thymidine rescue.

Medical Information:

Caution and Warning Statements:

Warning: PEMETREXED (ALIMTA®4) is a mutagen and may impair fertility. Furthermore, it may cause harm to the unborn child with possible risk of irreversible effects. PEMETREXED DISODIUM for injection alters genetic material and may be an irritant to the eyes and skin. Effects of exposure may include reproductive tissue changes, fetal changes, decreased fetal weight, decreased offspring survival, deceased blood cell counts, and lymphoid tissue and bone marrow changes.

Routes of Entry: Inhalation and skin contact.

Toxicological data is limited.

Target Organs/Systems: White blood cell counts, mild anemia, intestinal lesions, decreased testes weights with decreased sperm production and decreased red blood cells (animal studies)

Medical Conditions Generally Aggravated by Exposure: Not otherwise specified

Specific Medical Surveillance Information: Not otherwise specified

Occupational Exposure Level/Limit (OEL) & Sampling Methods:

Environmental Sentinel Contamination Action Level (ESCAL): Not otherwise specified

PEMETREXED (ALIMTA®4) exposure guide:

- 0.3 micrograms/m3 TWA for 8 or 12 hours
- 3.6 micrograms/m3 for no more than a total of 30 minutes (excursion limit)

Method: Not otherwise specified

Supplemental Response Information

Extinguishing Media: Use extinguishing agent which is the most appropriate to extinguish surrounding fire (carbon dioxide, foam, dry chemical or water fog as extinguishing media).

Solubility: PEMETREXED (ALIMTA®4) is water soluble.

Chemical Degradation/Neutralization Method: Not otherwise specified

Note: If a specific degradation or neutralization method is not provided in this section and you do not have other specific information that will guide you on how to clean up the specific material spilled, then follow the general spill procedure found in the introduction section of this handbook.

Incompatibility: ALTRETAMINE is incompatible with strong oxidizing agents (e.g., peroxides, permanganates, nitric acid, etc).

ALTRETAMINE (*al-TRET-a-mean*)
HEXALEN®5

Chemical Abstract Service (CAS) Registry Number: 645-05-6
Registry of Toxic Effects of Chemical Substances (RTECS): OS1050000
National Cancer Institute: NSC13875
$C_9H_{18}N_6$

Health & Safety Hazards/US Department of Transportation (DOT)/US Environmental Protection Agency (EPA)—Sources

Tumorigenic—Material Safety Data Sheet, Toxic—Material Safety Data Sheet, Mutagen—Material Safety Data Sheet, Reproductive Effector—Material Safety Data Sheet, Carcinogen—Material Safety Data Sheet, Pregnancy Category (D)—US Food and Drug Administration, Developmental Male—US California State Proposition 65, National Fire Protection Association Hazard Rating Health (2) Flammability (0) Instability/Reactivity (0)—Material Safety Data Sheet, Hazardous Materials Identification System (R) and/or US Department of Defense System Health (2★) with additional chronic hazard present Fire Hazard (0) Reactivity (0) Personal Protective Code (–) (None stated)—Material Safety Data Sheet.

ALTRETAMINE is available as 50 mg transparent capsules; a white crystalline powder.

ALTRETAMINE: Breastfeeding discontinue (facts and comparisons).

First Aid Medical Information/ Occupational Exposure Limits

First Aid Measures to include: Use general first aid measures.

Medical Information:

Caution and Warning Statements:

Toxic: Male reproductive toxicity. The Registry of Toxic Effects of Chemical Substances (RTECS) lists ALTRETAMINE as a suspected cardiovascular or blood toxicant; as a gastrointestinal or liver toxicant; and as a skin or sense organ toxicant. Used as a chemosterilant (pesticide).

Clinical/Therapeutic Levels: Protocol may cause anemia or other blood problems, fatigue, bleeding, bruising, fever and chills, anxiety, confusion, dizziness, weakness, and loss of balance or coordination, numbness or tingling in the arms and legs, diarrhea. Side effects that are more common are dizziness, drowsiness, mood changes, nausea, and vomiting.

ALTRETAMINE is an irritant; avoid contact with skin and mucous membranes (micromedex).

Caution: Females and males planning to have a child, pregnant women, and nursing mothers should exercise caution regarding potential occupational exposure to this cytotoxic drug. No information or not enough information exists or was provided concerning occupational exposures that may potentially occur while handling this drug and its affects on reproductive systems, the fetus, and/or if it is secreted along with breast milk, which may harm nursing infants. Staff members should consult with the occupational health physician monitoring workers' health in your facility to be apprised of potential hazards and should be advised to avoid becoming pregnant and/or breastfeeding or should be transferred in accordance with policy/procedures to other duties that do not involve preparation, handling, and administering this drug.

Therapeutic Levels: Protocol suggests ALTRETAMINE should not be used during pregnancy because it may cause birth defects. When using this drug, a reliable method of birth control is recommended. It is not recommended to breastfeed infants because ALTRETAMINE passes into breast milk and may harm the nursing infant.

Target Organs/Systems: Central nervous system, male reproductive systems, blood, bone marrow, immune system, and possibly fetus

Medical Conditions Generally Aggravated by Exposure:

- Clinical/therapeutic: Caution is advised when taking ALTRETAMINE. Consult your doctor if you have any of the following conditions: bone marrow depression, chicken pox, shingles, any infection, or reduced kidney function.
- Alcohol intake should be limited while taking this drug.
- Reproductive and pregnancy issues.

Specific Medical Surveillance Information: Reproductive and pregnancy counseling.

Clinical/therapeutic protocol suggests peripheral blood counts should be monitored at least monthly prior to the initiation of each course of (HEXALEN®5), and as clinically indicated. Because of the possibility of (HEXALEN®5) related neurotoxicity, neurological examination should be performed.

Occupational Exposure Level/Limit (OEL) & Sampling Methods: Not otherwise specified

Environmental Sentinel Contamination Action Level (ESCAL): Not otherwise specified

Supplemental Response Information

Extinguishing Media: Use extinguishing agent which is the most appropriate to extinguish surrounding fire (carbon dioxide, foam, dry chemical or water fog as extinguishing media).

Solubility: ALTRETAMINE (HEXALEN®5) (HEMEL) is insoluble in water but is increasingly soluble at pH 3 and below.

Chemical Degradation/Neutralization Method: Not otherwise specified

Note: If a specific degradation or neutralization method is not provided in this section and you do not have other specific information that will guide you on how to clean up the specific material spilled, then follow the general spill procedure found in the introduction section of this handbook.

Incompatibility: ALTRETAMINE is incompatible with strong oxidizing agents.

AMINOGLUTETHIMIDE

(ah-mee-no-gloo-TEH-tha-mide)
DL-AMINOGLUTETHIMIDE (CYTADREN®6)

Chemical Abstract Service (CAS) Registry
    Number: 125-84-8
Registry of Toxic Effects of Chemical Substances
    (RTECS): MA4026950
$C_{13}H_{16}N_2O_2$

Health & Safety Hazards/US Department of Transportation (DOT)/US Environmental Protection Agency (EPA)—Sources

Teratogen—University of Maryland at College Park, Suspect Teratogen—Sax's "Dangerous Properties of Industrial Materials," Administration Pregnancy Category (D)—US Navy, Developmental—US California State Proposition 65 and US California Environmental Protection Agency, National Fire Protection Association Hazard Rating Health (2) Flammability (0) Instability/Reactivity (0), Hazardous Materials Identification System (R) and/or US Department of Defense System Health (2★) with additional chronic hazard present Fire Hazard (0) Reactivity (0)—Material Safety Data Sheet.

AMINOGLUTETHIMIDE can cause fetal harm (facts and comparisons); breastfeeding discontinue; reproductive and developmental hazards (*A Guide for Occupational Health Professionals Technical Manual*, Navy Environmental Health Center [NEHC-TM-OEM 6260.01a]).

First Aid Medical Information/ Occupational Exposure Limits

First Aid Measures to include: Use general first aid measures.

Medical Information:

Caution and Warning Statements:

Caution: AMINOGLUTETHIMIDE toxicity has not been fully investigated. AMINOGLUTETHIMIDE is an irritant, irritating to eyes, respiratory

system, and skin. The Registry of Toxic Effects of Chemical Substances (RTECS) listed AMINOGLUTETHIMIDE as a suspected cardiovascular or blood toxicant and as a respiratory toxicant.

Masculinization of the female fetus has been reported.

Pregnancy: AMINOGLUTETHIMIDE has been shown to cause birth defects in humans and animals. However, this medicine may be needed in serious diseases or in other situations that threaten the mother's life. In addition, AMINOGLUTETHIMIDE has been shown to cause fertility problems in animals. Be sure you have discussed this with your doctor before being exposed to this medicine. Breastfeeding—it is not known whether AMINOGLUTETHIMIDE passes into breast milk. However, this medicine has not been reported to cause problems in nursing babies.

Target Organs/Systems: Adrenal cortex, blood, thyroid, eyes, respiratory system, fetus, and skin

Medical Conditions Generally Aggravated by Exposure:

- AMINOGLUTETHIMIDE blocks the synthesis of adrenal steroid hormones and the physiological conversion of androgens to estrogens
- Reproductive and pregnancy issues.

Specific Medical Surveillance Information: Reproductive and pregnancy counseling.

Occupational Exposure Level/Limit (OEL) & Sampling Methods: Not otherwise specified

Environmental Sentinel Contamination Action Level (ESCAL): Not otherwise specified

Supplemental Response Information

Extinguishing Media: Use extinguishing agent which is the most appropriate to extinguish surrounding fire (carbon dioxide, foam, dry chemical or water fog as extinguishing media).

Solubility: AMINOGLUTETHIMIDE is practically water insoluble, but freely soluble in most organic solvents (Merck).

Chemical Degradation/Neutralization Method: Not otherwise specified

Note: If a specific degradation or neutralization method is not provided in this section and you do not have other specific information that will guide you on how to clean up the specific material spilled, then follow the general spill procedure found in the introduction section of this handbook.

Incompatibility: AMINOGLUTETHIMIDE (CYTADREN®6) is incompatible with strong oxidizing agents.

AMSACRINE (*AM-sah-creen*)

AMSIDINE (M-AMSA)

AMSA P-D®7

ACRIDINYLANISIDIDE

Chemical Abstract Service (CAS) Registry
Number: 51264-14-3
Registry of Toxic Effects of Chemical Substances
(RTECS): PB1080000
$C_{21}H_{19}N_3O_3S$

AMSACRINE HCL (*AM-sah-creen*)

Chemical Abstract Service (CAS) Registry
Number: 54301-15-4
$C_{21}H_{19}N_3O_3S.HCL$
Registry of Toxic Effects of Chemical Substances
(RTECS): PB1081000

Health & Safety Hazards/US Department of Transportation (DOT)/US Environmental Protection Agency (EPA)—Sources

Carcinogen G2B—International Agency or Research on Cancer, Toxic—Material Safety Data Sheet, Cytotoxic—British Columbia Cancer Agency Canada, Mutagen—University of Maryland at College Park, Moderate Skin Irritant—Material Safety Data Sheet, Vesicant—British Columbia Cancer Agency Canada, National Fire Protection Association Hazard Rating Health (2) Flammability (0) Instability/Reactivity (0), Hazardous Materials Identification System (R) and/or US Department of Defense System Health (2★) with additional chronic hazard present Fire Hazard (0) Reactivity (0)—Material Safety Data Sheet, National Fire Protection Association Hazard Rating Health (3) Flammability (1) Instability/Reactivity (0)—Material Safety Data Sheet, Hazardous Materials Identification System (R) and/or US Department of Defense System Health (3) Fire Hazard (1) Reactivity (0) Personal Protective Code (E) (Safety Glasses, Chemical Gloves, Dust Respirator), UN 2811, CLASS 6.1, GROUP III.

AMSACRINE is an orange/red color fluid.

(UV Detection: 254 nm; Color Unknown, 265 nm)

First Aid Medical Information/ Occupational Exposure Limits

First Aid Measures to include: Use general first aid measures except for the following:

Dermal contact: After flushing skin for at least 20 minutes with water, cover the irritated skin with an emollient and seek medical assistance.

Medical Information:
Caution and Warning Statements:

Toxic: AMSACRINE is identified as a possible human carcinogen because of sufficient evidence from experimental studies. AMSACRINE may cause skin, eye, mucous membranes, and upper respiratory irritation. AMSACRINE is toxic if swallowed and harmful if inhaled. It is very hazardous to skin and is a permeator. The embryotoxicity have not been thoroughly investigated. British Columbia Cancer Agency lists AMSACRINE as a vesicant.

Signs and symptoms of exposure to AMSACRINE are moderate skin irritation (urticaria), headache, lightheadedness, nausea, and malaise. Gastrointestinal disturbances have occurred. This drug is toxic by inhalation. This drug is toxic by inhalation, in contact with skin, and if swallowed. This drug is irritating to eyes, respiratory system, and skin.

Caution: Females and males planning to have a child, pregnant women, and nursing mothers should exercise caution regarding potential occupational exposure to this cytotoxic drug. No information or not enough information exists or was provided concerning occupational exposure that may potentially occur while handling this drug and its affects on reproductive systems, the fetus, and/or if it is secreted along with breast milk, which may harm nursing infants. Staff members should consult with the occupational health physician monitoring workers' health in your facility to be apprised of potential hazards and should be advised to avoid becoming pregnant and/or breastfeeding or should be transferred in accordance with policy/procedures to other duties that do not involve preparation, handling, and administering this drug.

Therapeutic Levels: Pregnancy studies on effects in pregnancy have not been done in either humans or animals. Before receiving AMSACRINE make sure, your doctor knows if you are pregnant or if you may become pregnant. It is best to use some kind of birth control while you are receiving AMSACRINE. Tell your doctor right away if you think you have become pregnant while receiving AMSACRINE. Breastfeeding—AMSACRINE is not recommended during breast-feeding, because it may cause unwanted effects in nursing babies.

Target Organs/Systems: Liver, eyes, upper respiratory, GI tract, mucous membranes, skin, and fetus

Medical Conditions Generally Aggravated by Exposure:

- The toxicity of this drug has not been thoroughly investigated. Repeated exposure to a highly toxic material may produce general

deterioration of health by an accumulation in one or more human organs.
- Reproductive and pregnancy issues.

Specific Medical Surveillance Information: Reproductive and pregnancy counseling.

Occupational Exposure Level/Limit (OEL) &Sampling Methods: Not otherwise specified

Environmental Sentinel Contamination Action Level (ESCAL): Not otherwise specified

Supplemental Response Information

Extinguishing Media: Use extinguishing agent which is the most appropriate to extinguish surrounding fire (carbon dioxide, foam, dry chemical or water fog as extinguishing media).

Solubility: AMSACRINE is reported to be water insoluble and to be water soluble and dmso soluble (10 mg/ml).

Chemical Degradation/Neutralization Method: The International Agency for Research on Cancer recommends treating spill surfaces with a 5.25% sodium hypochlorite (bleach) solution after absorbing liquids with inert absorbent pads or removing any powder present: allow solution to stand for up to one hour, and then thoroughly wash spilled surfaces with soap and water; sample to determine if surface contamination is still present (if sampling method is available). If drug is still present, repeat above steps; dispose of wastes in accordance with your local procedures, state, and federal regulations.

Incompatibility: AMSACRINE is incompatible with strong oxidizing agents. Protect from light.

ANASTROZOLE (*an-AS-troe-zole*)
ARIMIDE
AMIMIDEX®8

Chemical Abstract Service (CAS) Registry
 Number: 120511-73-1
Registry of Toxic Effects of Chemical Substances
 (RTECS): CZ1465000
$C_{17}H_{19}N_5$

Health & Safety Hazards/US Department of Transportation (DOT)/US Environmental Protection Agency (EPA)—Sources

Non-cytotoxic—Material Safety Data Sheet, Fetotoxic—Material Safety Data Sheet, Pregnancy Category (D)—US Food and Drug Administration

ANASTROZOLE are available in white 1 mg tablets.

First Aid Medical Information/ Occupational Exposure Limits

First Aid Measures to include: Use general first aid measures except for the following:

Physician's note: Symptomatic treatment and supportive therapy as indicated. For additional information, consult the prescribing information.

Medical Information:

Caution and Warning Statements:

ANASTROZOLE: There is positive evidence of human fetal risk (Food and Drug Administration Pregnancy Category [D]). Breastfeeding is not recommended due to potential secretion into breast milk (British Columbia Cancer Agency Canada). (Occupational references are not available.)

Caution: Females and males planning to have a child, pregnant women, and nursing mothers should exercise caution regarding potential occupational exposure to this cytotoxic drug. No information or not enough information exists or was provided concerning occupational exposure that may potentially occur while handling this drug and its affects on reproductive systems, the fetus, and/or if it is secreted along with breast milk, which may harm nursing infants. Staff members should consult with the occupational health physician monitoring workers' health in your facility to be apprised of potential hazards and should be advised to avoid becoming pregnant and/or breastfeeding or should be transferred in accordance with policy/procedures to other duties that do not involve preparation, handling, and administering this drug.

Therapeutic Levels: There are no adequate and well-controlled studies in pregnant women using ARIMIDEX. ARIMIDEX (ANASTROZOLE) can cause fetal harm when administered to a pregnant woman. ANASTROZOLE has been found to cross the placental barrier following oral administration of 0.1 mg/kg in rats and rabbits (about 1 and 1.9 times the recommended human dose, respectively, on a mg/m² basis). Studies in both rats and rabbits at doses equal to or greater than 0.1 and 0.02 mg/kg/day, respectively (about 1 and 1/3, respectively, the recommended human dose on a mg/m² basis), administered during the period of organogenesis showed that ANASTROZOLE increased pregnancy loss (increased pre- and/or post-implantation loss, increased resorption, and decreased numbers of live fetuses); effects were dose related in rats. Placental weights were significantly increased in rats at doses of 0.1 mg/kg/day or more.

Evidence of fetotoxicity, including delayed fetal development (i.e., incomplete ossification [bone formation] and depressed fetal body weights), was observed in rats administered doses of 1 mg/kg/day (which produced plasma ANASTROZOLE C_{SSMAX} and $AUC_{0-24\,HR}$ that were 19 times and 9 times higher than the respective values found in postmenopausal volunteers at the recommended dose). There was no evidence of teratogenicity in rats administered doses up to 1.0 mg/kg/day. In rabbits, ANASTROZOLE caused pregnancy failure at doses equal to or greater than 1.0 mg/kg/day (about 16 times the recommended human dose on a mg/m^2 basis); there was no evidence of teratogenicity in rabbits administered 0.2 mg/kg/day (about 3 times the recommended human dose on a mg/m^2 basis).

Target Organs/Systems: Fetus

Medical Conditions Generally Aggravated by Exposure:

- Reproductive and pregnancy issues.

Specific Medical Surveillance Information: Reproductive and pregnancy counseling.

Occupational Exposure Level/Limit (OEL) & Sampling Methods:

Environmental Sentinel Contamination Action Level (ESCAL): Not otherwise specified
ANASTROZOLE Occupational Exposure Level/Limit (OEL): Astrazeneca Labs
0.0001 MG/M3 Time-Weighted Average (TWA) Company (Astrazeneca) Occupational Exposure Level/Limit (OEL)
(Method not listed or specified)

Supplemental Response Information

Extinguishing Media: Use extinguishing agent which is the most appropriate to extinguish surrounding fire (carbon dioxide, foam, dry chemical or water fog as extinguishing media).

Solubility: ANASTROZOLE has moderate aqueous solubility (0.5 mg/ml at 25°c); solubility is independent of pH in the physiological range. ANASTROZOLE is freely soluble in methanol, acetone, ethanol, and tetrahydrofuran, and very soluble in acetonitrile. (Water solubility unknown.)

Chemical Degradation/Neutralization Method: Not otherwise specified

Note: If a specific degradation or neutralization method is not provided in this section and you do not

have other specific information that will guide you on how to clean up the specific material spilled, then follow the general spill procedure found in the introduction section of this handbook.

Incompatibility: Not otherwise specified

ARSENIC TRIOXIDE
(*ar-se-nik tri-OX-side*)
TRISENOX®9

Chemical Abstract Service (CAS) Registry Number: 1327-53-3
Registry of Toxic Effects of Chemical Substances (RTECS): CG3325000
As_4O_3

Health & Safety Hazards/US Department of Transportation (DOT)/US Environmental Protection Agency (EPA)—Sources

Carcinogen G1—International Agency for Research on Cancer, Carcinogen C1—US National Toxicology Program–New Jersey Department of Health and Senior Services Hazardous Substances Fact Sheet and Material Safety Data Sheet, Carcinogen—Occupational Safety and Health Administration, Carcinogen TLV-G-A1—American Conference of Governmental Industrial Hygienists, Carcinogen—Occupational Safety and Health Administration, Carcinogen—US National Institute for Occupational Safety and Health, Carcinogen—Berkeley University Hazardous Chemical List, Teratogen—University of Maryland at College Park, Teratogen—Material Safety Data Sheet, Mutagen—Material Safety Data Sheet, Acute Toxic—University of Maryland at College Park, Highly Toxic—Material Safety Data Sheet, Fetotoxic—Material Safety Data Sheet, Sensitizer—Material Safety Data Sheet, Cytotoxic—Box Instructions, Pregnancy Category (D)—US Food and Drug Administration, United States, Carcinogen and Developmental—US California State Proposition 65—Mc, National Fire Protection Association Hazard Rating Health (3) Flammability (0) Instability/Reactivity (0), National Fire Protection Association Hazard Rating Health (3) Flammability (0) Instability/Reactivity (2), Hazardous Materials Identification System (R) and/or US Department of Defense System Health (3★) with additional chronic hazard present Fire Hazard (0) Reactivity (0), Personal Protective Code (-)(None stated), Hazardous Materials Identification System (R) and/or US Department of Defense System Health (3) Fire Hazard (0) Reactivity (0) Personal Protective Code (E) (Safety

Glasses, Chemical Gloves, Dust Respirator), US California State Environmental Protection Agency Listed, MIDI: HW01—(http://usaphcapps.amedd.army.mil/midi), UN 1561, Class 6.1, Group II, Poison B, SARA Title III 313, P012, Poison B.

TRISENOX®9 solution is available for injection (1 mg/ml).

ARSENIC TRIOXIDE is a white or transparent, glossy amorphous lumps or crystalline powder.

First Aid Medical Information/ Occupational Exposure Limits

First Aid Measures to include: Use general first aid except for the following:

Ingestion: Acute toxic; contact a poison control center if swallowed. Induce vomiting immediately as directed by medical personnel. Treat symptomatically and supportively. The estimated lethal dose is 120 milligrams.

Physician's note (A): If emesis if unsuccessful after two doses of ipecac, consider gastric lavage. Monitor urine ARSENIC level. Alkalization of urine may help prevent disposition of red cell breakdown products in renal tubular cells. If acute exposure is significant, maintain high urine output and monitor volume status, preferably with central venous pressure line. Abdominal x-rays should be done routinely for all ingestions. Chelation therapy with BAL, followed by n-penicillamine is recommended, but specific dosing guidelines are not clearly established.

Physician's note (B): The following antidote has been recommended. However, the decision as to whether the severity of poisoning requires administration of any antidote and actual dose required should be made by qualified medical personnel.

ARSENIC poisoning antidote: give Dimercaprol, 3 mg/kg (or 0.3 ml/kg) every 4 hours for 2 days and then 2 mg/kg every 2 hours for a total of 10 days. Dimercaprol is available as a 10% solution in oil for intramuscular administration. Next, give penicillamine, up to 100 mg/kg/day (maximum 1 g/day) divided into 4 doses for no longer than 1 week. If a longer administration period is warranted, dosage should not exceed 40 mg/kg/day. Give the drug orally half an hour before meals. Discontinue antidote when urine arsenic level falls below 50 ug/24 hr. (Dreisbach, *Handbook of Poisoning*, 12th ed.). Antidote should be administered by qualified medical personnel.

Physician's note (C): If swallowed, give gastric lavage followed by saline cathartic. Force fluids intake and give Dimercaprol (BAL) in recommended dosages as appropriate.

Medical Information:

Caution and Warning Statements: ARSENIC TRIOXIDE (TRISENOX®9) is considered a cancer hazard. Risk of cancer depends on duration and level of exposure. Material is considered super toxic. Ingestion is harmful and may be fatal. This drug is toxic by inhalation, and in contact with skin, may causes burns. Prolonged or repeated exposure may cause allergic reactions (sensitization) in certain sensitive individuals. Avoid prolonged or repeated exposure. Exposure may cause liver and kidney damage, and may cause blood abnormalities.

Exposure to ARSENIC TRIOXIDE may cause nausea, vomiting, paralysis, and gastrointestinal irritation. Inhalation of vapors may cause headache, nausea, dizziness, drowsiness, irritation of respiratory tract, and loss of consciousness.

Caution: Females and males planning to have a child, pregnant women, and nursing mothers should exercise caution regarding potential occupational exposure to this cytotoxic drug. No information or not enough information exists or was provided concerning occupational exposures that may potentially occur while handling this drug and its affects on reproductive systems, the fetus, and/or if it is secreted along with breast milk, which may harm nursing infants. Staff members should consult with the occupational health physician monitoring workers' health in your facility to be apprised of potential hazards and should be advised to avoid becoming pregnant and/or breastfeeding or should be transferred in accordance with policy/procedures to other duties that do not involve preparation, handling, and administering this drug.

Therapeutic Levels: ARSENIC TRIOXIDE (TRISENOX®9) may pass through the placental barrier in human and may affect genetic materials. Furthermore, this drug may cause adverse reproductive (paternal and maternal effects as well as fetotoxicity or post implantation mortality) and birth defects (Teratogen).

Target Organs/Systems: GI system, heart, liver kidneys, peripheral nervous system, skin, lungs, lymphatic system, bone marrow, fetus, and red blood cells

Medical Conditions Generally Aggravated by Exposure:

- Drinking alcohol can increase the liver damage caused from exposure to ARSENIC TRIOXIDE.
- Some scientists believe that skin changes such as thickening and pigment changes make those skin areas more susceptible to skin cancer.
- Repeated or prolonged exposure to the substance can produce target organs damage.

Repeated exposure to a highly toxic material may produce general deterioration of health by an accumulation in one or more human organs.
- Repeated exposure to a highly toxic material may produce general deterioration of health by an accumulation in one or more human organs.
- Reproductive and pregnancy issues.

Specific Medical Surveillance Information: Reproductive and pregnancy counseling.

Employees with frequent or potentially high exposure (half the TLV or greater), the following medical tests are recommended:

- Examination of the nose, eyes, nails and nervous system. Test urine for arsenic levels (this is most accurate at the end of a workday). Eating shellfish or fish may elevate arsenic levels for up to two days. National Institute for Occupational Safety And Health recommends arsenic levels in urine should not be greater than 100 micrograms per liter of urine.
- Medical surveillance of nervous system; test for urine ARSENIC levels (National Institute for Occupational Safety and Health recommends exposure levels, urine ARSENIC should not be greater than 100 micrograms per liter of urine), liver and kidney functions test, and examination of your skin periodically for abnormal growths.
- Liver and kidney functions tests.
- Examination of abnormal skin growths by a trained specialist.

Occupational Exposure Level/Limit (OEL) & Sampling Methods:

Environmental Sentinel Contamination Action Level (ESCAL): Not otherwise specified
US Occupational Safety and Health Administration (OSHA):
0.010 mg/m3 (AS)
Action level 5 µg/m3 Time-Weighted Average (TWA) 8-hrs (AS)
(Refer to 29 CFR 1910.1018)
US National Institute for Occupational Safety and Health (NIOSH) Recommended Exposure Limit:
Ceiling 0.002 mg/m3 (AS)/15 min; CARCINOGEN
US National Institute for Occupational Safety and Health (NIOSH) Immediately Dangerous to Life or Health:

5 mg/m3 inorganic AG compounds CARCINOGEN
US Department of Energy's (DOE) Temporary Emergency Exposure Limits (s):
TEEL3: 9.1 mg/m3
Canada: Time-Weighted Average (TWA) 0.05 (mg(AS)/m3)
US American Conference of Governmental Industrial Hygienists (ACGIH):
TLV: 0.01 mg/m3 Time-Weighted Average (TWA); CARCINOGEN—Confirmed Human CA)
Biological Exposure Indices issued (2004)
UK MEL (Maximum Exposure Limit): 0.1 mg/m3 Time-Weighted Average (TWA)
MAK: CARCINOGEN Category 1; germ cell mutagen group: 3A
(DFG 2004)(Germany)
Measurement Method: Particulate filter; acid; hydride generation atomic absorption spectrometry; National Institute for Occupational Safety and Health IV #7900; also #7300, elements.
US Occupational Exposure Level/Limit (OEL)—US Environmental Protection Agency (EPA) AEGLS:
ARSENIC TRIOXIDE. 0.1 mg/m3 AG3 TRK (Inhalable Dust Fraction)

Acute Exposure Guideline Levels (AEGLS) (Proposed)

(mg/m3)

	10 min	30 min	60 min	4 hr	8 hr
AEGL 1	NR	NR	NR	NR	NR
AEGL 2	3.7	3.7	3.0	1.9	1.2
AEGL 3	11	11	9.1	5.7	3.7

NR = not recommended due to insufficient data.
(Some of the above methods are not listed or specified.)

Supplemental Response Information

Extinguishing Media: Use extinguishing agent which is the most appropriate to extinguish surrounding fire (carbon dioxide, foam, dry chemical or water fog as extinguishing media).

Solubility: ARSENIC TRIOXIDE (TRIS-ENOX®9) is slightly to partially water soluble (18 g/l at 20 deg C) with a pH range from 7.5 to 8.5.

Chemical Degradation/Neutralization Method: Not otherwise specified

Note: If a specific degradation or neutralization method is not provided in this section and you do not have other specific information that will guide you on how to clean up the specific material spilled, then follow the general spill procedure found in the introduction section of this handbook.

Incompatibility: ARSENIC TRIOXIDE and sodium chlorate will produce a spontaneously flammable mixture; hydrogen fluoride and ARSENIC TRIOXIDE react with incandescence. ARSENIC TRIOXIDE and zinc on heating may explode. Keep away from incompatibles such as oxidizing agents, metals, and acids. Can generate arsine, which is an extremely poisonous gas, when arsenic compounds contact acid, alkalis, or water in the presence of an active metal (zinc, aluminum, manganese, sodium, iron, etc.). Furthermore, this drug is incompatible with halogens and metal carbide.

ASPARAGINASE (1)

(a-SPARE-a-ji-naze)
L-ASPARAGINASE
ELSPAR®10
LEUNASE®11

Chemical Abstract Service (CAS) Registry Number: 9015-68-3 (mixture)
Registry of Toxic Effects of Chemical Substances (RTECS): CI9000000
C_{1377}-H_{2208}-N_{382}-O_{442}-S_{17}

ERWINASE

(Two Degradation Methods)

Health & Safety Hazards/US Department of Transportation (DOT)/US Environmental Protection Agency (EPA)—Sources

Teratogen—University of Maryland at College Park, Teratogen—Material Safety Data Sheet, Reproductive Effector—Registry of Toxic Effects of Chemical Substances (RTECS), Sensitizer—Material Safety Data Sheet, Mutagen—Registry of Toxic Effects of Chemical Substances (RTECS), Cytotoxic—British Columbia Cancer Agency Canada, Nonvesicant—British Columbia Cancer Agency Canada, Lactation Avoid Breastfeeding (World Health Organization), Pregnancy Category (C)—US Food and Drug Administration, National Fire Protection Association Hazard Rating

Health (3) Flammability (0) Instability/Reactivity (0), Hazardous Materials Identification System (R) and/or US Department of Defense System (3★) with additional chronic hazard present Fire Hazard (0) Reactivity (0) Personal Protective Code (-) (None stated).

CRISANTASPASE (ERWINASE) is a colorless fluid from powder.

ASPARAGINASE (USAN) is an enzyme isolated from Escherichia Coli, or obtained from other sources. See also colaspase, PEGASPARGASE, and CRISANTASPASE.

L-ASPARAGINASE (ELSPARION)

White lyophilized plug or powder. When reconstituted, ELSPAR®10 should be a clear, colorless solution. If the solution becomes cloudy, discard (odorless).

L-ASPARAGINASE (ELSPAR®10) is a powder available as an injection after reconstitution occurs.

First Aid Medical Information/ Occupational Exposure Limits

First Aid Measures to include: Use general first aid measures except for the following:

Ingestion: Do not induce vomiting. May dilute with water, and then get medical attention:

Medical Information:

Caution and Warning Statements: May cause sensitization by inhalation and skin contact. Exposure may cause allergic respiratory reaction. There is a possible risk of harm to the unborn child. Exposure may cause skin and eye irritation.

Signs and symptoms of exposure are CNS depression, nausea, headache, and vomiting. Other symptoms may include anorexia, chills, fever, weight loss, adnominal cramps, hyperglycemia, pancreatitis, and bone marrow depression, a decrease in blood concentration of fibrinogen depressing the clotting mechanisms, and liver and kidney damage

In clinical uses, the adverse reactions following intravenous administration are skin rashes, joint pain, respiratory distress, and anaphylaxis. Rare serious reactions include hemorrhage due to low fibrinogen, pancreatitis, liver dysfunction, bone marrow suppression, and CNS effects.

Caution: Females and males planning to have a child, pregnant women, and nursing mothers should exercise caution regarding potential occupational exposure to this cytotoxic drug. No information or not enough information exists or was provided concerning occupational exposures that may potentially occur while handling this drug and its affects on reproductive systems, the fetus, and/or if it is secreted along with breast milk, which may harm nursing infants. Staff members should consult with the occupational health physician monitoring workers' health in your facility to be apprised of potential hazards and should be advised to avoid becoming pregnant and/or breastfeeding or should be transferred in accordance with policy/procedures to other duties that do not involve preparation, handling, and administering this drug.

Therapeutic Levels: The Food and Drug Administration lists this dug as a Pregnancy Category (C); (ELSPAR®10) should be used during pregnancy only if the potential benefit justifies the potential risk to the fetus. For nursing mothers, it is not known whether this drug is secreted in human milk. Because many drugs are secreted in human milk and because of the potential for serious adverse reactions in nursing infants from (ELSPAR®10), a decision should be made whether to discontinue nursing or to discontinue the drug, taking into account the importance of the drug to the mother.

Target Organs/Systems: Liver and kidneys, pancreas, bone marrow, blood, reproductive systems, fetus, and skin

Medical Conditions Generally Aggravated by Exposure:

- Medical conditions generally aggravated by exposure are hypersensitivity to L-ASPARAGINASE, pancreatitis or liver impairment. ASPARAGINASE is also contraindicated in patients who have had previous anaphylactic reactions to it, and asthma.
- Reproductive and pregnancy issues.

Specific Medical Surveillance Information: Reproductive and pregnancy counseling.

Occupational Exposure Level/Limit (OEL) & Sampling Methods:

> *Environmental Sentinel Contamination Action Level (ESCAL)*: Not otherwise specified
> Occupational Exposure Level/Limit (OEL): Merck 10 μ/m3 8-hr Time-Weighted Average (TWA) (Method not listed or specified)

Supplemental Response Information

Extinguishing Media: Use extinguishing agent which is the most appropriate to extinguish surrounding fire (carbon dioxide, foam, dry chemical or water fog as extinguishing media).

Solubility: L-ASPARAGINASE (ELSPAR®10) is freely water soluble, while being practically insoluble in methanol, acetone, and chloroform.

Chemical Degradation/Neutralization Method: There are two or more recommended procedures for L-ASPARAGINASE. See below for optional method.

A manufacturer's Material Data Safety Sheet recommends treating spill surfaces with a ~2 mol/liter (~8g/100 ml), aqueous caustic soda (sodium hydroxide) solution after absorbing liquids with inert absorbent pads or removing any powder present: allow solution to stand for up to one hour, and then thoroughly wash spilled surfaces with soap and water; sample to determine if surface contamination is still present (if sampling method is available). If drug is still present, repeat above steps; dispose of wastes in accordance with your local procedures, state, and federal regulations.

Incompatibility: L-ASPARAGINASE is incompatible with strong oxidizing agents.

ASPARAGINASE (2)

(a-SPARE-a-ji-naze)
L-ASPARAGINASE
ELSPAR®10
LEUNASE®11

> Chemical Abstract Service (CAS) Registry Number: 9015-68-3 (mixture)
> Registry of Toxic Effects of Chemical Substances (RTECS): C19000000
> C_{1377}-H_{2208}-N_{382}-O_{442}-S_{17}

ERWINASE

(Two Degradation Methods)

Health & Safety Hazards/US Department of Transportation (DOT)/US Environmental Protection Agency (EPA)—Sources

Teratogen—University of Maryland at College Park, Teratogen—Material Safety Data Sheet, Reproductive Effector—Registry of Toxic Effects of Chemical Substances (RTECS), Sensitizer—Material Safety Data Sheet, Mutagen—Registry of Toxic Effects of Chemical Substances (RTECS), Cytotoxic—British Columbia Cancer Agency Canada, Nonvesicant—British Columbia Cancer Agency Canada, Pregnancy Category (C)—US Food and Drug Administration, National Fire Protection Association Hazard Rating Health (3) Flammability (0) Instability/Reactivity (0), Hazardous Materials Identification System (R) and/or US Department of Defense System (3★) with additional chronic hazard present Fire Hazard (0) Reactivity (0) Personal Protective Code (–) (None stated).

CRISANTASPASE (ERWINASE) is a colorless fluid from powder.

ASPARAGINASE (USAN) is an enzyme isolated from escherichia coli or obtained from other sources. See also colaspase, PEGASPARGASE, and CRISANTASPASE.

L-ASPARAGINASE (ELSPAR®10) is a powder available as an injection.

White lyophilized plug or powder. When reconstituted, ELSPAR®10 should be a clear, colorless solution. If the solution becomes cloudy, discard (odorless).

L-ASPARAGINASE (ELSPAR®10) is a powder available as an injection after reconstitution occurs.

First Aid Medical Information/ Occupational Exposure Limits

First Aid Measures to include: Use general first aid measures except for the following:

Ingestion: Do not induce vomiting. May dilute with water, and then get medical attention:

Medical Information:

Caution and Warning Statements: May cause sensitization by inhalation and skin contact. Exposure may cause allergic respiratory reaction. There is a possible risk of harm to the unborn child. Exposure may cause skin and eye irritation.

Signs and symptoms of exposure are CNS depression, nausea, headache, and vomiting. Other symptoms may include anorexia, chills, fever, weight loss, adnominal cramps, hyperglycemia, pancreatitis, and bone marrow depression, a decrease in blood concentration of fibrinogen depressing the clotting mechanisms, and liver and kidney damage.

In clinical uses, the adverse reactions following intravenous administration are skin rashes, joint pain, respiratory distress, and anaphylaxis. In rare serous reactions include hemorrhage due to low fibrinogen, pancreatitis, liver dysfunction, bone marrow suppression, and CNS effects.

Caution: Females and males planning to have a child, pregnant women, and nursing mothers should exercise caution regarding potential occupational exposure to this cytotoxic drug. No information or not enough information exists or was provided concerning occupational exposures that may potentially occur while handling this drug and its affects on reproductive systems, the fetus, and/or if it is secreted along with breast milk, which may harm nursing infants. Staff members should consult with the occupational health physician monitoring workers' health in your facility to be apprised of potential hazards and should be advised

to avoid becoming pregnant and/or breastfeeding or should be transferred in accordance with policy/procedures to other duties that do not involve preparation, handling, and administering this drug.

Therapeutic Levels: The Food and Drug Administration lists this drug as a Pregnancy Category (C); ELSPAR®10 should be used during pregnancy only if the potential benefit justifies the potential risk to the fetus. For nursing mothers, it is not known whether this drug is secreted in human milk. Because many drugs are secreted in human milk and because of the potential for serious adverse reactions in nursing infants from ELSPAR®10, a decision should be made whether to discontinue nursing or to discontinue the drug, taking into account the importance of the drug to the mother.

Target Organs/Systems: Liver and kidneys, pancreas, bone marrow, blood, reproductive systems, fetus, and skin

Medical Conditions Generally Aggravated by Exposure:

- Medical conditions generally aggravated by exposure are hypersensitivity to L-ASPARAGINASE, pancreatitis or liver impairment. ASPARAGINASE is also contraindicated in patients who have had previous anaphylactic reactions to it, and asthma.
- Reproductive and pregnancy issues.

Specific Medical Surveillance Information: Reproductive and pregnancy counseling.

Occupational Exposure Level/Limit (OEL) & Sampling Methods:

Environmental Sentinel Contamination Action Level (ESCAL): Not otherwise specified
Occupational Exposure Level/Limit (OEL): Merck 10 μ/m3 8-hr TWA
(Method not listed or specified)

Supplemental Response Information

Extinguishing Media: Use extinguishing agent which is the most appropriate to extinguish surrounding fire (carbon dioxide, foam, dry chemical or water fog as extinguishing media).

Solubility: L-ASPARAGINASE (ELSPAR®10) is freely water soluble, while being practically insoluble in methanol, acetone, and chloroform.

Chemical Degradation/Neutralization Method: There are two or more recommended procedures for L-ASPARAGINASE. See below and above for optional method:

- The international agency for research on cancer (International Agency for Research on Cancer) recommended degradation method for L-ASPARAGINASE:
- The International Agency for Research on Cancer recommends treating spill surfaces with a 5.25% sodium hypochlorite bleach) solution after absorbing liquids with inert absorbent pads or removing any powder present: allow solution to stand for up to one hour, and then thoroughly wash spilled surfaces with soap and water; sample to determine if surface contamination is still present (if sampling method is available). If drug is still present, repeat above steps; dispose of wastes in accordance with your local procedures, state, and federal regulations.

Incompatibility: L-ASPARAGINASE is incompatible with strong oxidizing agents.

AVASTIN®12
BEVACIZUMAB (*be-va-SIZ-yoo-mab*)
BEVACIZUMABUM

Chemical Abstract Service (CAS) Registry Number: 216974-75-3
C_8-H_{10}-N_4-O_2

Health & Safety Hazards/US Department of Transportation (DOT)/US Environmental Protection Agency (EPA)—Sources

Cytotoxic British Columbia Cancer Agency Canada, Nonvesicant—British Columbia Cancer Agency Canada, Possible Sensitizer—Material Safety Data Sheet, Pregnancy Category (C)—US Food and Drug Administration, Reproductive Effector—Material Safety Data Sheet, Fetotoxic—Material Safety Data Sheet.

BEVACIZUMAB is available as an injection.

AVASTIN®12 is a clear to slightly opalescent, colorless to pale brown sterile solution for intravenous (IV) infusion. AVASTIN®12 is available in 100 mg and 400 mg single dose vials containing 4 ml and 16 ml, respectively of BEVACIZUMAB (25 mg/ml).

First Aid Medical Information/ Occupational Exposure Limits

First Aid Measures to include: Use general first aid measures except for the following:

Ingestion: Drink moderate amount (8–12 oz or 250 ml) of water. Do not induce vomiting. Seek medical assistance.

Medical Information:
Caution and Warning Statements: AVASTIN®12 toxicity, particularly as it pertains to occupational exposure, is not fully known.

AVASTIN®12 may cause a systemic allergic reaction. In a study with monkeys, AVASTIN®12 was associated with physeal dysplasia (abnormal development of growth plate cartilage). AVASTIN®12 may impair fertility. Hemoptysis (coughing up of blood or bloody sputum from the lungs or airway) has occurred in patients with non-small cell lung cancer treated with chemotherapy and AVASTIN®12.

Caution: Females and males planning to have a child, pregnant women, and nursing mothers should exercise caution regarding potential occupational exposure to this cytotoxic drug. No information or not enough information exists or was provided concerning occupational exposures that may potentially occur while handling this drug and its affects on reproductive systems, the fetus, and/or if it is secreted along with breast milk, which may harm nursing infants. Staff members should consult with the occupational health physician monitoring workers' health in your facility to be apprised of potential hazards and should be advised to avoid becoming pregnant and/or breastfeeding or should be transferred in accordance with policy/procedures to other duties that do not involve preparation, handling, and administering this drug.

Food and Drug Administration Pregnancy Category (C); it is not known whether AVASTIN®12 is secreted in human milk.

Clinical drug tests (not occupational exposures) may cause impaired wound healing, holes in colon, bleeding leading to disability strokes or death. Other possible side effects are heart failure, kidney damage, high blood pressure, tiredness/weakness, thrombophlebitis, diarrhea, decrease in white blood cells, headache, and mouth sores.

Target Organs/Systems: Reproductive systems and fetus

Medical Conditions Generally Aggravated by Exposure:

- Reproductive and pregnancy issues.

Specific Medical Surveillance Information: Reproductive and pregnancy counseling.

Occupational Exposure Level/Limit (OEL) & Sampling Methods: Not otherwise specified

Environmental Sentinel Contamination Action Level (ESCAL): Not otherwise specified

Supplemental Response Information

Extinguishing Media: Use extinguishing agent which is the most appropriate to extinguish surrounding fire (carbon dioxide, foam, dry chemical or water fog as extinguishing media).

Solubility: AVASTIN®12 is water soluble.

Chemical Degradation/Neutralization Method: A manufacturer's Material Safety Data Sheet recommends using alkaline soap/detergent and water to clean spill surfaces after absorbing liquids with inert absorbent pads or removing any powder present: repeat using soap and water; sample to determine if surface contamination is still present (if sampling method is available). If drug is still present, repeat above steps; dispose of wastes in accordance with your local procedures, state, and federal regulations.

Incompatibility: Not otherwise specified

AZACYTIDINE (*ay-za-SYE-ti-deen*)
5-AZACYTIDINE

> Chemical Abstract Service (CAS) Registry
> Number: 320-67-2
> Registry of Toxic Effects of Chemical Substances
> (RTECS): XZ3017500

VIDAZA®13

$C_8H_{12}N_4O_5$
National Cancer Institute: NSC 102816

Health & Safety Hazards/US Department of Transportation (DOT)/US Environmental Protection Agency (EPA)—Sources

Carcinogen G2A—International Agency for Research on Cancer, Carcinogen C2—US National Toxicology Program, Carcinogen—Berkeley University Hazardous Chemical List, Carcinogen—Material Safety Data Sheet, Carcinogen—University of Maryland at College Park, Possible Carcinogen—US Occupational Safety and Health Administration, Reproductive Effector—US National Institute of Environmental Health Sciences (NIEHS), Teratogen—University of Maryland at College Park, Mutagen—Material Safety Data Sheet, Mutagen—University of Maryland at College Park, Toxic—Material Safety Data Sheet, Pregnancy Category (D)—US Food and Drug Administration, Carcinogen—US California State Proposition 65, National Fire Protection Association Hazard Rating Health (1) Flammability (0) Instability/Reactivity (1), National Fire Protection Association Hazard Rating Health (1) Flammability (1) Instability/Reactivity (0), Hazardous Materials Identification System (R) and/or US Department of Defense System (1★) with additional chronic hazard present Fire Hazard (0) Reactivity (1) Personal Protective Code (-)(None stated), US California State Protection Agency Listed.

(UV Fluorescence at 210 nm; Color Unknown, ~ 242 nm)

First Aid Medical Information/ Occupational Exposure Limits

First Aid Measures to include: Use general first aid measures except for the following:

Ingestion: If swallowed, if victim is conscious and alert, rinse mouth out and give 2–4 cups of milk or water. Seek medical assistance.

Medical Information:

Caution and Warning Statements: 5-AZACYTIDINE (AZACYTIDINE) is toxic. Exposure may cause cancer and may cause heritable genetic damage. Harmful if swallowed (ingested). Exposure or ingestion may cause gastrointestinal irritation with nausea, vomiting, and diarrhea. Furthermore, may cause blood abnormalities. Inhalation of dust may cause respiratory tract irritation. Signs and symptoms of exposure are nausea, headache, and vomiting. May cause eye and skin irritation. AZACYTIDINE may alter genetic material and may be a mutagen.

Caution: Females and males planning to have a child, pregnant women, and nursing mothers should exercise caution regarding potential exposure to 5-AZACYTIDINE (AZACYTIDINE). No information or not enough information was provided concerning if the drug and/or metabolites are potentially secreted into human breast milk. Staff who are pregnant and/or breastfeeding should be transferred in accordance with policy/procedures to other duties that do not involve handling 5-AZACYTIDINE (AZACYTIDINE). Exposure to this drug may cause heritable genetic damage. Staff members should consult with the occupational health physician monitoring workers' health in your facility to be apprised of potential hazards and should be advised to avoid becoming pregnant and/or breastfeeding or should be transferred in accordance with policy/procedures to other duties that do not involve preparation, handling, and administering this drug.

Target Organs/Systems: Blood, bone marrow, immune system, liver, fetus, and GI system

Medical Conditions Generally Aggravated by Exposure:

- Reproductive and pregnancy issues.

Specific Medical Surveillance Information: Reproductive and pregnancy counseling.

Occupational Exposure Level/Limit (OEL) & Sampling Methods: Not otherwise specified

Environmental Sentinel Contamination Action Level (ESCAL): Not otherwise specified

Supplemental Response Information

Extinguishing Media: Use extinguishing agent which is the most appropriate to extinguish surrounding fire (carbon dioxide, foam, dry chemical or water fog as extinguishing media).

Solubility: 5-AZACYTIDINE is water soluble (0.5–1.0 g/100 ml at 21C).

Chemical Degradation/Neutralization Method: Not otherwise specified

Note: If a specific degradation or neutralization method is not provided in this section and you do not have other specific information that will guide you on how to clean up the specific material spilled, then follow the general spill procedure found in the introduction section of this handbook.

Incompatibility: 5-AZACYTIDINE is incompatible with strong oxidizing agents.

AZATHIOPRINE (1)

(ay-za-THYE oh preen)
IMURAN® 14

Chemical Abstract Service (CAS) Registry
Number: 446-86-6
Registry of Toxic Effects of Chemical Substances
(RTECS): UO8925000
$C_9H_7N_7O_2S$
(Two Degradation Methods)

Health & Safety Hazards/US Department of Transportation (DOT)/US Environmental Protection Agency (EPA)—Sources

Carcinogen G1—International Agency for Research on Cancer, Carcinogen C1—US National Toxicology Program, Toxic—Material Safety Data Sheet, Mutagen—Material Safety Data Sheet, Teratogen—University of Maryland at College Park, Carcinogen—University of Maryland at College Park, Reproductive Effector—Material Safety Data Sheet, Sensitizer—Material Safety Data Sheet, Skin Sensitizer—US National Library of Medicine Haz Map, Pregnancy Category

(D)—US Food and Drug Administration, Developmental and Carcinogen—US California State Proposition 65 (0.0004 Mg/Day(Value)), National Fire Protection Association Hazard Rating Health (1) Flammability (1) Instability/Reactivity (0)—Material Safety Data Sheet, National Fire Protection Association Hazard Rating Health (2) Flammability (0) Instability/Reactivity (1)—Material Safety data Sheet, Hazardous Materials Identification System (R) and/or US Department of Defense System Health (1) Fire Hazard (1) Reactivity (0) Personal Code (E) (Safety Glasses, Chemical Gloves, Dust Respirator)—Material Safety Data Sheet, Hazardous Materials Identification System (R) and/or US Department of Defense System Health (2★) with additional chronic hazards present Fire Hazard (0) Reactivity (1).

IMURAN®14 (AZATHIOPRINE) is available as an injection and 100 mg and 50 mg tablet form.

AZATHIOPRINE—Breastfeeding: discontinue (drug and its metabolites transmitted in breast milk at low level [facts and comparisons]) (*A Guide for Occupational Health Professionals Technical Manual*, Navy Environmental Health Center [NEHC-TM-OEM 6260.01a]).

Note: AZATHIOPRINE is insoluble in water, but may be dissolved with addition of one molar equivalent of alkali. The sodium salt of AZATHIOPRINE is sufficiently soluble to make a 10 mg/ml water solution which is stable for 24 hours at 59° to 77° F (15° to 25° C).

First Aid Medical Information/Occupational Exposure Limits

First Aid Measures to include: Use general first aid measures except for the following:

Physician's note (A): Treat according to locally accepted protocols. For additional guidance, refer to the current prescribing information or to the local poison control information center. Medical treatment in cases of overexposure should be treated as an overdose of immunosuppressive agent. In allergic individuals, exposure to this material may require treatment for initial or delayed allergic symptoms and signs. This may include immediate and/or delayed treatment of anaphylactic reactions. No specific antidotes are recommended.

Physician's note (B): If overexposure is expected, daily watch of the blood count should continue for at least two weeks or longer if necessary.

Medical Information:
Caution and Warning Statements:
Toxic: Exposure to AZATHIOPRINE (IMURAN®14) may cause cancer, adverse reproductive

effects, and birth defects (teratogenic). Exposure may affect genetic materials (mutagenic). This drug may cause heritable genetic damage. Dermal and eye contact may cause irritation. Inhalation may cause upper respiratory tract and mucous membrane irritation. Symptoms may include coughing and hoarseness. Ingestion is harmful and can cause gastrointestinal tract disturbances, slightly bitter taste in mouth, nausea, vomiting, hypermotility, and diarrhea. May affect urinary system/kidneys (renal failure, acute tubular necrosis), blood (leucopenia, thrombocytopenia, macrocytic anemia, changes in white blood cell count), cardiovascular system, liver (elevation in liver enzymes), and musculoskeletal system. Other symptoms may include rash or red spots on skin, unusual bleeding or bruising, blood in urine or stools, infection, and death. Prolonged or repeated exposure may cause allergic reactions (dermatitis or asthma) in certain sensitive individuals if inhaled, ingested or in contact with skin.

Caution: Females and males planning to have a child, pregnant women, and nursing mothers should exercise caution regarding potential occupational exposure to this cytotoxic drug. No information or not enough information exists or was provided concerning occupational exposure that may potentially occur while handling this drug and its affects on reproductive systems, the fetus, and/or if it is secreted along with breast milk, which may harm nursing infants. Staff members should consult with the occupational health physician monitoring workers' health in your facility to be apprised of potential hazards and should be advised to avoid becoming pregnant and/or breastfeeding or should be transferred in accordance with policy/procedures to other duties that do not involve preparation, handling, and administering this drug.

Following assessment, if the risk of exposure is considered significant then exposed individuals should undergo appropriate health surveillance that may include symptom enquiry, clinical examination, and monitoring of lead organ effects (e.g., full blood counts). In the event of overexposure, individuals should receive post exposure health surveillance focused on the most likely health effects (e.g., full blood counts).

Target Organs/Systems: Blood, liver, kidneys, bladder, cardiovascular system, immune system, bone marrow, fetus, cancer, and possible sensitizer

Medical Conditions Generally Aggravated by Exposure:

- Persons with allergy to one or more drug components. Developing offspring during pregnancy.

Specific Medical Surveillance Information: Reproductive and pregnancy counseling.

Occupational Exposure Level/Limit (OEL) & Sampling Methods:

Environmental Sentinel Contamination Action Level (ESCAL): Air

Occupational Exposure Level/Limit (OEL) Glaxo Wellcome:

IMURAN®14 (AZATHIOPRINE) 3 µ/m3 (15 min Time-Weighted Average (TWA)

Occupational Exposure Level/Limit (OEL) GSK 3 mg/m3 (8 hr Time-Weighted Average [TWA])★

Carcinogen, reproductive hazard, skin sensitizer

★Occupational hygiene air monitoring methods: An occupational/industrial hygiene monitoring method has been developed for this material. For advice on suitable monitoring methods, consult your local occupational or industrial hygiene specialist, health and safety department, or the health and safety group identified.

Occupational Exposure Level/Limit (OEL): UK Maximum Exposure Limit (MEL): 5 µ/m3 (Ceiling limit; not Time-Weighted) (Method not listed or specified)

Supplemental Response Information

Extinguishing Media: Use extinguishing agent which is the most appropriate to extinguish surrounding fire (carbon dioxide, foam, dry chemical or water fog as extinguishing media).

Solubility: AZATHIOPRINE is insoluble in water (0.11 g/l) with a pH range of 4.9 to 5 (at 10% suspension at 21 deg. C). AZATHIOPRINE is soluble in aqueous bases and slightly soluble in alcohol (ethanol).

AZATHIOPRINE (IMURAN®14) salt is sufficiently soluble in water (10 mg/ml water solution at neutral or acid pH) (refer to note in health and safety hazards column).

Chemical Degradation/Neutralization Method: There are two or more recommended procedures (bleach [sodium hypochlorite] solution method) and dilute caustic soda and sodium hypochlorite solution method) for AZATHIOPRINE (IMURAN®14) see below.

The International Agency for Research on Cancer recommends treating spill surfaces with a 5.25% sodium hypochlorite (bleach) solution after absorbing liquids with inert absorbent pads or removing any powder present: allow solution to stand for up to one hour, and then thoroughly wash spilled surfaces with soap and water; sample to determine if surface contamination is still present (if sampling method is available). If drug is still present, repeat above steps; dispose of wastes in accordance with your local procedures, state, and federal regulations.

Incompatibility: AZATHIOPRINE is incompatible with strong oxidizing agents and strong bases. Avoid heat and ignition sources; protect from light.

AZATHIOPRINE (2)
(*ay-za-THYE-oh-preen*)
IMURAN®14

$C_9H_7N_7O_2S$
Chemical Abstract Service (CAS) Registry
  Number: 446-86-6
Registry of Toxic Effects of Chemical Substances
  (RTECS): UO8925000
(Two Degradation Methods)

Health & Safety Hazards/US Department of Transportation (DOT)/US Environmental Protection Agency (EPA)—Sources

Carcinogen G1—International Agency for Research on Cancer, Carcinogen C1—US National Toxicology Program, Toxic—Material Safety Data Sheet, Mutagen—Material Safety Data Sheet, Teratogen—University of Maryland at College Park, Carcinogen—University of Maryland at College Park, Reproductive Effector—Material Safety Data Sheet, Sensitizer—Material Safety Data Sheet, Skin Sensitizer—US National Library of Medicine Haz Map, Pregnancy Category (D)—US Food and Drug Administration, Developmental and Carcinogen—US California State Proposition 65 ((0.0004 Mg/Day)(Value)), National Fire Protection Association Hazard Rating Health (1) Flammability (1) Instability/Reactivity (0)—Material Safety Data Sheet, National Fire Protection Association Hazard Rating Health (2) Flammability (0) Instability/Reactivity (1)—Material Safety Data Sheet, Hazardous Materials Identification System (R) and/or US Department of Defense System Health (1) Fire Hazard (1) Reactivity (0) Personal Protective Code (E) (Safety Glasses, Chemical Gloves, Dust Respirator)—Material Safety Data Sheet, Hazardous Materials Identification System (R) and/or US Department of Defense System (2★) with additional chronic hazards present Fire Hazard (0) Reactivity (1) Personal Protective Code (None stated)—Material Safety Data Sheet.

IMURAN®14 (AZATHIOPRINE) is available as an injection and in 100 mg and 50 mg tablet form.

AZATHIOPRINE—Breastfeeding: discontinue (drug and its metabolites transmitted in breast milk at low level).

Note: AZATHIOPRINE is insoluble in water, but may be dissolved with addition of one molar equivalent of alkali. The sodium salt of AZATHIOPRINE is sufficiently soluble to make a 10 mg/ml water solution which is stable for 24 hours at 59° to 77° F (15° to 25° C).

First Aid Medical Information/ Occupational Exposure Limits

First Aid Measures to include: Use general first aid measures except for the following:

Overexposure: If overexposure is expected, daily watch of the blood count should continue for at least two weeks or longer if necessary.

Medical Information:

Caution and Warning Statements: Exposure to AZATHIOPRINE (IMURAN®14) may cause cancer, adverse reproductive effects and birth defects (teratogenic). Exposure may affect genetic materials (mutagenic). Dermal and eye contact may cause irritation. Inhalation may cause upper respiratory tract and mucous membrane irritation. Symptoms may include coughing and hoarseness. Ingestion is harmful and can cause gastrointestinal tract disturbances, slightly bitter taste in mouth, nausea, vomiting, hypermotility, and diarrhea. This drug may affect urinary system/kidneys (renal failure, acute tubular necrosis), blood (leucopenia, thrombocytopenia, macrocytic anemia, changes in white blood cell count), cardiovascular system, liver (elevation in liver enzymes), musculoskeletal system. Other symptoms may include rash or red spots on skin, unusual bleeding or bruising, blood in urine or stools, infection, and death. Prolonged or repeated exposure may cause allergic reactions (dermatitis or asthma) in certain sensitive individuals if inhaled, ingested, or in contact with skin.

Caution: Females and males planning to have a child, pregnant women, and nursing mothers should exercise caution regarding potential occupational exposure to this cytotoxic drug. No information or not enough information exists or was provided concerning occupational exposure that may potentially occur while handling this drug and its affects on reproductive systems, the fetus, and/or if it is secreted along with breast milk, which may harm nursing infants. Staff members should consult with the occupational health physician monitoring workers' health in your facility to be apprised of potential hazards and should be advised to avoid becoming pregnant and/or breastfeeding or should be transferred in accordance with policy/procedures to other duties that do not involve preparation, handling, and administering this drug.

Target Organs/Systems: Blood, liver, kidneys, bladder, cardiovascular system, immune system, fetus, and bone marrow

Medical Conditions Generally Aggravated by Exposure:

- Allergy to one or more substances found in the drug that may increase the sensitivity to occupational exposure. Developing offspring during pregnancy.

Specific Medical Surveillance Information: Reproductive and pregnancy counseling.

Occupational Exposure Level/Limit (OEL) & Sampling Methods: Not otherwise specified

Environmental Sentinel Contamination Action Level (ESCAL): Air

Supplemental Response Information

Extinguishing Media: Use extinguishing agent which is the most appropriate to extinguish surrounding fire, e.g., carbon dioxide, foam, dry chemical or water fog as extinguishing media, but do not use a water jet.

Solubility: AZATHIOPRINE is insoluble in water (0.11 g/l) with a pH range of 4.9 to 5 (at 10% suspension at 21 deg. C). AZATHIOPRINE is soluble in aqueous bases and slightly soluble in alcohol (ethanol).

AZATHIOPRINE (IMURAN®14) salt is sufficiently soluble in water (10 mg/ml water solution at neutral or acid pH) (refer to note in health and safety hazards column).

Chemical Degradation/Neutralization Method: There are two or more recommended procedures (bleach [sodium hypochlorite] solution method and dilute caustic soda/sodium hypochlorite solution method) for AZATHIOPRINE (IMURAN®14); see below and above.

A manufacturer's Material Safety Data Sheet recommends treating spill surfaces with dilute caustic soda and sodium hypochlorite solution after absorbing liquids with inert absorbent pads or removing any powder present: allow solution to stand for up to one hour, and then thoroughly wash spilled surfaces with soap and water; sample to determine if surface contamination is still present (if sampling method is available at your facility). If drug is still present, repeat above steps; dispose of wastes in accordance with your local procedures, state, and federal regulations.

Incompatibility: AZATHIOPRINE is incompatible with strong oxidizing agents and strong bases. Avoid heat and ignition sources; protect from light.

B

BEXAROTENUM
BEXAROT.ENE *(beks-AIR-o-teen)*
TARGRETIN®15

　　Chemical Abstract Service (CAS) Registry
　　　　Number: 153559-49-0
　　$C_{24}-H_{28}-O_2$

Health & Safety Hazards/US Department of Transportation (DOT)/US Environmental Protection Agency (EPA)—Sources

Teratogen—Box Instructions, Reproductive Effector—Box Instructions, Pregnancy Category (X)—US Food and Drug Administration.

BEXAROTENE is available in capsules (75 mg) and as a skin topical gel (1%); white powder or clear gel.

First Aid Medical Information/ Occupational Exposure Limits

First Aid Measures to include: Use general first aid measures.

Medical Information:

Caution and Warning Statements:

Note: BEXAROTENUM (TARGRETIN®15) therapeutic dose information was extrapolated below.

Caution: The toxicity of most cytotoxic drugs has not been fully investigated, particularly as it pertains to occupational exposure. BEXAROTENUM (TARGRETIN®15) is one of the drugs that has little occupational hazards information available. Therefore, therapeutic dose information was extrapolated below to assist in determining occupational toxicity, and signs and symptoms of overexposure. Furthermore, it is prudent to minimize occupational exposure to BEXAROTENUM (TARGRETIN®15).

Exposure to BEXAROTENUM (TARGRETIN®15) may increase the skin sensitivity to sunlight or sunlamp. The most common side effect is an increase in blood lipids (fats in the blood). Another common side effect is underactive thyroid. An infrequent side effect of TARGRETIN®15 is pancreatitis (inflamed pancreas). Symptoms of pancreatitis include persistent nausea, vomiting, and abdominal or back pain.

Avoid skin contact, eye contact, inhalation, and ingestion. Use appropriate prudent practices and administrative procedures to prevent opportunities for direct contact with the skin, eyes and/or to prevent inhalation.

Caution: Females and males planning to have a child, pregnant women, and nursing mothers should exercise caution regarding potential occupational exposure to this cytotoxic drug. No information or not enough information exists or was provided concerning occupational exposure that may potentially occur while handling this drug and its affects on reproductive systems, the fetus, and/or if it is secreted along with breast milk, which may harm nursing infants. Staff members should consult with the occupational health physician monitoring workers' health in your facility to be apprised of potential hazards and should be advised to avoid becoming pregnant and/or breastfeeding or should be transferred in accordance with policy/procedures to other duties that do not involve preparation, handling, and administering this drug.

Target Organs/Systems: Blood, thyroid, pancreas, and possibly fetus

Medical Conditions Generally Aggravated by Exposure:

- The following medical conditions are generally aggravated by exposure to BEXAROTENUM; if currently or previously had an inflamed pancreas (pancreatitis), liver or kidney disease, gall bladder disease, and/or diabetes; if you have or ever had high triglyceride (a fatty substance) levels in your blood; and if you are taking a medication to reduce high triglyceride and cholesterol levels in the blood. Furthermore, notify your occupational health staff if allergic to retinoid medications (e.g., ACCUTANE [ISOTRETINOIN], SORIATANE [ACITRETIN], TEGISON [ETRETINATE], and VESINOID [TRETINOIN]).
- Previously chemotherapy or radiation medicines may increase the effects of the exposure to BEXAROTENUM (TARGRETIN®15) in the blood.
- Alcohol consumption may increase the effects of the drug to harm your body.
- Reproductive and pregnancy issues.

Specific Medical Surveillance Information: Reproductive and pregnancy counseling.

Recommended therapeutic blood testing, which is needed to check levels of lipids, including triglycerides and cholesterol, and blood tests to detect thyroid activity.

Occupational Exposure Level/Limit (OEL) & Sampling Methods: Not otherwise specified

Environmental Sentinel Contamination Action Level (ESCAL): Not otherwise specified

Supplemental Response Information

Extinguishing Media: Use extinguishing agent which is the most appropriate to extinguish surrounding fire (carbon dioxide, foam, dry chemical or water fog as extinguishing media).

Solubility: TARGRETIN®15 (BEXAROTENE) is insoluble in water and slightly soluble in vegetable oils and ethanol.

Chemical Degradation/Neutralization Method: Not otherwise specified

Note: If a specific degradation or neutralization method is not provided on this table and you do not have other specific information that will guide you on how to clean up the specific material spilled, then follow the general spill procedure found in the introduction section of this handbook.

Incompatibility: Not otherwise specified

BICALUTAMIDE (*bye-kah-LOO-tah-mide*)
CASODEX®16

Chemical Abstract Service (CAS) Registry Number: 90357-06-5
Registry of Toxic Effects of Chemical Substances (RTECS): TX1413500
C_{18}-H_{14}-F_4-N_2-O_4-S

Health & Safety Hazards/US Department of Transportation (DOT)/US Environmental Protection Agency (EPA)—Sources

Pregnancy Category (X)—US Food and Drug Administration, Teratogen—Material Safety Data Sheet, Reproductive Effector—Material Safety Data Sheet, Probable Carcinogen—Material Safety Data Sheet, UN 3077, Group III.

CASODEX®16 (BICALUTAMIDE) is available as 50 mg tablets.

First Aid Medical Information/ Occupational Exposure Limits

First Aid Measures to include: Use general first aid measures.

Medical Information:
Caution and Warning Statements:
BICALUTAMIDE—Studies in animals have shown that repeated doses produce cancer. May impair fertility and cause harm to the unborn child. Male rats' reproductive performance was reduced but was reversible after cessation of dosing.

Caution: Females and males planning to have a child, pregnant women, and nursing mothers should exercise caution regarding potential occupational exposure to this cytotoxic drug. No information or not enough information exists or was provided concerning occupational exposures that may potentially occur while handling this drug and its affects on reproductive systems, the fetus, and/or if it is secreted along with breast milk, which may harm nursing infants. Staff members should consult with the occupational health physician monitoring workers' health in your facility to be apprised of potential hazards and should be advised to avoid becoming pregnant and/or breastfeeding or should be transferred in accordance with policy/procedures to other duties that do not involve preparation, handling, and administering this drug.

Therapeutic Levels: May impair fertility and cause harm to the unborn child. Nursing mothers, CASODEX®16 is not indicated for use in women. It is not known whether this drug is excreted in human milk.

Target Organs/Systems: Reproductive systems, blood, bone marrow, and possibly fetus
Medical Conditions Generally Aggravated by Exposure:

- Pregnancy.

Specific Medical Surveillance Information: Reproductive and pregnancy counseling.
Occupational Exposure Level/Limit (OEL) & Sampling Methods:

Environmental Sentinel Contamination Action level
  (ESCAL): Air
BICALUTAMIDE (CASODEX®16)
  Occupational Exposure Level/Limit (OEL):
  Astrazeneca
0.01 mg/m3 COM
(Method not listed or specified)

Supplemental Response Information
Extinguishing Media: Use extinguishing agent which is the most appropriate to extinguish surrounding fire (carbon dioxide, foam, dry chemical or water fog as extinguishing media).

Solubility: BICALUTAMIDE is practically insoluble in water at 37°C (5 mg per 1000 ml), slightly soluble in chloroform and absolute ethanol, sparingly soluble in methanol, and soluble in acetone and tetrahydrofuran.
Chemical Degradation/Neutralization Method: Not otherwise specified

If a specific degradation or neutralization method is not provided on this table and you do not have other specific information that will guide you on how to clean up the specific material spilled, then follow the general spill procedure found in the introduction section of this handbook.
Incompatibility: Not otherwise specified

BISANTRENE HYDROCHLORIDE

Chemical Abstract Service (CAS) Registry
  Number: 71439-68-4
CL 216942
National Cancer Institute: NSC 337766

ADAH
ORANGE CRUSH

$C_{22}-H_{22}-N_8.2CI-H$
$C_{22}H_{23}ClN_8$

BISANTRENE

Chemical Abstract Service (CAS) Registry
  Number: 78186-34-2
Registry of Toxic Effects of Chemical Substances
  (RTECS): CA9647000
$C_{22}H_{22}N_8$

Health & Safety Hazards/US Department of Transportation (DOT)/US Environmental Protection Agency (EPA)—Sources
Pregnancy Category (None stated)—US Food and Drug Administration, Mutagen—University of Maryland at College Park, Mutagen—Toxic Material Safety Data Sheet.

First Aid Medical Information/ Occupational Exposure Limits
First Aid Measures to include: Use general first aid measures.
Medical Information:
Caution and Warning Statements: Not otherwise specified
Target Organs/Systems: Not otherwise specified

Medical Conditions Generally Aggravated by Exposure: Not otherwise specified

Specific Medical Surveillance Information: Not otherwise specified

Occupational Exposure Level/Limit (OEL) & Sampling Methods: Not otherwise specified

Environmental Sentinel Contamination Action Level (ESCAL): Not otherwise specified

Supplemental Response Information

Extinguishing Media: Use extinguishing agent which is the most appropriate to extinguish surrounding fire (carbon dioxide, foam, dry chemical or water fog as extinguishing media).

Solubility: BISANTRENE HYDROCHLORIDE: Not otherwise specified

Chemical Degradation/Neutralization Method: Not otherwise specified

Note: If a specific degradation or neutralization method is not provided in this section and you do not have other specific information that will guide you on how to clean up the specific material spilled, then follow the general spill procedure found in the introduction section of this handbook.

Incompatibility: Not otherwise specified

BLEOMYCIN (*blee-o-MYE-sin*)
BLEOMYCIN SULFATE

Registry of Toxic Effects of Chemical Substances (RTECS): EC5988000
Chemical Abstract Service (CAS) Registry Number: 9041-93-4

BLENOXANE®17

Chemical Abstract Service (CAS) Registry Number: 11056-06-7
National Cancer Institute: NSC125066

BLEOCIN

Chemical Abstract Service (CAS) Registry Number: 67763-87-5
$C_{55}H_{84}N_{17}O_{21}S_3$

Health & Safety Hazards/US Department of Transportation (DOT)/US Environmental Protection Agency (EPA)—Sources

Carcinogen G2B—International Agency for Research on Cancer, Carcinogen—University of Maryland at College Park, Mutagen—University of Maryland at College Park, Teratogen—University of Maryland at College Park, Reproductive Effector—Material Safety Data Sheet, Mutagen—Material Safety Data Sheet, Tumorigenic—Material Safety Data Sheet, Toxic—Material Safety Data Sheet, Teratogen—Material Safety Data Sheet, Cytotoxic—Material Safety Data Sheet, Cytotoxic—British Columbia Cancer Agency Canada, Nonvesicant—British Columbia Cancer Agency Canada, Sensitizer—Material Safety Data Sheet, Irritant—Toxic Material Safety Data Sheet, Lactation Avoid Breastfeeding (World Health Organization), Pregnancy Category (D)—US Food and Drug Administration, National Fire Protection Association Hazard Rating Health (1) Flammability (1) Instability/Reactivity (0)—Material Safety Data Sheet, National Fire Protection Association Hazard Rating Health (2) Flammability (1) Instability/Reactivity (0)—Material Safety Data Sheet, National Fire Protection Association Hazard Rating Health (2) Flammability (0) Instability/Reactivity (1)—Material Safety Data Sheet, Hazardous Materials Identification System (R) and/or US Department of Defense System Health (3) Fire Hazard (1) Reactivity (0) Personal Protective Code (X) (Ask Supervisor)—Material Safety Data Sheet, Hazardous Materials Identification System (R) and/or US Department of Defense System Health (2★) with additional chronic hazard present Fire Hazard (1) Reactivity (0) Personal Protective Code (E) (Safety Glasses, Chemical Gloves, Dust Respirator)—Material Safety Data Sheet, Hazardous Materials Identification System (R) and/or US Department of Defense System Health (2★) with additional chronic hazard present Fire Hazard (0) Reactivity (0) Personal Protective Code (-) (None stated)—Material Safety Data Sheet, National Fire Protection Association Hazard Rating Health (2) Flammability (0) Instability/Reactivity (0)—Material Safety Data Sheet.

BLEOMYCIN SULFATE

BLEOMYCIN is a clear fluid for injection (15,000 international units) after being dissolved from powder.

BLEOMYCIN SULFATE is an odorless, colorless or white or yellowish white or cream colored amorphous hygroscopic powder.

BLEOMYCIN: Breastfeeding is contraindicated.

First Aid Medical Information/ Occupational Exposure Limits

First Aid Measures to include: Use general first aid measures except for the following.

Ingestion: If victim is conscious and alert, drink water, milk, or egg whites, and seek medical attention. Never drink alcoholic beverages.

Physician's note: Overdose treatment—Treatment of idiosyncratic reactions is symptomatic and may consist of volume expansion, pressor agents, antihistamines, and corticosteroids. Treat symptomatically. Up to 40% of the dose is excreted unchanged in the urine within 24 hours.

Medical Information:

Caution and Warning Statements:

Caution: BLEOMYCIN has not been fully characterized. Therefore, it is prudent to minimize occupational exposure and environmental releases.

BLEOMYCIN is identified as being a potential carcinogen and a cytotoxic drug. Mutagenic potential was documented in animals' studies. BLEOMYCIN has an important dose-dependent effects following injection including lung, skin, and mucous membrane changes. Toxic if absorbed through skin, with significant degree of absorption in workers with skin diseases. Possible risk of irreversible effects exists. BLEOMYCIN causes heritable genetic damage and possible sensitizer.

Exposure may cause skin rash (allergic skin reaction). Contact with eye may cause conjunctivitis. Exposure may lead to a possible allergic reaction (sensitization) if inhaled, ingested, or in contact with skin. If injection occurs, symptoms are fever, chills, hypotension and wheezing. BLEOMYCIN is readily absorbed through skin.

Caution: Females and males planning to have a child, pregnant women, and nursing mothers should exercise caution regarding potential occupational exposure to this cytotoxic drug. No information or not enough information exists or was provided concerning occupational exposure that may potentially occur while handling BLEOMYCIN and its affects on reproductive systems, the fetus, and/or if it is secreted along with breast milk, which may harm nursing infants. Staff members should consult with the occupational health physician monitoring workers' health in your facility to be apprised of potential hazards and should be advised to avoid becoming pregnant and/or breastfeeding or should be transferred in accordance with policy/procedures to other duties that do not involve preparation, handling, and administering this drug.

Target Organs/Systems: Lungs, reproductive systems, skin, eyes, mucous membranes, blood, fetus, cardiovascular system, and GI tract

Medical Conditions Generally Aggravated by Exposure:

- Pregnancy.
- Toxic if absorbed through skin, with significant degree of absorption in workers with skin

diseases. Therapeutic doses of this material may aggravate renal disease or pulmonary impairment. Pre-existing kidney, liver, audiometric system, and central nervous system disorders may be aggravated by exposure to this product. Other organs that undergo rapid cellular division may also be targets after systemic exposure.

- Repeated exposure to a highly toxic material may produce general deterioration of health by an accumulation in one or more human organs.

Specific Medical Surveillance Information: Reproductive and pregnancy counseling.

Pre-employment and periodic examinations should be done at least annually. A complete blood count, including differential should be taken to provide a baseline. Keep a permanent registry of all staff involved with this drug. Hypersensitivity to BLEOMYCIN may occur because of exposure to previous cytotoxic drugs and/or radiation therapy.

Occupational Exposure Level/Limit (OEL) & Sampling Methods:

Environmental Sentinel Contamination Action Level (ESCAL): Not otherwise specified
BLEOMYCIN Occupational Exposure Level/ Limit (OEL): Bedford Labs
50 ng/m3
(Method not listed or specified)

Supplemental Response Information

Extinguishing Media: Use extinguishing agent which is the most appropriate to extinguish surrounding fire (carbon dioxide, foam, dry chemical or water fog as extinguishing media).

Solubility: BLEOMYCIN is completely water soluble (14–20 mg/ml) with a range of pH of 4.5–6.

BLEOMYCIN SULFATE is very water soluble, slightly soluble in dehydrate alcohol, and practically insoluble in acetone and ether.

Chemical Degradation/Neutralization Method: A manufacturer's Material Safety Data Sheet (MSDS) recommends treating spill surfaces with a 10% sodium hypochlorite (bleach) solution after absorbing liquids with inert absorbent pads or removing any powder present: allow solution to stand for up to one hour, and then thoroughly wash spilled surfaces with soap and water; sample to determine if surface contamination is still present (if sampling method is available). If drug is still present, repeat above steps; dispose of wastes in accordance with your local procedures, state, and federal regulations.

Incompatibility: BLEOMYCIN is incompatible with strong oxidizing agents, acids and caustic chemicals. BLEOMYCIN is incompatible with amino-acids, aminophylline, ascorbic acid, dexamethasone, frusemide, riboflavin, and sulfhydryl-containing reagents.

BUSULFAN (*bu-SUL-fan*)
MYLERAN®78

Chemical Abstract Service (CAS) Registry
    Number: 55-98-1
Registry of Toxic Effects of Chemical Substances
    (RTECS): EK1750000
$C_6H_{14}O_6S_2$
$CH_3-SO_2-0(CH_2)4-0S0_2-CH_3$

1,4-BUTANEDIOL, DIMETHANESULFONATE

Health & Safety Hazards/US Department of Transportation (DOT)/US Environmental Protection Agency (EPA)—Sources

Carcinogen G1—International Agency for Research on Cancer, Carcinogen C1—US National Toxicology Program and Material Safety Data Sheet, Carcinogen—University of Maryland at College Park, Carcinogen—Berkeley University Hazardous Chemical List, Teratogen—University of Maryland at College Park, Teratogen—Material Safety Data Sheet, Toxic—Material Safety Data Sheet, Reproductive Effector—Material Safety Data Sheet, Mutagen—US New Jersey State Department of Health and Senior Services Hazardous Substances Fact Sheet, Mutagen—Material Safety Data Sheet, Cytotoxic—Material Safety Data Sheet, Cytotoxic—British Columbia Cancer Agency Canada, Vesicant—British Columbia Cancer Agency Canada, Pregnancy Category (D)—US Food and Drug Administration, Developmental and Carcinogen—US California State Proposition 65, US California State Environmental Protection Agency Listed, UN 2811 (Toxic), Class 6.1, Group III, Na 1759.

BUSULFAN is manufactured as a 2 mg tablets or colorless liquid dissolved from a white powder.

BULSULFAN may cause fetal harm; breastfeeding: discontinue; and reproductive/developmental hazards (*A Guide for Occupational Health Professionals Technical Manual*, Navy Environmental Health Center [NEHC-TM-OEM 6260.01a]).

BULSULFAN is a white crystalline powder.

First Aid Medical Information/ Occupational Exposure Limits

First Aid Measures to include: Use general first aid measures except for the following:

Ingestion: If victim is conscious and alert, give 2–4 cups of milk or water. Never give anything by mouth to an unconscious person. Get medical aid immediately.

Physician's note: Treat according to locally accepted protocols. For additional guidance, refer to the current prescribing information or to the local poison control information center. Treatment in cases of overexposure should be treated as an overdose of a cytotoxic agent. Antidotes: no specific antidotes are recommended.

Medical Information:

Caution and Warning Statements: BUSULFAN is a carcinogen in humans. It has been shown to cause leukemia and kidney and uterine cancer. BUSULFAN is toxic and an irritant. BUSULFAN is toxic by inhalation, ingestion and by skin contact. BUSULFAN has powerful cytotoxic properties. It is moisture sensitive. BUSULFAN is mutagenic in mouse and possibly in man. BUSULFAN may cause heritable genetic damage and may cause fetal harm. Exposure to BUSULFAN may cause irritation to eyes, respiratory system, and skin to include blistering of the skin. Eye contact may cause irreversible eye damage, which is seen as corneal opacity. The Registry of Toxic Effects of Chemical Substances (RTECS) listed BUSULFAN as a suspected cardiovascular or blood toxicant; as a gastrointestinal or as a liver toxicant; or kidney toxicant; as a neurotoxicant and as a skin or sense organ toxicant.

Exposure to BUSULFAN can cause irritation to the skin, eyes and lungs, nausea, vomiting, diarrhea, and seizures. Damage to bone marrow and liver may occur. British Columbia Cancer Agency lists BUSULFAN as a cytotoxic drug and a vesicant.

Caution: Females and males planning to have a child, pregnant women, and nursing mothers should exercise caution regarding potential occupational exposure to this cytotoxic drug. No information or not enough information exists or was provided concerning occupational exposure that may potentially occur while handling this drug and its affects on reproductive systems, the fetus, and/or if it is secreted along with breast milk, which may harm nursing infants. Staff members should consult with the occupational health physician monitoring workers' health in your facility to be apprised of potential hazards and should be advised to avoid becoming pregnant and/or breastfeeding or should be transferred in accordance with policy/procedures to other duties that do not involve preparation, handling, and administering this drug.

Therapeutic Levels: BUSULFAN interferes with spermatogenesis in experimental animals. There have been clinical reports of sterility, azoospermia, and testicular atrophy in male patients receiving this drug. Exposure to females has reduced fertility in females.

Entry to the working area should be controlled. New or expectant mothers are at greater risk if exposed to the active ingredient, which is readily absorbed through the skin. They should not handle unpackaged or packaged product.

Target Organs/Systems: Bone marrow, blood, GI tract, liver, eyes, respiratory system, mucous membrane, and fetus

Medical Condition Generally Aggravated by Exposure:

- Alcohol consumption may increase the liver damage caused by BUSULFAN exposure.
- Pregnancy.

Specific Medical Surveillance Information: Reproductive and pregnancy counseling

Recommended medical surveillance for staff working with BUSULFAN is a complete blood cell count, a chest x-ray, lung function tests, and liver function tests.

Occupational Exposure Level/Limit (OEL) & Sampling Methods:

Environmental Sentinel Contamination Action Level (ESCAL): Not otherwise specified

BUSULFA (MYLERAN®78) Occupational Exposure Level/Limit (OEL) GW Occupational Exposure Level/Limit (OEL) GSK (SAME)

1.0 μ/m3 (Occupational Exposure Level/Limit (OEL) GW/GSK 2005)

(Method not listed or specified)

Supplemental Response Information

Extinguishing Media: Use extinguishing agent which is the most appropriate to extinguish surrounding fire (foam, dry chemical or water fog as extinguishing media).

Warning: Carbon dioxide extinguishers may be ineffective.

Solubility: BUSULFAN is water insoluble to very slightly soluble in water, but decomposes in water. BUSULFAN is very slightly soluble in alcohol; freely soluble in acetone (soluble 1 in 45) and in acetronirile.

Chemical Degradation/Neutralization Method: A manufacturer's Material Safety Data Sheet (MSDS) recommended using a dilute caustic soda and sodium hypochlorite (bleach) solution to neutralize BUSULFAN and spill surfaces.

Incompatibility: BUSULFAN is incompatible with strong oxidizing agents.

C

CAMPTOSAR®18

Chemical Abstract Service (CAS) Registry Number: 100286-90-6

IRINOTECAN HYDROCHLORIDE TRIHYDRATE

Chemical Abstract Service (CAS) Registry Number: 136572-09-3

$C_{33}H_{39}ClN_4O_6$

IRINOTECAN (eye-rye-no-TEE-can)

Chemical Abstract Service (CAS) Registry Number: 97682-44-5

IRINOTECAN HCL

Chemical Abstract Service (CAS) Registry Number: 689-03-4

CPT

CPT-11

$C_{33}-H_{38}-N_4-O_6.CL-H$

$C_{33}H_{38}N_4O_6.HCl.3H_2O$

CAMPTOTHECIN
S(+)-CAMPTOTHECIN
CAMPTOTHECIN

Chemical Abstract Service (CAS) Registry Number: 7689-03-4 (mixture)

Registry of Toxic Effects of Chemical Substances (RTECS): UQ0492000

$C_{20}-H_{16}-N_2-0_4$

CAMPTOTHECIN

Chemical Abstract Service (CAS) Registry Number: 97682-44-5

Registry of Toxic Effects of Chemical Substances (RTECS): DW1061000

Health & Safety Hazards/US Department of Transportation (DOT)/US Environmental Protection Agency (EPA)—Sources

Mutagen—Material Safety Data Sheet, Reproductive Effector—Toxic Material Safety Data Sheet, Highly Toxic—Material Safety Data Sheet, Cytotoxic—British Columbia Cancer Agency Canada, Nonvesicant—British Columbia Cancer Agency Canada, Pregnancy Category (D)—US Food and Drug Administration, National Fire Protection Association Hazard Rating Health (2) Flammability (1) Instability/Reactivity (0)—Material Safety Data Sheet, Hazardous Materials Identification System (R) and/or US Department of Defense System Health (2) Fire Hazard (1) Reactivity (0) Personal Protective Code (E) (Safety Glasses, Chemical Gloves, Dust Respirator)—Material Safety Data Sheet, National Fire Protection Association Hazard Rating Health (2) Flammability (0) Instability/Reactivity (0)—Material Safety Data Sheet, Hazardous Materials Identification System (R) and/or US Department of Defense System Health (2) Fire Hazard (0) Reactivity (0) Personal Protective Code (-) (None stated)—Material Safety Data Sheet, National Fire Protection Association Health (3) Flammability (1) Instability/Reactivity (0)—Material Safety Data Sheet, Hazardous Materials Identification System (R) and/or US Department of Defense System Health (3★) Fire Hazard (1) Reactivity (0) Personal Protective Code (E) (Safety Glasses, Chemical Gloves, Dust Respirator)—Material Safety Data Sheet, UN 1544, Class 6.1, Group III; UN 2811, Toxic Solid, Class 6.1 (Toxic).

CAMPTOSAR®18 (IRINOTECAN) is available as an injection (20 mg/ml).

First Aid Medical Information/ Occupational Exposure Limits

First Aid Measures to include: Use general first aid measures.

Medical Information:

Caution and Warning Statements: Highly toxic, may cause heritable genetic damage, irritating to eyes, respiratory system, and causes skin burns. Exposure to CAMPTOSAR®18 may result in rare side effects—decreased platelet count with increased risk of bleeding.

Caution: The toxicities of most cytotoxic drugs have not been fully investigated, particularly as it pertains to occupational exposure. CAMPTOSAR®18 is one of the drugs that has little occupational hazards information available. Therefore, therapeutic dose information was extrapolated below to assist in determining occupational toxicity, and signs and symptoms of overexposure. Therefore, it is prudent to minimize occupational exposure to CAMPTOSAR®18.

Exposure to CAMPTOSAR®18 may produce nausea, vomiting and diarrhea, extreme fatigue, and mouth sores. May cause harm to fetus (unborn child). CAMPTOSAR®18 may cause heritable genetic damage. Exposure may cause fetal harm.

Carcinogenesis, mutagenesis, and impairment of fertility long-term carcinogenicity studies with IRINOTECAN (CAMPTOSAR®18) were not conducted.

Caution: Females and males planning to have a child, pregnant women, and nursing mothers should exercise caution regarding potential occupational exposure to this cytotoxic drug. No information or not enough information exists or was provided concerning occupational exposure that may potentially occur while handling this drug and its affects on reproductive systems, the fetus, and/or if it is secreted along with breast milk, which may harm nursing infants. Staff members should consult with the occupational health physician monitoring workers' health in your facility to be apprised of potential hazards and should be advised to avoid becoming pregnant and/or breastfeeding or should be transferred in accordance with policy/procedures to other duties that do not involve preparation, handling, and administering this drug.

Target Organs/Systems: Blood and fetus

Medical Conditions Generally Aggravated with Exposure:

- Repeated exposure to a highly toxic material may produce general deterioration of health by an accumulation in one or more human organs.
- Reproductive and pregnancy issues.

Specific Medical Surveillance Information: Reproductive and pregnancy counseling.

Therapeutic laboratory tests careful monitoring of the white blood cell count with differential, hemoglobin, and platelet count is recommended before each dose of CAMPTOSAR®18.

Occupational Exposure Level/Limit (OEL) & Sampling Methods: Not otherwise specified

Environmental Sentinel Contamination Action Level (ESCAL): Air, surface

Supplemental Response Information

Extinguishing Media: Use extinguishing agent which is the most appropriate to extinguish surrounding fire (carbon dioxide, foam, dry chemical or water fog as extinguishing media). (Do not use water jet.)

Solubility:

CAMPTOSAR®18
(IRINOTECAN HCL):
S(+)-CAMPTOTHECIN:
CAMPTOSAR ®18 (IRINOTECAN HCL) is
    slightly to freely soluble in water and organic
    solvents.
S(+)-CAMPTOTHECIN is water insoluble.

Chemical Degradation/Neutralization Method: Not otherwise specified

Note: If a specific degradation or neutralization method is not provided in this section and you do not have other specific information that will advise you on how to clean up the specific material spilled, then follow the general spill procedure found in the introduction section of this handbook.

Incompatibility: CAMPTOTHECIN is incompatible with strong oxidizing agents. Avoid heat, flames, sparks, and other sources of ignition.

CAPECITABINE *(KAP-e-SYE-ta-been)*
XELODA®19

Chemical Abstract Service (CAS) Registry
    Number: 154361-50-9
Registry of Toxic Effects of Chemical Substances
    (RTECS):HA3852500
$C_{15}-H_{22}-F-N_3-0_6$

5'-DEOXY-5-FLUOROCYTISINE

Chemical Abstract Service (CAS) Registry
    Number: 158798-73-3

Health & Safety Hazards/US Department of Transportation (DOT)/US Environmental Protection Agency (EPA)—Sources

Toxic—Material Safety Data Sheet, Teratogen—Material Safety Data Sheet, Pregnancy Category (D)—US Food and Drug Administration, Hazardous Materials Identification System (R) and/or US Department of Defense System: Health (1) Fire Hazard (1) Reactivity (0) Personal Protective Code (D)(Face Shield, Chemical Gloves, Chemical Apron), National Fire Protection Association Hazard Rating: Health (1) Flammability (1) Instability/Reactivity (0)—Material Safety Data Sheet.

CAPECITABINE (XELODA®19) is a peach color 500 mg and 150 mg tablet.

First Aid Medical Information/ Occupational Exposure Limits

First Aid Measures to include: Use general first aid measures except for the following:

Ingestion: Drink plenty of water and induce vomiting only if conscious; repeat several times. Seek medical assistance.

Physician's note (A): In case of accidental exposure, treat symptomatically and supportively and keep a sample of urine in order to determine the content of fluoro-b-alanine.

Physician's note (B): Treat symptoms and eliminate overexposure. Consult the package insert for additional information that can assist with treatment of overexposure.

Medical Information:

Caution and Warning Statements: CAPECITABINE may cause birth defects based on animal data. Exposure may cause reproductive systems effects. Toxic exposure may occur by inhalation, in contact with skin, and if swallowed.

Caution: Females and males planning to have a child, pregnant women, and nursing mothers should exercise caution regarding potential occupational exposure to this cytotoxic drug. No information or not enough information exists or was provided concerning occupational exposure that may potentially occur while handling this drug and its affects on reproductive systems, the fetus, and/or if it is secreted along with breast milk, which may harm nursing infants. Staff members should consult with the occupational health physician monitoring workers' health in your facility to be apprised of potential hazards and should be advised to avoid becoming pregnant and/or breastfeeding or should be transferred in accordance with policy/procedures to other duties that do not involve preparation, handling, and administering this drug.

Target Organs/Systems: Skin, eyes, gastrointestinal, kidney/liver, hematopoietic/blood, immune systems, possibly reproductive system, and fetus

Medical Conditions Generally Aggravated with Exposure:

- Hypersensitivity reactions may occur in individuals who have exhibited hypersensitivity to 5-fluorouracil.
- Reproductive and pregnancy issues.

Specific Medical Surveillance Information: Reproductive and pregnancy counseling.

Pre-existing gastrointestinal system conditions, kidney disorders, liver disorders, and other disorders involving the target organs of this product may be aggravated by exposures to this product (especially in doses approaching therapeutic levels for this product).

Occupational Exposure Level/Limit (OEL) & Sampling Methods:

Environmental Sentinel Contamination Action Level (ESCAL): Not otherwise specified
XELODA®19 Occupational Exposure Level/Limit (OEL) & Sampling Methods:
Occupational Exposure Level/Limit (OEL): Hoffmann-La Roche Inc.
0.01 mg/m3 Time-Weighted Average (TWA)

Occupational Exposure Level/Limit (OEL): Pharmacia & Upjohn
Occupational Exposure Level/Limit (OEL): CAMTOSAR
0.4 µg/m3 Time-Weighted Average (TWA)
(Method not listed or specified)

Supplemental Response Information

Extinguishing Media: Use extinguishing agent which is the most appropriate to extinguish surrounding fire (carbon dioxide, foam, dry chemical or water fog as extinguishing media).

Solubility: CAPECITABINE is water soluble.

Chemical Degradation/Neutralization Method: Not otherwise specified

Note: If a specific degradation or neutralization method is not provided in this section and you do not have other specific information that will guide you on how to clean up the specific material spilled, then follow the general spill procedure found in the introduction section of this handbook.

Incompatibility: XELODA®19 is incompatible with strong oxidizers and strong acids.

CARBOPLATIN (*car-bo-PLA-tin*)
PARAPLATIN®20

Chemical Abstract Service (CAS) Registry Number: 41575-94-4
Registry of Toxic Effects of Chemical Substances (RTECS): TP2300000
$C_6H_{12}N_2O_4Pt_2$

1,1-CYCLOBUTANEDICARB-OXYLATODIAM-MINEPL

Chemical Abstract Service (CAS) Registry Number: 7440-06-4 (Platinum) (Mixture)

Health & Safety Hazards/US Department of Transportation (DOT)/US Environmental Protection Agency (EPA)—Sources

Mutagen—University of Maryland at College Park, Mutagen—Material Safety Data Sheet, Embryotoxic—Material Safety Data Sheet, Carcinogen—Material Safety Data Sheet, Teratogen—Material Safety Data Sheet, Reproductive Effector—Material Safety Data Sheet, Highly Toxic—Material Safety Data Sheet, Cytotoxic—Material Safety Data Sheet, Ototoxic—T. C. Hain, Sensitizer—Material Safety Data Sheet, Cytotoxic—British Columbia Cancer Agency Canada, Nonvesicant—British Columbia Cancer Agency Canada, Pregnancy Category (D)—US Food and Drug Administration, Developmental—US California State Proposition 65, National Fire Protection Association Hazard Rating Health (3) Flammability (1) Instability/Reactivity (0)—Material Safety Data Sheet, National Fire Protection Association Hazard Rating Health (2) Flammability (1) Instability/Reactivity (0)—Material Safety Data Sheet, National Fire Protection Association Hazard Rating Health (2) Flammability (0) Instability/Reactivity (0)—Material Safety Data Sheet, Hazardous Materials Identification System (R) and/or US Department of Defense System Health (2) Fire Hazard (1) Reactivity (0) Personal Protective Code (E) (Safety Glasses, Chemical Gloves, Dust Respirator), Material Safety Data Sheet, Hazardous Materials Identification System (R) and/or US Department of Defense System Health (3) Flammability (1) Reactivity (0) Personal Protective Code (X) (Ask Supervisor), UN 2811, Class 6.1, Group III, US California State Environmental Protection Agency Listed.

CARBOPLATIN is a white solid or a colorless fluid.

First Aid Medical Information/ Occupational Exposure Limits

First Aid Measures to include: Use general first aid measures except for the following:

Ingestion: If swallowed, induction of vomiting, if person is conscious, alert, and not experiencing convulsions. Seek medical assistance.

Eye contact: Do not use an eye ointment. Seek medical attention. Follow general first aid measures.

Physician's notes: CARBOPLATIN should be treated as potentially carcinogenic, and may be mutagenic, teratogenic, or allergenic. If respiratory distress occurs after inhalation of airborne droplets, administer emergency airway support and 100% humidified supplemental oxygen with the assisted ventilation, if needed. If coughing or difficulty in breathing develops, evacuating for respiratory tract irritation, bronchitis or pneumonitis. Treatment is symptomatic. There is no specific antidote.

Medical Information:

Caution and Warning Statements: CARBOPLATIN is listed as a possible carcinogen. CARBOPLATIN is highly toxic if ingested. May cause harm to the unborn child. Exposure may cause heritable genetic damage. This drug may cause sensitization by inhalation and skin contact (permeator). CARBOPLATIN is harmful by inhalation, in contact with skin, and if ingested. Inhalation: transient bronchial irritation, conjunctivitis, injection-reversible blood effects, hepatic toxicity, kidney, abnormalities, and electrolyte loss. Exposure may produce allergic reactions (sensitizer). Eye contact may cause conjunctivitis and ringing of the ears, which may lead to hearing loss.

Caution: Females and males planning to have a child, pregnant women, and nursing mothers should exercise caution regarding potential occupational exposure to this cytotoxic drug. No information or not enough information exists or was provided concerning occupational exposure that may potentially occur while handling this drug and its affects on reproductive systems, the fetus, and/or if it is secreted along with breast milk, which may harm nursing infants. Staff members should consult with the occupational health physician monitoring workers' health in your facility to be apprised of potential hazards and should be advised to avoid becoming pregnant and/or breastfeeding or should be transferred in accordance with policy/procedures to other duties that do not involve preparation, handling, and administering this drug.

Target Organs/Systems: Bone marrow, blood, kidneys, reproductive systems (male and female organs), hearing (inner ear), skin (hair loss), embryo/fetus, gastrointestinal system, nervous system, lungs, and liver

Medical Conditions Generally Aggravated by Exposure:

- Exposure to CARBOPLATIN may aggravate kidney disease, liver, nervous system, hearing disorders, neurological diseases, anemia and other forms of bone marrow suppression (as platinum, soluble salt), a hearing disorder, kidney disorders, hearing loss, and pregnancy.
- CARBOPLATIN is a toxicologically synergistic product. Certain other cytotoxic oncology drugs, which have similar targets as CARBOPLATIN, especially myelosuppressive drugs should be cautioned.

Specific Medical Surveillance Information: Reproductive and pregnancy counseling.

Baseline testing would include a urine analysis, a complete blood count with differential, a blood test for renal function, and for liver function.

Supplemental testing may include hearing test, lung function test, and chest x-ray. Based on opportunity for exposure and duration of exposure a periodic follow-up examination may be considered. This exam is overseen by a physician thoroughly knowledgeable about both the toxicity of this compound and the extent of workplace exposure. It is recommended that the content be similar to the pre-placement exam.

Occupational Exposure Level/Limit (OEL) & Sampling Methods:

Environmental Sentinel Contamination Action Level (ESCAL): Not otherwise specified
US Occupational Safety and Health Administration (OSHA) PLATINUM:
Permissible Exposure Limit (PEL) (OSHA) 2 μg/m3 Time-Weighted Average (8-hours TWA)

US American Conference of Governmental Industrial Hygienists (ACGIH):
TLV 2 μg/m3 Time-Weighted Average (TWA)

US National Institute for Occupational Safety and Health
Recommended Exposure Limit 2 μg/m3 Time-Weighted Average (TWA)
IDLH: Cannot be established

Bristol-Myers Squibb
2 μg/m3 (Sensitizer)
Bristol-Myers Squibb exposure guidelines summary: adherence to this guideline should protect employees from experiencing the therapeutic and/or adverse effects of this drug. Recommended industrial hygiene monitoring methods: contact the Bristol-Myers Squibb AIHA accredited industrial hygiene laboratory at 732-227-7368.
(Some of the above methods are not available)

Supplemental Response Information

Extinguishing Media: Use extinguishing agent which is the most appropriate to extinguish surrounding fire (carbon dioxide, foam, dry chemical or water fog as extinguishing media). Do not use water jet.

Solubility: CARBOPLATIN is miscible in water (15 mg/ml).

CARBOPLATIN is water soluble (14 mg/ml) with a pH range of 5.0–7.0 (1 % solution).

CARBOPLATIN is virtually insoluble in ethanol, acetone, and dimethylacetamide.

Chemical Degradation/Neutralization Method: There are two recommended procedures (alkaline detergent/water solution; and a 3m sulphuric acid and 0.3m potassium or 5% sodium hypochlorite) for CARBOPLATIN. See below for optional methods.

A manufacturer's Material Safety Data Sheet recommends using alkaline soap/detergent and water to clean spill surfaces after absorbing liquids with inert absorbent pads or removing any power present: repeat using soap and water; sample to determine if surface contamination is still present (if sampling method is available). If drug is still present, repeat above steps; dispose of wastes in accordance with your local procedures, state, and federal regulations.

Incompatibility: CARBOPLATIN is incompatible with strong oxidizing agents, acids, and caustics chemicals.

Warning: Formation of a platinum precipitate when precipitation comes in to contact with aluminum.

CARBOPLATIN (*kar-boe-PLAH-tin*)
PARAPLATIN®20

Chemical Abstract Service (CAS) Registry
Number: 41575-94-4
Registry of Toxic Effects of Chemical Substances
(RTECS): TP2300000

DIAMMINE
C_6-H_{12}-N_2-O_4-PT

1,1-CYCLOBUTANEDICARB-OXYLATODIAM-MINEPL

Chemical Abstract Service (CAS) Registry
Number: 7440-06-4 (mixture)
C_4-$H_6(CO_2)_2$
$PT(NH_3)_2$

Health & Safety Hazards/US Department of Transportation (DOT)/US Environmental Protection Agency (EPA)—Sources

Mutagen—University of Maryland at College Park, Mutagen—Material Safety Data Sheet, Embryotoxic—Material Safety Data Sheet, Carcinogen—Material Safety Data Sheet, Teratogen—Material Safety Data Sheet, Reproductive Effector—Material Safety Data Sheet, Highly Toxic—Material Safety Data Sheet, Cytotoxic—Material Safety Data Sheet, Ototoxic—T. C. Hain, Sensitizer—Material Safety Data Sheet, Cytotoxic—British Columbia Cancer Agency Canada, Nonvesicant—British Columbia Cancer Agency Canada, Pregnancy Category (D)—US Food and Drug Administration, Developmental—US California State Proposition 65, National Fire Protection Association Hazard Rating Health (3) Flammability (1) Instability/Reactivity (0)—Material Safety Data Sheet, National Fire Protection Association Hazard Rating Health (2) Flammability (1) Instability/Reactivity (0)—Material Safety Data Sheet, National Fire Protection Association Hazard Rating Health (2) Flammability (0) Instability/Reactivity (0)—Material Safety Data Sheet, Hazardous Materials Identification System (R) and/or US Department of Defense System Health (2) Fire Hazard (1) Reactivity (0) Personal Protective Code (E) (Safety Glasses, Chemical Gloves, Dust Respirator), Material Safety Data Sheet, Hazardous Materials Identification System (R) and/or US Department of Defense System Health (3) Fire Hazard (1) Reactivity (0) Personal Protective Code (X) (Ask Supervisor), UN 2811, Class 6.1, Group III, US California State Environmental Protection Agency Listed.

CARBOPLATIN (PARAPLATIN®20) is available as an injection (50 mg, 150 mg, and 450 mg).

First Aid Medical Information/Occupational Exposure Limits

First Aid Measures to include: Use general first aid measures except for the following:

Ingestion: If swallowed, induction of vomiting, if person is conscious, alert, and not experiencing convulsions. Seek medical assistance.

Eye contact: Do not use an eye ointment. Seek medical attention. Follow general first aid measures.

Physician's notes: CARBOPLATIN should be treated as potentially carcinogenic, and may be mutagenic, teratogenic, or allergenic. If respiratory distress occurs after inhalation of airborne droplets, administer emergency airway support and 100% humidified supplemental oxygen with the assisted ventilation, if needed. If coughing or difficulty in breathing develops, evacuating for respiratory tract irritation, bronchitis, or pneumonitis. Treatment is symptomatic. There is no specific antidote.

Medical Information:

Caution and Warning Statements: CARBOPLATIN is listed as a possible carcinogen. CARBOPLATIN is highly toxic if ingested. May cause harm to the unborn child. Exposure may cause heritable genetic damage. This drug may cause sensitization by inhalation and skin contact (permeator). CARBOPLATIN is harmful by inhalation, in contact with skin, and if ingested. Inhalation—transient bronchial irritation, conjunctivitis, injection—reversible blood effects, hepatic toxicity, kidney, abnormalities, and electrolyte loss. Exposure may produce allergic reactions (sensitizer). Eye contact may cause conjunctivitis and ringing of the ears, which may lead to hearing loss.

Caution: Females and males planning to have a child, pregnant women, and nursing mothers should exercise caution regarding potential occupational exposure to this cytotoxic drug. No information or not enough information exists or was provided concerning occupational exposure that may potentially occur while handling this drug and its affects on reproductive systems, the fetus, and/or if it is secreted along with breast milk, which may harm nursing infants. Staff members should consult with the occupational health physician monitoring workers' health in your facility to be apprised of potential hazards and should be advised to avoid becoming pregnant and/or breastfeeding or should be transferred in accordance with policy/procedures to other duties that do not involve preparation, handling, and administering this drug.

Target Organs/Systems: Bone marrow, blood, kidneys, reproductive systems (male and female organs), hearing (inner ear), skin (hair loss), embryo/fetus, gastrointestinal system, nervous system, lungs, and liver

Medical Conditions Generally Aggravated by Exposure:

- Exposure to CARBOPLATIN may aggravate kidney disease, liver, nervous system, hearing disorders, neurological diseases, anemia and other forms of bone marrow suppression (as platinum, soluble salt), and a hearing disorder. Kidney disorders, hearing loss, and pregnancy.
- CARBOPLATIN is a toxicological synergistic product, certain other cytotoxic oncology drugs, which have similar targets as CARBOPLATIN; especially myelosuppressive drugs should be cautioned.

Specific Medical Surveillance Information: Reproductive and pregnancy counseling.

Baseline testing would include a urine analysis, a complete blood count with differential, and a blood test for renal function and a test for liver function.

Supplemental testing may include hearing test, lung function test, and chest x-ray. Based on opportunity for exposure and duration of exposure a periodic follow-up examination may be considered. This exam is overseen by a physician thoroughly knowledgeable about both the toxicity of this compound and the extent of workplace exposure. It is recommended that the content be similar to the pre-placement exam.

Occupational Exposure Level/Limit (OEL) & Sampling Methods:

> *Environmental Sentinel Contamination Action Level (ESCAL)*: Air, surface, personal
> US Occupational Safety and Health Administration (OSHA) PLATINUM:
> Permissible Exposure Limit (PEL) (OSHA) 2 μg/m3 Time-Weighted Average (8-hours TWA)
>
> US American Conference of Governmental Industrial Hygienists (ACGIH):
> TLV 2 μg/m3 Time-Weighted Average (TWA)
>
> US National Institute for Occupational Safety and Health
> Recommended Exposure Limit 2 μg/m3 Time-Weighted Average (TWA)
> *IDLH*: Cannot be established

Bristol-Myers Squibb
2 μg/m3 (Sensitizer)
Bristol-Myers Squibb exposure guidelines summary: adherence to this guideline should protect employees from experiencing the therapeutic and/or adverse effects of this drug. Recommended industrial hygiene monitoring methods: contact the Bristol-Myers Squibb AIHA accredited industrial hygiene laboratory at 732-227-7368.
(Some of the above methods are not available)

Supplemental Response Information

Extinguishing Media: Use extinguishing agent which is the most appropriate to extinguish surrounding fire (carbon dioxide, foam, dry chemical or water fog as extinguishing media). Do not use water jet.

Solubility: CARBOPLATIN is miscible in water (15 mg/ml).

CARBOPLATIN is water soluble (14 mg/ml) with a pH range of 5.0–7.0 (1 % solution).

CARBOPLATIN is virtually insoluble in ethanol, acetone, and dimethylacetamide.

Chemical Degradation/Neutralization Method: There are two recommended procedures (alkaline detergent/water solution; and a 3m sulphuric acid and 0.3m potassium or 5% sodium hypochlorite) for CARBOPLA-TIN. See below and above for optional methods.

A manufacturer's Material Safety Data Sheet recommends treating spill surfaces with a 3m sulphuric acid and 0.3m potassium or 5% sodium hypochlorite after absorbing liquids with inert absorbent pads or removing any powder present allow the solution to stand for up to one hour, and then thoroughly wash spilled surfaces with soap and water; repeat using soap and water; sample to determine if surface contamination is still present (if sampling method is available). If drug is still present, repeat above steps; dispose of wastes in accordance with your local procedures, state, and federal regulations.

Incompatibility: CARBOPLATIN is incompatible with strong oxidizing agents, acids and caustics chemicals.

Warning: Formation of a platinum precipitate when precipitation comes in to contact with aluminum.

CARMUSTINE (*kar-MUS-teen*)
BCNU
BiCNU®21
BISCHLOROETHYL NITROSOUREA

Chemical Abstract Service (CAS) Registry
Number: 154 93 8 (ethyl alcohol is used as a diluents, only CARMUSTINE hazards were evaluated and listed)
Registry of Toxic Effects of Chemical Substances (RTECS): YS2625000
$C_5H_9Cl_2N_3O_2$

Health & Safety Hazards/US Department of Transportation (DOT)/US Environmental Protection Agency (EPA)—Sources

Carcinogen G2A—International Agency for Research on Cancer, Highly Toxic—Material Safety Data Sheet, Carcinogen C2—US National Toxicology Program-Material Safety Data Sheet, Carcinogen—US National Institutes of Health (NIH) and Material Safety Data Sheet, Carcinogen—University of Maryland at College Park, Teratogen—University of Maryland at College Park, Teratogen—US National Institutes of Health (NIH) and Material Safety Data Sheet, Mutagen—US National Institutes of Health (NIH) and Material Safety Data Sheet, Embryotoxic—US National Institutes of Health (NIH) and Material Safety Data Sheet, Cytotoxic—British Columbia Cancer Agency Canada, Vesicant—British Columbia Cancer Agency

Canada, Pregnancy Category (D)—US Food and Drug Administration, Carcinogen and Developmental—US California State Proposition 65, US California State Environmental Protection Agency Listed, UN 1992, UN 2811.

CARMUSTINE (BICNU®21) is a colorless fluid (~100 mg) after being dissolved from a powder.

BISCHLOROETHYL NITROSOUREA (CARMUSTINE) (BLENOXANE®17): Breastfeeding is contraindicated.

First Aid Medical Information/ Occupational Exposure Limits

First Aid Measures to include: Use general first aid measures except for the following.

Dermal contact: Avoid rubbing of skin or increasing its temperature.

Medical Information:

Caution and Warning Statements: Exposure to CARMUSTINE may cause cancer (listed as probable human carcinogen), heritable genetic damage, and may cause harm to the unborn child.

Exposure may also cause impair fertility and is considered to be a very toxic if swallowed. CARMUSTINE is irritating to the skin, eyes, and respiratory system.

CARMUSTINE (BISCHLOROETHYL NITROSOUREA) can cause nausea, vomiting, and diarrhea, while repeated exposure may cause eye damage with loss of vision. CARMUSTINE (BISCHLOROETHYL NITROSOUREA) may damage the liver and kidneys. Inhalation can cause scarring of the lungs (fibrosis) with coughing and shortness of breath. High exposure can damage bone marrow, which will reduce resistance to infections. British Columbia Cancer Agency lists CARMUSTINE as a vesicant.

Caution: Females and males planning to have a child, pregnant women, and nursing mothers should exercise caution regarding potential occupational exposure to this cytotoxic drug. No information or not enough information exists or was provided concerning occupational exposure that may potentially occur while handling this drug and its affects on reproductive systems, the fetus, and/or if it is secreted along with breast milk, which may harm nursing infants. Staff members should consult with the occupational health physician monitoring workers' health in your facility to be apprised of potential hazards and should be advised to avoid becoming pregnant and/or breastfeeding or should be transferred in accordance with policy/procedures to other duties that do not involve preparation, handling, and administering this drug.

Target Organs/Systems: Reproductive systems, blood, bone marrow, gastrointestinal system, lungs, eyes, liver, kidneys, and skin

Medical Conditions Generally Aggravated by Exposure:

- CARMUSTINE is toxic, carcinogenic, teratogenic, mutagenic, and embryotoxic. It is a reproductive hazard for males and females. It is absorbed by various body tissues, through the skin and respiratory and intestinal tracts, and transplacentally. Alcohol consumption can increase the liver damage caused by exposure from BISCHLOROETHYL NITROSOUREA (CARMUSTINE).
- Reproductive and pregnancy issues.

Specific Medical Surveillance Information: Reproductive and pregnancy counseling.

A complete blood count, including differential, a lung function test, may be taken to provide a baseline. If symptoms develop and/or overexposure is suspected, an examination of the eyes and vision can be performed along with liver and kidney functions tests, and another complete set of blood counts.

Occupational Exposure Level/Limit (OEL) & Sampling Methods: Not otherwise specified

Environmental Sentinel Contamination Action Level (ESCAL): Not otherwise specified

Supplemental Response Information

Extinguishing Media: Use extinguishing agent which is the most appropriate to extinguish surrounding fire (carbon dioxide, foam, dry chemical or water fog as extinguishing media).

Solubility: CARMUSTINE is 0.4% by weight soluble in water (poorly water soluble), 50% by weight soluble in alcohol, and highly soluble in lipids.

Chemical Degradation/Neutralization Method: Not otherwise specified

Note: If a specific degradation or neutralization method is not provided in this section and you do not have other specific information that will guide you on how to clean up the specific material spilled, then follow the general spill procedure found in the introduction section of this handbook.

Incompatibility: CARMUSTINE is incompatible with acids, bases, and polyvinyl chloride containers. Protect from moisture.

CHLORAMBUCIL (*klor-AM-bu-cil*)
LEUKERAN®22

Chemical Abstract Service (CAS) Registry
  Number: 305-03-3
Registry of Toxic Effects of Chemical Substances
  (RTECS): ES7525000
$C_{14}H_{19}Cl_2NO_2$

Health & Safety Hazards/US Department of Transportation (DOT)/US Environmental Protection Agency (EPA)—Sources

Human Carcinogen—Material Safety Data Sheet, Carcinogen C1—US National Toxicology Program, Carcinogen G1 -International Agency for Research on Cancer, Carcinogen—Berkeley University Hazardous Chemical List, Carcinogen—University of Maryland at College Park, Carcinogen—US National Institutes of Health (NIH) and Material Safety Data Sheet, Teratogen—University of Maryland at College Park, Teratogen—US National Institutes of Health (NIH) and Material Safety Data Sheet, Probable Teratogen—Material Safety Data Sheet, Reproductive Effector—US National Institute of Environmental Health Sciences (NIEHS), Reproductive Effector—Material Safety Data Sheet, Toxic—US National Institutes of Health (NIH) and Material Safety Data Sheet, Mutagen—US National Institutes of Health (NIH) and Material Safety Data Sheet, Probable Mutagen—Material Safety Data Sheet, Cytotoxic—Material Safety Data Sheet, Skin Sensitizer—Material Safety Data Sheet, Vesicant—Material Safety Data Sheet, Pregnancy Category (D)—US Food and Drug Administration, Carcinogen and Developmental—US California State Proposition 65, National Fire Protection Association Hazard Rating Health (2) Flammability (0) Instability/Reactivity (0)—Material Safety Data Sheet, U035, UN 2811, Class 6.1, MIDI: HW01—(http://usaphcapps.amedd.army.mil/midi/) .

CHLORAMBUCIL (LEUKARAN) is supplied in 2 mg brown tablets.

CHLORAMBUCIL is a white to pale beige crystalline or granular powder with a slight odor.

CHLORAMBUCIL is a white, crystalline powder.

(CHLORAMBUCIL) Males: reversible sterility, permanent sterility, azoospermia; females: reversible sterility, permanent sterility, amenorrhea; can cause fetal harm; breastfeeding should be discontinued.

First Aid Medical Information/ Occupational Exposure Limits

First Aid Measures to include: Use general first aid measures except for the following:

Ingestion: Flush out mouth with water. Drink plenty of water and induce vomiting only if conscious and alert. Seek medical assistance. Ipecac-induced vomiting is not recommended because of the potential of seizures.

Physician's note: In case of accidental exposure, treat symptomatically and supportively. Gastric lavage and administer charcoal if ingestion was recent. Control of hyperactivity or convulsions will require sedation; diazepam is suitable, the route being dictated by the condition. Daily blood counts are necessary for three weeks or until bone marrow function has recovered. Transfusions of fresh blood and barrier nursing would be required if bone marrow suppression occurs.

Medical treatment in cases of overexposure should be treated as an overdose of a cytotoxic agent. Treat according to locally accepted protocols. For additional guidance, refer to the current prescribing information or to the local poison control information center.

Antidotes: No specific antidotes are recommended.

Medical Information:

Caution and Warning Statement: CHLORAMBU-CIL (CCNU) exposure produces human infertility and is toxic. CHLORAMBUCIL is probably mutagenic and teratogenic in humans. This drug may cause cancer and may cause heritable genetic damage. This drug may cause a possible risk of harm to the unborn child. Acute: central nervous system (CNS) toxicity. Chronic: can severely suppress bone marrow function. Exposure to CHLORAMBUCIL (CCNU) may cause skin, eye, mucous membranes, and upper respiratory tract irritation. Exposure can cause fever, myelosuppression, hepatotoxicity, infertility, seizures, and GI toxicity. The Registry of Toxic Effects of Chemical Substances (RTECS) listed CHLORAMBUCIL as a cardiovascular or blood toxicant, as a neurotoxicant, and as a respiratory toxicant.

Caution: Females and males planning to have a child, pregnant women, and nursing mothers should exercise caution regarding potential occupational exposure to this cytotoxic drug. No information or not enough information exists or was provided concerning occupational exposure that may potentially occur while handling this drug and its affects on reproductive systems, the fetus, and/or if it is secreted along with breast milk, which may harm nursing infants. Staff members should consult with the occupational health physician monitoring workers' health in your facility to be apprised of potential hazards and should be advised to avoid becoming pregnant and/or breastfeeding or should be transferred in accordance with policy/procedures to other duties that do not involve preparation, handling, and administering this drug.

Therapeutic Levels: The Food and Drug Administration lists this drug as a Pregnancy Category (D); CHLORAMBUCIL can cause fetal harm when administered to a pregnant woman. Unilateral renal agenesis has been observed in two offspring whose mothers received CHLORAMBUCIL during the first trimester. Urogenital malformations, including absence of a kidney, were found in fetuses of rats given CHLORAMBUCIL. There are no adequate and well-controlled studies in pregnant women. For nursing mothers, it is not known whether this drug is excreted in human milk because many drugs are excreted in human milk and because of the potential for serious adverse reactions in nursing infants from CHLORAMBUCIL.

New or expectant mothers are at greater risk if exposed to the active ingredient, which is readily absorbed through the skin. They should not handle packaged or unpackaged cytotoxic product.

Target Organs/Systems: Bone marrow, blood, eyes, CNS, skin, GI tract, liver, reproductive systems, upper respiratory tract, and possibly fetus

Medical Condition Generally Aggravated by Exposure: Reproductive and pregnancy issues.

Furthermore, CHLORAMBUCIL is toxic, carcinogenic, mutagenic, and teratogenic. It is absorbed through the intestinal tract. Drinking alcohol may increase the liver damage caused by CHLORAMBUCIL, especially if more than light alcohol consumption.

Specific Medical Surveillance Information:

- Reproductive and pregnancy counseling.
- Observe for delayed vesicant effects; consider ophthalmological consultation if eye contact occurs. If exposure occurs, the recommended medical tests are liver and kidney functions tests, lung function tests, and complete blood cell count.

Occupational Exposure Level/Limit (OEL) & Sampling Methods:

Environmental Sentinel Contamination Action Level (ESCAL): Air

CHLORAMBUCIL *OCCUPATIONAL EXPOSURE LEVEL/LIMIT (OEL)*:
GSK
0.5 µ/m3 Time-Weighted Average (8 Hour TWA)
(Method not listed or specified)

Supplemental Response Information

Extinguishing Media: Use extinguishing agent which is the most appropriate to extinguish surrounding fire (foam, dry chemical or water fog as extinguishing media) (carbon dioxide extinguishers may be ineffective).

Solubility: CHLORAMBUCIL is very slightly to slightly water soluble. CHLORAMBUCIL solubility/miscibility: tablets is <0.1 mg/ml in water, >/=100 mg/ml in DMSO, >/=100 mg/ml in 95% ethanol, and >/=100 mg/ml in 95% acetone.

Chemical Degradation/Neutralization Method: A manufacturer's Material Safety Data Sheet recommends treating spill surfaces with a ~2 mol/liter (~8g/100 ml), aqueous caustic soda (sodium hydroxide) solution after absorbing liquids with inert absorbent pads with inert absorbent pads or removing any powder present: allow solution to stand for up to one hour, and then thoroughly wash spilled surfaces with soap and water; sample to determine if surface contamination is still present (if sampling method is available). If drug is still present, repeat above steps; dispose of wastes in accordance with your local procedures, state, and federal regulations.

Incompatibility: Protect CHLORAMBUCIL from light.

CHLORMETHINE (1)

MECHLORETHANMINE *(me-KLOR-eth-a-meen)*

Chemical Abstract Service (CAS) Registry Number: 51-75-2
Registry of Toxic Effects of Chemical Substances (RTECS): IA1750000

NITROGEN MUSTARD
Chemical Abstract Service (CAS) Registry Number: 55-86-7

CHLORMETHINE HYDROCHLORIDE
MUSTARGEN®76

$C_5H_{11}Cl_2N$
HN-2
(Two Degradation Methods)

Health & Safety Hazards/US Department of Transportation (DOT)/US Environmental Protection Agency (EPA)—Sources

Carcinogen G2A—International Agency for Research on Cancer, Carcinogen G1—International Agency for Research on Cancer, Carcinogen C2—US National Toxicology Program and New Jersey Depart of Health and Senior Services Hazardous Substances Fact Sheet, Carcinogen—Berkeley University Hazardous Chemical List, Carcinogen—University of Maryland at College Park, Teratogen—University of Maryland at College Park, Vesicant—Wikipedia, Ototoxic—US Environmental Protection Agency (EPA) CEPP, Ototoxic—Drugs.com, Pregnancy Category (D)—US Food and Drug Administration, Carcinogen and Developmental—US California State Proposition 65, National Fire Protection Association Hazard Rating Health (4) Flammability (1) Instability/Reactivity (0)—Material Safety Data Sheet, Superfund Amendments and Reauthorization Act (SARA) Listed—United States Environmental Protection Agency; US California State Environmental Protection Agency Listed, Title III.

MECHLORETHAMINE is available as an injection.

MECHLORETHAMINE can cause fetal harm; breastfeeding: incompatible, reproductive and developmental hazard (*A Guide for Occupational Health Professionals Technical Manual*, Navy Environmental Health Center, [NEHC-TM-OEM 6260.01a]).

MECHLORETHAMINE is a white or almost white, hydroscopic, vesicant, crystalline powder or mass.

First Aid Medical Information/ Occupational Exposure Limits

First Aid Measures to include: Use general first aid measures except for the following:

Ingestion:

Physician's note: Do not induce emesis. There is no evidence that activated charcoal is beneficial. Administer nothing by mouth (NPO).

Dermal contact: In case of contact with material, immediately flush skin for 20 minutes. Speed in removing materials from skin is of extreme importance.

Medical Information:

Caution and Warning Statements: CHLORMETHINE is listed as a carcinogen and developmental toxicant. It is also a suspected cardiovascular or blood toxicant, reproductive toxicant (EPA-SARA), and skin or sense organ toxicant (Registry of Toxic Effects of Chemical Substances [RTECS]).

Nitrogen mustard agents are absorbed by the skin causing erythema and blisters. Ocular exposure to these agents may cause incapacitating injury to the cornea and conjunctiva. Inhaled, nitrogen mustard damages the respiratory tract epithelium and may cause death. Nitrogen mustard may decrease fertility. There is no antidote for nitrogen mustard toxicity.

Signs and symptoms of exposure: Nausea, vomiting, nose irritation, skin lesions, ringing in the ears (tinnitus), and menstrual irregularities.

Caution: Females and males planning to have a child, pregnant women, and nursing mothers should exercise caution regarding potential occupational exposure to this cytotoxic drug. No information or not enough information exists or was provided concerning occupational exposure that may potentially occur while handling this drug and its affects on reproductive systems, the fetus, and/or if it is secreted along with breast milk, which may harm nursing infants. Staff members should consult with the occupational health physician monitoring workers' health in your facility to be apprised of potential hazards and should be advised to avoid becoming pregnant and/or breastfeeding or should be transferred in accordance with policy/procedures to other duties that do not involve preparation, handling, and administering this drug.

Target Organs/Systems: CNS, respiratory, GI tract, eyes, dermal (skin), fetus, and hematopoietic, and immune systems

Medical Conditions Aggravated by Exposure:

- May damage fetus in pregnant women (EPA profile—Gilman 1980)

Specific Medical Surveillance Information: Reproductive and pregnancy counseling.

Recommended medical surveillance may consist of a complete blood count, and a hearing test (audiogram).

Occupational Exposure Level/Limit (OEL) & Sampling Methods:

Environmental Sentinel Contamination Action Level (ESCAL): Not otherwise specified
MECHLORETHANMINE *Occupational Exposure Level/Limit (OEL)*:
The Surgeon General's working group
0.01 mg/m3 Time-Weighted Average (TWA)

US Department of Energy's (DOE) Temporary Emergency Exposure Limits (TEELs):
TEEL-0: 1.25 mg/m3
TEEL-1: 4 mg/m3
TEEL-2: 29 mg/m3
TEEL-3: 29 mg/m3

US Environmental Protection Agency Acute Exposure Guideline Levels (AEGLS) (mg/m3):

	10 min	30 min	60 min	4 hr	8 hr
AEGL 1	NR	NR	NR	NR	NR
AEGL 2	0.13	0.044	0.022	0.0056	0.0028
AEGL 3	2.2	0.74	0.37	0.093	0.047

NR = not recommended due to insufficient data (Method not listed or specified)

Supplemental Response Information

Extinguishing Media: Use extinguishing agent which is the most appropriate to extinguish surrounding fire (carbon dioxide, foam, dry chemical or water fog as extinguishing media) (avoid methods that cause splashing or spreading).

Solubility: Nitrogen mustard solubility range is from water soluble to practically water insoluble (pH = 3.0 to 5.0 in a 0.2% solution of water).

Chemical Degradation/Neutralization Method: There are two recommended methods (sodium thiosulfate/ sodium bicarbonate solution or sodium hypochlorite 5% and water solution) for nitrogen mustards. See below for optional methods.

A manufacturer's product label recommends treating spill surfaces by mixing with an equal volume of sodium thiosulfate/sodium bicarbonate solution after absorbing liquids with inert absorbent pads with inert absorbent pads or removing any powder present: allow solution to stand for up to one hour, and then thoroughly wash spilled surfaces with soap and water; sample to determine if surface contamination is still present (if sampling method is available). If drug is still present, repeat above steps; dispose of wastes in accordance with your local procedures, state, and federal regulations.

Incompatibility: HN-2 and HN-3 do not have any incompatible actions on metals or other materials.

CHLORMETHINE (2)
MECHLORETHANMINE *(me-KLOR-eth-a-meen)*

Chemical Abstract Service (CAS) Registry Number: 51-75-2
Registry of Toxic Effects of Chemical Substances (RTECS): IA1750000

NITROGEN MUSTARD

Chemical Abstract Service (CAS) Registry
Number: 55-86-7

CHLORMETHINE HYDROCHLORIDE MUSTARGEN®76

$C_5H_{11}Cl_2N$
HN-2
(Two Degradation Methods)

Health & Safety Hazards/US Department of Transportation (DOT)/US Environmental Protection Agency (EPA)—Sources

51-75-2, Carcinogen G2A—International Agency for Research on Cancer, Carcinogen G1—International Agency for Research on Cancer, Carcinogen C2—US National Toxicology Program and US New Jersey State Department of Health and Senior Services Hazardous Substances Fact Sheet, Carcinogen—Berkeley University Hazardous Chemical List, Carcinogen—University of Maryland at College Park, Teratogen—University of Maryland at College Park, Vesicant—Wikipedia.org, Ototoxic—US Environmental Protection Agency (EPA) CEPP, Pregnancy Category (D)—US Food and Drug Administration, Carcinogen and Developmental—US California State Proposition 65, National Fire Protection Association Hazard Rating Health (4) Flammability (1) Instability/Reactivity (0), US California State Environmental Protection Agency Listed, US Title III, Superfund Amendments and Reauthorization Act (SARA) Listed—US Environmental Protection Agency.

MECHLORETHAMINE (MUSTARD) can cause fetal harm; breastfeeding: incompatible; reproductive and developmental hazards (*A Guide for Occupational Health Professionals Technical Manual*, Navy Environmental Health Center [NEHC-TM-OEM 6260.01a]).

First Aid Medical Information/ Occupational Exposure Limits

First Aid Measures to include: Use general first aid measures except for the following:

Ingestion:

Physician's note: Do not induce emesis. There is no evidence that activated charcoal is beneficial. Administer nothing by mouth (NPO).

Dermal contact: In case of contact with material, immediately flush skin for 20 minutes. Speed in removing materials from skin is of extreme importance.

Medical Information:

Caution and Warning Statements: CHLORMETHINE is listed as a carcinogen and developmental toxicant. It is also a suspected cardiovascular or blood toxicant, reproductive toxicant (EPA-SARA), and skin or sense organ toxicant (Registry of Toxic Effects of Chemical Substances [RTECS]).

Nitrogen mustard agents are absorbed by the skin causing erythema and blisters. Ocular exposure to these agents may cause incapacitating injury to the cornea and conjunctiva. Inhaled, nitrogen mustard damages the respiratory tract epithelium and may cause death. Nitrogen mustard may decrease fertility. There is no antidote for nitrogen mustard toxicity.

Signs and Symptoms of Exposure: Nausea, vomiting, nose irritation, skin lesions, ringing in the ears (tinnitus), and menstrual irregularities.

Caution: Females and males planning to have a child, pregnant women, and nursing mothers should exercise caution regarding potential occupational exposure to this cytotoxic drug. No information or not enough information exists or was provided concerning occupational exposure that may potentially occur while handling this drug and its affects on reproductive systems, the fetus, and/or if it is secreted along with breast milk, which may harm nursing infants. Staff members should consult with the occupational health physician monitoring workers' health in your facility to be apprised of potential hazards and should be advised to avoid becoming pregnant and/or breastfeeding or should be transferred in accordance with policy/procedures to other duties that do not involve preparation, handling, and administering this drug.

Target Organs/Systems: CNS, respiratory, GI tract, eyes, dermal (skin), fetus, hematopoietic, and immune systems

Medical Conditions Aggravated by Exposure:

- May damage fetus in pregnant women (EPA profile—Gilman 1980)

Specific Medical Surveillance Information: Reproductive and pregnancy counseling. Recommended medical surveillance may consist of a complete blood count, and a hearing test (audiogram).

Occupational Exposure Level/Limit (OEL) & Sampling Methods:

Environmental Sentinel Contamination Action Level (ESCAL): Not otherwise specified
MECHLORETHANMINE *Occupational Exposure Level/Limit (OEL)*:

The Surgeon General's Working Group
0.01 mg/m3 Time-Weighted Average (TWA)

US Department of Energy's (DOE) Temporary
Emergency Exposure Limits (TEELs):
TEEL-0: 1.25 mg/m3
TEEL-1: 4 mg/m3
TEEL-2: 29 mg/m3
TEEL-3: 29 mg/m3

US Environmental Protection Agency Acute Exposure
Guideline Levels (AEGLS)
(mg/m3):

	10 min	30 min	60 min	4 hr	8 hr
AEGL 1	NR	NR	NR	NR	NR
AEGL 2	0.13	0.044	0.022	0.0056	0.0028
AEGL 3	2.2	0.74	0.37	0.093	0.047

NR = not recommended due to insufficient data
(Method not listed or specified)

Supplemental Response Information

Extinguishing Media: Use extinguishing agent which is the most appropriate to extinguish surrounding fire (carbon dioxide, foam, dry chemical or water fog as extinguishing media) (avoid methods that cause splashing or spreading).

Solubility: Nitrogen mustards solubility range is from water soluble to practically water insoluble.

Chemical Degradation/Neutralization Method: There are two recommended methods for nitrogen mustards. See below and above for optional methods.

Several government agencies recommends treating spill surfaces with sodium hypochlorite 5% and water solution after absorbing liquids with inert absorbent pads with inert absorbent pads or removing any powder present: allow solution to stand for up to one hour, and then thoroughly wash spilled surfaces with soap and water; sample to determine if surface contamination is still present (if sampling method is available). If drug is still present, repeat above steps; dispose of wastes in accordance with your local procedures, state, and federal regulations.

Incompatibility: HN-2 and HN-3 do not have any incompatible actions on metals or other materials.

CHLOROZOTOCIN
DCNU

Chemical Abstract Service (CAS) Registry
Number: 54749-90-5

Registry of Toxic Effects of Chemical Substances
(RTECS): LZ5758000
National Cancer Institute: NSC 178248
$C_9H_{16}ClN_3O_7$

Health & Safety Hazards/US Department of Transportation (DOT)/US Environmental Protection Agency (EPA)—Sources

Carcinogen—US National Institutes of Health (NIH) and Material Safety Data Sheet, Carcinogen C2—US National Toxicology Program, Carcinogen G2A—International Agency for Research on Cancer, Carcinogen—Berkeley University Hazardous Chemical List, Carcinogen—University of Maryland at College Park, Mutagen—University of Maryland at College Park, Mutagen—US National Institutes of Health (NIH) and Material Safety Data Sheet, Tumorigenic—Toxic Material Safety Data Sheet, Carcinogen—US California State Proposition 65 and Scorecard®.

First Aid Medical Information/ Occupational Exposure Limits

First Aid Measures to include: Use general first aid measures except for the following:

Ingestion: Do not induce vomiting. If conscious and alert, rinse mouth out and drink 2-4 cups of milk or water. Refer for gastric lavage. Seek medical assistance.

Dermal contact: Avoid rubbing of skin or increasing its temperature. Do not rinse with organic solvents.

Medical Information:

Caution and Warning Statements: CHLOROZOTOCIN is toxic, carcinogenic and mutagenic. CHLOROZOTOCIN is readily absorbed through the intestinal tract. CHLOROZOTOCIN is a suspected gastrointestinal or liver toxicant (Registry of Toxic Effects of Chemical Substances [RTECS]).

Human systemic effects by IV route: anorexia, leukopenia, nausea or vomiting, and thrombocytopenia. (Lewis, R.J., *Sax's Dangerous Properties of Industrial Materials*, 9th ed., vols. 1–3 [New York: Van Nostrand Reinhold, 1996], 844.)

Target Organs/Systems: Skin, liver, and kidneys
Medical Conditions Generally Aggravated by Exposure:

- If preexisting skin, liver, and kidney medical problems.

Specific Medical Surveillance Information: Consider treatment for liver or kidney involvement.

Occupational Exposure Level/Limit (OEL) & Sampling Methods: Not otherwise specified

Environmental Sentinel Contamination Action Level (ESCAL): Not otherwise specified

Supplemental Response Information

Extinguishing Media: Use extinguishing agent which is the most appropriate to extinguish surrounding fire (carbon dioxide, foam, dry chemical or water fog as extinguishing media).

Solubility: CHLOROZOTOCIN is highly water soluble.

Chemical Degradation/Neutralization Method: A manufacturer's Material Safety Data Sheet recommends treating spill surfaces with a ~2 mol/liter (~8 g/100 ml), aqueous caustic soda (sodium hydroxide) solution after absorbing liquids with inert absorbent pads or removing any powder present: allow solution to stand for up to one hour, and then thoroughly wash spilled surfaces with soap and water; sample to determine if surface contamination is still present (if sampling method is available). If drug is still present, repeat above steps; dispose of wastes in accordance with your local procedures, state, and federal regulations.

Incompatibility: CHLORZOTOZIN is incompatible with strong acid and strong alkali.

CIDOFOVIR *(si-DOF-o-veer)*
VISTIDE®25

Chemical Abstract Service (CAS Registry)
    Number: 149394-66-1
$C_8H_{14}N_3O_6P$

ANHYDROUS CIDOFOVIR OR CIDOFOVIR DIHYDRATE

Chemical Abstract Service (CAS) Registry
    Number: 113852-37-2

ANHYDROUS CIDOFOVIR

Health & Safety Hazards/US Department of Transportation (DOT)/US Environmental Protection Agency (EPA)—Sources

Experimental Teratogen—Material Safety Data Sheet, Teratogen—Material Safety Data Sheet, Experimental Reproductive Effector—Material Safety Data Sheet, Experimental Embryotoxic—Material Safety Data Sheet, Pregnancy Category (C)—US Food and Drug Administration, Carcinogen and Developmental Male and Female—US California Proposition 65, National Fire Protection Association Health (1) Flammability (1) Instability/Reactivity/Reactivity (0)—Material Safety Data Sheet.

CIDOFOVIR is available for injection.

CIDOFOVIR: Males: inhibition of spermatogenesis in rats and monkeys; recommends not given to nursing mothers because of potential for reproductive and developmental harm (*A Guide for Occupational Health Professionals Technical Manual*, Navy Environmental Health Center [NEHC-TM-OEM 6260.01a]).

First Aid/Medical Information/ Occupational Exposure Limits

First Aid Measures to include: Use general first aid measures.

Medical Information:

Caution and Warning Statements:

Warning: CIDOFOVIR should be considered a potential human carcinogen.

Caution: VISTIDE®25 (CIDOFOVIR) toxicological properties of this drug have not been fully characterized. Therefore, it is suggested that conservative handling practices be employed at all times. This drug may be harmful if swallowed. Exposure to skin may result in minimal effects such as skin irritation. Eye contact may cause eye irritation. Reproductive, teratogenic, and embryotoxic effects have been reported in animal data.

Caution: Females and males planning to have a child, pregnant women, and nursing mothers should exercise caution regarding potential occupational exposure to this cytotoxic drug. No information or not enough information exists or was provided concerning occupational exposure that may potentially occur while handling this drug and its affects on reproductive systems, the fetus, and/or if it is secreted along with breast milk, which may harm nursing infants. Staff members should consult with the occupational health physician monitoring workers' health in your facility to be apprised of potential hazards and should be advised to avoid becoming pregnant and/or breastfeeding or should be transferred in accordance with policy/procedures to other duties that do not involve preparation, handling, and administering this drug.

Target Organs/Systems: Skin, reproductive (fetus), and eyes

Medical Conditions Generally Aggravated by Exposure:

- Pregnancy.

Specific Medical Surveillance: Reproductive and pregnancy counseling.

Evaluate renal function including urinalysis for proteinuria with all suspected overdoses.

Obtain CBC with differential following a sign overdose or as indicated. Neutropenia has been reported during routine use of CIDOFOVIR.

Decreases in serum bicarbonate and phosphate, polyuria, and severe vomiting have occurred. Monitor electrolytes and status following a significant exposure.

Occupational Exposure Level/Limit (OEL) & Sampling Methods: Not otherwise specified

Environmental Sentinel Contamination Action Level (ESCAL): Not otherwise specified

Supplemental Response Information

Extinguishing Media: Use extinguishing agent which is the most appropriate to extinguish surrounding fire (carbon dioxide, foam, dry chemical or water fog as extinguishing media).

Solubility: CIDOFOVIR (VISTIDE®25) has an aqueous solubility of >=170 mg/ml @ pH 6–8 (HSDB) (Drugbank.com).

Chemical Degradation/Neutralization Method: A manufacturer's MSDS recommends using alkaline soap/detergent and water to clean spill surfaces after absorbing liquids with inert absorbent pads or removing any powder present; repeat using soap and water; sample to determine if surface contamination is still present (if sampling method is available). If the drug is still present, repeat above steps; dispose of wastes in accordance with your local procedures, state, and federal regulations.

Incompatibility: CIDOFOVIR is incompatible with strong oxidizing materials.

CISPLATIN (*sis-PLA-tin*)
CIS-PLATIN

Chemical Abstract service (CAS) Registry
Number: 15663-27-1 (mixture)
RTECS: TP2450000

PLATINOL®26
CIS-DICHLORO-DIAMMINE-PLATIN (II)

$Cl_2H_6N_2Pt$
Cl2-H4-N2Pt 15663-27-1

Health & Safety Hazards/ US Department of Transportation (DOT)/US Environmental Protection Agency (EPA)—Sources

Acutely Toxic—US National Institute of Health (NIH)—Material Safety Data Sheet, Carcinogen—Occupational Safety and Health Administration and a Material Safety Data Sheet, Carcinogen—US National Institute of Health (NIH) and Material Safety Data Sheet, Carcinogen C2—US National Toxicology Program, Carcinogen G2A—International Agency for Research on Cancer, Carcinogen—University of Maryland at College Park, Teratogen—University of Maryland at College Park, Reproductive—Material Safety Data Sheet, Embryotoxic—US National Institute of Health (HIH) and Material Safety Data Sheet, Fetotoxic—Material Safety Data Sheet, Mutagen—US National Institute of Health (NIH) and Material Safety Data Sheet, Cytotoxic—Material Safety Data Sheet, Ototoxic—T. C. Hain, Ototoxic—Material Safety Data Sheet, Sensitizing—Material Safety Data Sheet, Corrosive—Material Safety Data Sheet, Cytotoxic—British Columbia Cancer Agency Canada, Irritant—British Columbia Cancer Agency Canada, Pregnancy Category (D)—US Food and Drug Administration, Carcinogen—US California Proposition 65, National Fire Protection Association Health (2) Flammability (0) Instability/Reactivity (0)—Material Safety Data Sheet, National Fire Protection Association Health (3) Flammability (0) Instability/Reactivity (0), Hazardous Materials Identification System (R) and/or US Department of Defense System (3★) with additional Chronic hazard present Fire Hazard (0) Reactivity (0) Personal Protective Code (E) (Safety Glasses, Chemical Gloves, Dust Respirator), Hazardous Materials Identification System (R) and/or US Department of Defense System Health (3) Fire Hazard (0) Reactivity (0) Personal Protective Code (X) (Ask Supervisor), Hazardous Materials Identification System (R) and/or US Department of Defense System Health (3★) with additional chronic hazard present Fire Hazard (1) Reactivity (0) Personal Protective Code (E) (Safety Glasses, Chemical Gloves, Dust Respirator)—Material Safety Data Sheet, UN 2811, CLASS 6.1, GROUP II.

CISPLATIN is a colorless fluid.

CISPLATIN can cause fetal harm; recommends no breastfeeding (found in human milk) but controversy exists.

CISPLATIN (PLATINOL®26)—Breastfeeding: excreted into human breast milk. The American Academy of Pediatrics has classified CISPLATIN as a drug "usually compatible with breastfeeding." The World Health Organization (WHO) working group on human lactation does not recommend nursing during CISPLATIN chemotherapy.

CISPLATIN is a yellow powder or yellow or orange-yellow crystals.

(CIS-PLATIN: VU absorption in 0.1 NHC, lambda max = 301 +− 2 nm, epsilon = 124–145 nm)

First Aid/Medical Information/ Occupational Exposure Limits

First Aid Measures to include: Use general first aid measures except for the following:

Ingestion: Acute toxic: contact a poison control center if swallowed. Drink milk or water, if conscious and alert; only induce vomiting if directed by medical personnel.

Dermal contact: Avoid rinsing skin with organic solvents or scanned with UV light. Avoid rubbing of skin or increasing its temperature.

Eye contact: Immediately check for contact lenses and remove any contact lenses. Irrigate immediately with sodium bicarbonate solution, followed by copious quantities of running water for at least 15 minutes, occasionally lifting the upper and lower lids. Obtain ophthalmologic evaluation.

Inhalation: During post exposure, consider treating for pulmonary irritation.

Physician's note (A): Treatment is supportive and symptomatic. Patients should be monitored for at least three to four weeks in case of delayed toxicity. Anticipated complications include phytotoxicity, ototoxicity, neurotoxicity, and hematotoxicity. There is no specific antidote for CISPLATIN toxicity. Hydration with 3 to 6l intravenous fluids/day and intravenous mannitol, which increases the urinary volume and thus decreases the effective urinary concentration of platinum and its metabolites, is recommended. Monitor vital signs, renal, hepatic, ECG, hematological, OTIC, and neurological functions. Serum electrolyte concentrations and fluid requirements should be monitored and corrected, if necessary. Peripheral blood counts should be monitored since the hematological effects can be slow in manifestation. Monitoring should continue for 3 to 4 weeks after exposure. Although not life threatening, ototoxicity can be cumulative and persistent. This drug may cause skin irritation and corrosive burns upon contact. BC Cancer Agency lists CISPLATIN as an irritant.

Physician's note (B): For ingestion, consider gastric lavage, activated charcoal slurry, and catharsis.

Physician's note (C): Treat symptomatically and supportively.

Medical Information:

Caution and Warning Statements: Danger, if CISPLATIN is swallowed (ingested). It may be fatal. Exposure to CISPLATIN may cause cancer in humans. This drug may cause loss of hearing. Exposure may cause liver and kidney damage. Exposure may cause allergic respiratory and skin reaction. May cause damage to fetus and may damage the testes (male reproductive glands). Inhalation exposure may cause transient bronchial irritant. Skin contact may cause mild irritant. Eyes contact may cause conjunctivitis. Intravenous exposure may cause anaphylactic reactions. This drug may cause kidney toxicity, peripheral neuropathy, and irreversible hematological effects. RTECS listed as a suspected gastrointestinal or liver toxicant. Exposure may result in anaphylactic reaction.

Caution: Females and males planning to have a child, pregnant women, and nursing mothers should exercise caution regarding potential occupational exposure to this cytotoxic drug. No information or not enough information exists or was provided concerning occupational exposure that may potentially occur while handling this drug and its affects on reproductive systems, the fetus, and/or if it is secreted along with breast milk, which may harm nursing infants. Staff members should consult with the occupational health physician monitoring workers' health in your facility to be apprised of potential hazards and should be advised to avoid becoming pregnant and/or breastfeeding or should be transferred in accordance with policy/procedures to other duties that do not involve preparation, handling, and administering this drug.

Target Organs/Systems: Liver, kidneys, nervous system, hearing (inner ear), CNS, skin, eyes, blood, bone marrow, gastrointestinal tract, respiratory and reproductive systems

Medical Conditions Generally Aggravated by Exposure:

- Persons suffering asthma or other related respiratory disorders may be more susceptible to anaphylactic reaction to CISPLATIN. Disorders including the target organs of this product can be aggravated by exposure to CISPLATIN, especially in doses approaching therapeutic levels for this product. Pre-existing renal impairment, myelosuppression, hearing impairment or previous history of allergic reaction to CISPLATIN or other platinum containing compounds, and pregnancy.

Specific Medical Surveillance Information: Reproductive and pregnancy counseling.

Recommended medical testing for CISPLATIN is obtaining an audiogram, complete blood count, and kidney function tests. If exposure occurs, recommended that blood levels of CISPLATIN and an exam of the nervous system be performed. Routine procedures: a pre-placement physical examination and history (noting any risk factors) for employees with potential exposure to (PLATINOL®26) is recommended. A complete blood count, including differential, may be taken to provide a baseline. Periodic follow-up examinations should be given in accordance with institutional policy, overseen by a physician thoroughly knowledgeable about both the toxicity of the substance and the extent of workplace exposure. A permanent registry of all staff that routinely prepare or administer (PLATINOL®26) should be considered.

Occupational Exposure Level/Limit (OEL) & Sampling Methods:

> *Environmental Sentinel Contamination Action Level (ESCAL)*: Surface
> CISPLATIN Occupational Exposure Level/Limit:
> US Occupational Safety Health Administration (OSHA)
> Permissible Exposure Limit (PEL): 0.002 mg/m3 Time-Weighted Average (TWA)(as pt)
>
> US American Conference of Governmental Industrial Hygienists (ACGIH):
> TLV 0.002 mg/m3 Time-Weighted Average (TWA) (Soluble salt of platinum)
>
> US National Institute for Safety and Health (NIOSH).
> Recommended Exposure Limit (REL) 0.002 mg/ m3 Time-Weighted Average (TWA) 10 hours (as pt)
>
> OEL—Australia: TWA 1 mg/m3
> OEL—UK: 0.002 mg/m3 TWA OES UK
>
> OEL—Bristol-Myers Squib
> PLATINOL®26 (CISPLATIN) (2005) 0.00002 mg/m3 Time-Weighted Average (8 Hour TWA)
> Monitoring methods and references: NIOSH Methods S191 or 7300; measurement method: particulate filter; acid/reagent; graphite furnace atomic absorption spectrometry; NIOSH II (7) # S191.
> (Some of the above methods were not available)

Supplemental Response Information

Extinguishing Media: Use extinguishing agent which is the most appropriate to extinguish surrounding fire (carbon dioxide, foam, dry chemical or water fog as extinguishing media).

Solubility: CISPLATIN is slightly water soluble to water soluble and soluble in saline with a pH range of 3.2 to 4.5 (1% solution). CISPLATIN is very soluble in acetone. CISPLATIN is practically insoluble in alcohol.

Chemical Degradation/Neutralization Method: A manufacturer's MSDS recommends treating spill surfaces with a ~2 mol/liter (~8g/100 ml) (5% sodium hydroxide), aqueous caustic soda (sodium hydroxide) solution after absorbing liquids with inert absorbent pads or removing any powder present: allow solution to stand for up to one hour, and then thoroughly wash spilled surfaces with soap and water; sample to determine if surface contamination is still present (if sampling method is available). If still present, repeat above steps; dispose of wastes in accordance with your local procedures, state, and federal regulations.

Incompatibility: CISPLATIN is incompatible with oxidizing agents, bleach, aluminum, sodium bicarbonate, sodium bisulfate, sodium metabisulfate, and antioxidants. Furthermore, the drug should not be administered through an aluminum needle, since aluminum reacts with and inactivates the drug. Avoid heat, flames, sparks, and other sources of ignition.

CLADRIBINE (*KLA-drih-bean*)

LEUSTATIN(®27
2-CHLORO-2'-DEOXYADENO-SINE
CLABRIBINE NOVAPLUS®28
LEUSTAT
2-CDA

> Chemical Abstract Service (CAS) Number: 4291-63-8 (MIXTURE)
> RTECS: AU7357760
> RWJ26251
> $C_{10}H_{12}ClN_5O_3$

Health & Safety Hazards/US Department of Transportation (DOT)/US Environmental Protection Agency (EPA)—Sources

Teratogen—Material Safety Data Sheet, Mutagen—Material Safety Data Sheet, Fetotoxic—Material Safety Data Sheet, Cytotoxic—British Columbia Cancer Agency Canada, Nonvesicant—British Columbia Cancer Agency Canada, Pregnancy Category (D)—US Food and Drug Administration, Developmental—US California Proposition 65, National Fire Protection Association Health (3) Flammability (-) Instability/Reactivity (-)—Material Safety Data Sheet.

CLADRIBINE (LEUSTAT) is a colorless fluid from powder (8 and 10 ml vials).

CLADRIBINE (DEOYADENOSINE): Breast-feeding should be discontinued because of reproductive and developmental harm (*A Guide for Occupational Health Professionals Technical Manual*, Navy Environmental Health Center [NEHC-TM-OEM 6260.01a]).

First Aid/Medical Information/ Occupational Exposure Limits

First Aid Measures to include: Use general first aid measures except for the following:

Ingestion: If ingested, flush mouth with water and seek medical assistance. If person is conscious and medical assistance is not available, induce vomiting.

Medical Information:

Caution and Warning Statements: CLADRIBINE is a possible human teratogen and mutagenic (DNA damage and cause suppression of rapidly generating cells). Absorption occurs via inhalation, ingestion, or skin contact. CLADRIBINE exposure may cause irritation to eyes, respiratory system or dermatitis to skin. This drug may cause fatigue, nausea, vomiting and dizziness, and a variety of other systemic effects. Neurologic toxicity is possible with high exposure/dose. CLADRIBINE is fetotoxic.

Caution: Females and males planning to have a child, pregnant women, and nursing mothers should exercise caution regarding potential occupational exposure to this cytotoxic drug. No information or not enough information exists or was provided concerning occupational exposure that may potentially occur while handling this drug and its affects on reproductive systems, the fetus, and/or if it is secreted along with breast milk, which may harm nursing infants. Staff members should consult with the occupational health physician monitoring workers' health in your facility to be apprised of potential hazards and should be advised to avoid becoming pregnant and/or breastfeeding or should be transferred in accordance with policy/procedures to other duties that do not involve preparation, handling, and administering this drug.

Target Organs/Systems: Digestive, central nervous systems, eyes, liver, kidneys, blood forming system, skin, fetus, and heart

Medical Conditions Generally Aggravated by Exposure:

- Individuals who are hypersensitive to CLADRIBINE or any of its components. Individuals with severe bone marrow suppression, neutropenia, anemia,

thrombocytopenia, fever, and peripheral polyneuropathy, and medical conditions of the digestive system, CNS, and pregnancy.

Specific Medical Surveillance Information: Reproductive and pregnancy counseling.

Occupational Exposure Level/Limit (OEL) & Sampling Methods:

Environmental Sentinel Contamination Action Level (ESCAL): Not otherwise specified

Occupational Exposure Level/Limit (OEL): Bedford Lab and Ben Venue Laboratories, Inc.
2.5 µ/m3 TWA
(Method not listed or specified)

Occupational Exposure Level/Limit: Pharmaceutical Research Institute and J&J 1996 OEL
0.0025 mg/m3 Time-Weighted Average (TWA)
(Method not listed or specified)

Supplemental Response Information

Extinguishing Media: Use extinguishing agent which is the most appropriate to extinguish surrounding fire (carbon dioxide, foam, dry chemical or water fog as extinguishing media).

Solubility: CLADRIBINE is water soluble with a pH range of 5.5–8.0.

Chemical Degradation/Neutralization Method: Not otherwise specified

Note: If a specific degradation or neutralization method is not provided on this table and you do not have other specific information that will guide you on how to clean up the specific material spilled, then follow the general spill procedure found at the introduction section of this table.

Incompatibility: CLADRIBINE is incompatible with strong oxidizers or water reactive oxidizers.

CYCLOPHOSPHAMIDE (1)
(SYE-kloe-FOS-fa-mide)
Chemical Abstract Service (CAS) Registry Number: 50-18-0
NSC 26271
$C_7H_{15}Cl_2N_2O_2P$

CYTOXAN ANHYDROUS FORM
CYCLOPHOSPHAMIDE HYDRATE/MONO-HYDRATE (*SYE-kloe-FOS-fa-mide*)
CTX
PROCYTOX®37

CAS Registry Number: 6055-19-2

C_7-H_{15}-CL_2-N_2-O_2-$P.H_2O$

CYCLOPHOSPHAMIDE MONOHYDRATE

CAS Registry Numbers: 60007-96-7, 60030-72-0, 6007-95-6

RTECS: RP6157750
CYCLOPHOSPHAMIDE

CAS Registry Number: 50-18-0
RTECS: RP5950000
NSC 26271
$C_7H_{15}Cl_2N_2O_2P$
(Two Degradation Methods)
(Mixture)

Health & Safety Hazards/US Department of Transportation (DOT)/US Environmental Protection Agency (EPA)—Sources

Carcinogen G1—International Agency for Research on Cancer, Carcinogen—US National Toxicology Program and Material Safety Data Sheet, Carcinogen C1—US National Toxicology Program, Carcinogen—Berkeley University Hazardous Chemical List, Carcinogen—University of Maryland at College Park, Carcinogen—Material Safety Data Sheet, Mutagen—Material Safety Data Sheet, Teratogen—University of Maryland at College Park, Teratogen—Material Safety Data Sheet, Reproductive Effector—Centre College, Embryotoxic—Material Safety Data Sheet, Acutely Toxic—Material Safety Data Sheet, Irritant—Material Safety Data Sheet, Pregnancy Category (D)—US Food and Drug Administration, Carcinogen and Developmental Male and Female—US California Proposition 65, Cytotoxic—Material Safety Data Sheet, Cytotoxic—British Columbia Cancer Agency Canada, Nonvesicant—British Columbia Cancer Agency Canada, Ototoxic—Wikipedia, National Fire Protection Association Health (2) Flammability (0) Instability/Reactivity (0)—Material Safety Data Sheet, National Fire Protection Association Health (3) Flammability (1) Instability/Reactivity (1)—Material Safety Data Sheet, National Fire Protection Association Health (2) Flammability (1) Instability/Reactivity (0)—Material Safety Data Sheet, Hazardous Materials Identification System (R) and/or US Department of Defense System Health (2) Fire Hazard (1) Reactivity (0) Personal Protection Code (E) (Safety Glasses, Chemical Gloves, Dust Respirator)—Material Safety Data Sheet, Hazardous Materials Identification System (R) and/or US Depart-

ment of Defense System Health (2★) with additional chronic hazard present Fire Hazard (0) Reactivity (0) Personal Protection Code (-) (None stated), MIDI: HW01—(http://usaphcapps.amedd.army.mil/midi/), U058, UN 2811, Class 6.1, Group III; US California Environmental Protection Agency Listed,

CYCLOPHOSPHAMIDE is a colorless fluid from powder and 50 mg pink or 50 mg white tablets.

CYCLOPHOSPHAMIDE: 25 mg tablets (light blue) and 50 mg tablets (light blue).

CYCLOPHOSPAMIDE (CYTOXAN): Breast-feeding—The American Academy of Pediatrics classified CYCLOPHOSPHAMIDE as contraindicated during breastfeeding in 1994 and listed it as a cytotoxic drug that may interfere with cellular metabolism of the nursing infant in 2001. Neonatal side effects: possible immune suppression.

CYCLOPHOSPAMIDE: Breastfeeding is contraindicated because of possible immune suppression, association with carcinogenesis, and neutropenia. Breastfeeding is not recommended because this drug may be distributed into breast milk.

First Aid/Medical Information/ Occupational Exposure Limits

First Aid Measures to include: Use the general first aid measures except for the following:

Dermal contact: Skin should not be rinsed with organic solvent or scanned with UV light. Avoid rubbing skin or increasing its temperature. Irritated skin can be covered with emollient. Seek medical attention.

Ingestion: Drink milk or water and induce vomiting only if conscious and alert. Seek medical assistance.

Physicians note (A): In case of accidental exposure, treat symptomatically and supportively.

Physician's note (B): Overdose treatment; since there is no known antidote for CYCLOPHOSPHAMIDE overdose, treatment should be supportive and include appropriate treatment for any concurrent infection, myelosuppression, or cardiac toxicity, should it occur. Liberal fluid intake and frequent urination are advised to reduce the risk of cystitis, but care must be taken to avoid water retention and intoxication.

Medical Information:

Caution and Warning Statements: CYCLOPHOSPAMIDE MONOHYDRATE is a human carcinogen. Acutely toxic if swallowed. Exposure may cause heritable genetic damage and may cause harm to the unborn child. Exposure may cause skin irritation (permeator) and severe eye irritation. Material may be irritating to mucous membranes and upper respiratory tract. Male and female reproductive toxicity has been documented. CYTOXAN ANHYDROUS may be a cardiotoxic substance. CYTOXAN may cause delayed bone marrow suppression and possibly cardiotoxicity substance. RTECS lists CYTOXAN as a suspected cardiovascular or blood toxicant; as a gastrointestinal or liver toxicant; as a kidney toxicant and as a neurotoxicant.

Exposure may cause nausea, vomiting, anorexia, headache, dizziness, rash, conjunctivitis, GI effects, cystitis, genito-urinary, kidney damage, alopecia, pulmonary fibrosis, changes in metabolism, and permanent sterility.

Caution: Females and males planning to have a child, pregnant women, and nursing mothers should exercise caution regarding potential occupational exposure to this cytotoxic drug. No information or not enough information exists or was provided concerning occupational exposure that may potentially occur while handling this drug and its affects on reproductive systems, the fetus, and/or if it is secreted along with breast milk, which may harm nursing infants. Staff members should consult with the occupational health physician monitoring workers' health in your facility to be apprised of potential hazards and should be advised to avoid becoming pregnant and/or breastfeeding or should be transferred in accordance with policy/procedures to other duties that do not involve preparation, handling, and administering this drug.

Target Organs/Systems: Eyes, bone marrow, bladder, upper respiratory tract, skin, reproductive, and cardiovascular system (heart)

Medical Conditions Generally Aggravated by Exposure:

- Low platelet, leukocyte counts, coagulation disorders, renal, pulmonary, cardiac diseases, recent radiation, chemotherapy, reproductive and pregnancy issues.

Specific Medical Surveillance Information:
Bladder cancer

1. Nmp22@bladderchek (nuclear matrix protein) to detect elevated levels of tumor markers in the urine (reported to be more accurate than below)
2. Urinalysis to detect microscopic heamaturia
3. Urine cytology
4. Urine culture to rule out urinary tract infection

Occupational Exposure Level/Limit (OEL) & Sampling Methods: Not otherwise specified

Environmental Sentinel Contamination Action Level (ESCAL): Air, surface

Supplemental Response Information

Extinguishing Media: Use extinguishing agent which is the most appropriate to extinguish surrounding fire (carbon dioxide, foam, dry chemical or water fog as extinguishing media).

Solubility: CYTOXAN ANHYDROUS is water solubility (40 g/l water). It is freely soluble in alcohol. (1% solution has a pH of 4.5)

Chemical Degradation/Neutralization Method: There are two recommended methods (bleach [sodium hypochlorite] solution method and potassium hydroxide in methanol solution method) for CYCLOPHOSPHAMIDE (see below).

The IARC recommends treating spill surfaces with a 5.25% sodium hypochlorite (bleach) solution after absorbing liquids with inert absorbent pads or removing any powder present: allow solution to stand for up to one hour, and then thoroughly wash spilled surfaces with soap and water; sample to determine if surface contamination is still present (if sampling method is available). If drug is still present, repeat above steps; dispose of wastes in accordance with your local procedures, state, and federal regulations.

Incompatibility: CYTOXAN ANHYDROUS is incompatible with strong bases, strong acids, alkalis and strong oxidizing agents. Benzyl alcohol preserved diluents. Avoid exposure to heat.

CYTARABINE (sye-TARE-a-been)
UDICIL
CYTOSAR-U®31
CYTOSAR
TARABINE PFS®32
ARABINOCYTIDINE
ARA-C

> Chemical Abstract Service (CA) Registry Number: 147-94-4
> RTECS: HA5425000
> $C_9H_{13}N_3O_5$

CYTARABINE HYDROCHLORIDE

Health & Safety Hazards/US Department of Transportation (DOT)/US Environmental Protection Agency (EPA)—Sources

Suspected Carcinogen—Material Safety Data Sheet, Teratogen—University of Maryland at College Park, Mutagen—Material Safety Data Sheet, Teratogen—Material Safety Data Sheet, Cytotoxic—British Columbia Cancer Agency Canada, Irritant—Material

Safety Data Sheet, Nonvesicant—British Columbia Cancer Agency Canada, Pregnancy Category (D)—US Food and Drug Administration, Pregnancy Category (X)—US Food and Drug Administration, Developmental—US California Proposition 65, US California Environmental Protection Agency Listed, National Fire Protection Association Health (2) Flammability (0) Instability/Reactivity (0)—Material Safety Data Sheet, National Fire Protection Association Health (2) Flammability (1) Instability/Reactivity (0)—Material Safety Data Sheet, Hazardous Materials Identification System (R) and/or US Department of Defense System Health (2) with additional chronic hazard present Fire Hazard (1) Reactivity (0) Personal Protection code (E) (Safety Glasses, Chemical Gloves, Dust Respirator), Hazardous Materials Identification System (R) and/or US Department of Defense System Health (2) with additional chronic hazard present Fire Hazard (0) Reactivity (0) Personal Protection Code (-) (None stated), TOXIC SOLID, ORGANIC, Not otherwise specified (DACTINOMYCIN), UN281, CLASS 6.1, GROUP II.

CYTARABINE is an odorless fluid from powder.

CYTARABINE can cause fetal harm; breastfeeding should be discontinued.

CYTARABINE is an odorless white or almost white, crystalline powder.

First Aid/Medical Information/ Occupational Exposure Limits

First Aid Measures to include: Use general first aid measures except for the following:

Note: Medical attention should be sought immediately after the initial first aid measures are taken.

Physician's note (A): The time of onset and duration of symptoms from accidental overexposure to CYTOSAR has not been determined. The intravenous half-life of CYTARABINE ranges between 1 and 3 hours. The extent of skin absorption has not been measured, but is probably insignificant. CYTARABINE is known to be teratogenic. The primary toxic effects of chronic overexposure are bone marrow depression and immunosuppressant. Massive overdosage has been reported to irreversibly damage the central nervous system. This drug may be allergenic.

Physician's note (B): CYTARABINE should be treated as potentially carcinogenic, and may be mutagenic, teratogenic, or allergenic. If respiratory distress occurs after inhalation of airborne droplets, administer emergency airway support and 100% humidified supplemental oxygen with assisted ventilation if needed. If

coughing or difficulty in breathing develops, evacuating for respiratory tract irritation, bronchitis or pneumonitis. Treatment is symptomatic. Medical attention should be sought immediately after the preceding first aid measures are taken.

Medical Information:

Caution and Warning Statements: CYTOSAR®30 (CYTARABINE) is known to be a teratogenic agent. Animal studies have produced some evidence of genotoxicity. Exposure may cause eyes, skin, mucous membranes and upper respiratory tract irritation. Primary toxic effect (poison) of CYTARABINE is bone marrow suppression and loss of immune response. Signs and symptoms of overexposure: irritation, anorexia, nausea, vomiting, diarrhea, prolonged bleeding, maculopapular rash, conjunctivitis, and infections.

Caution: Females and males planning to have a child, pregnant women, and nursing mothers should exercise caution regarding potential occupational exposure to this cytotoxic drug. No information or not enough information exists or was provided concerning occupational exposure that may potentially occur while handling this drug and its affects on reproductive systems, the fetus, and/or if it is secreted along with breast milk, which may harm nursing infants. Staff members should consult with the occupational health physician monitoring workers' health in your facility to be apprised of potential hazards and should be advised to avoid becoming pregnant and/or breastfeeding or should be transferred in accordance with policy/procedures to other duties that do not involve preparation, handling, and administering this drug.

Therapeutic Levels: CYTARABINE is listed by the Food and Drug Administration as a Pregnancy Category (D) drug; breastfeeding is not recommended due to the potential secretion of CYTARABINE into breast milk.

Target Organs/Systems: Nerves (CNS), bone marrow, immune system, eyes, skin, fetus, and upper respiratory tract

Medical Condition Generally Aggravated by Exposure:

- Individuals who are hypersensitive to CYTARABINE or have preexisting bone marrow suppression, chickenpox (including recent exposure), herpes zoster, impaired liver function, infection, previous cytotoxic drug or radiation therapy, and pregnancy.

Specific Medical Surveillance Information: Reproductive and pregnancy counseling.

CYTATABINE delivered intravenously has a half-life that ranges between 1 to 3 hours. A reported massive over-dosage has cause irreversible CNS damage to the exposed person.

Occupational Exposure Level/Limit (OEL) & Sampling Methods:

> *Environmental Sentinel Contamination Action Level (ESCAL)*: Not otherwise specified
> *Occupational Exposure Level/Limit (OEL)*: Pharmacia & Up John
> 2 µg/m3 TWA
> (Method not listed or specified)

Supplemental Response Information

Extinguishing Media: Use extinguishing agent which is the most appropriate to extinguish surrounding fire (carbon dioxide, foam, dry chemical or water fog as extinguishing media).

Solubility: CYTARABINE (CYTOSAR-U®31) is completely (freely) water soluble and slightly soluble in alcohol and in chloroform (pH 7.7).

Chemical Degradation/Neutralization Method: A manufacturer's Material Safety Data Sheet (MSDS) recommends treating spill surfaces with a ~2 mol/liter (~8 g/100 ml), aqueous caustic soda (sodium hydroxide) solution after absorbing liquids with inert absorbent pads or removing any powder present: allow solution to stand for up to one hour, and then thoroughly wash spilled surfaces with soap and water; sample to determine if surface contamination is still present (if sampling method is available). If the drug is still present, repeat above steps; dispose of wastes in accordance with your local procedures, state, and federal regulations.

Incompatibility: CYTARABINE is incompatible with oxidizing agents, strong acids, strong bases, and exposure to light.

CYTOSINE ARABINOSIDE
CYTOSINE ARABINOSIDE HYDROCHLORIDE
ALEXAN®33

Chemical Abstract Service (CAS) Registry
Number: 71-30-7
RTECS: HA5500000
$C_9H_{14}ClN_3O_5$

CYTOSINE

Chemical Abstract Service (CAS) Registry
Number: 69-74-9

RTECS: UW7350150
$C_4H_5N_3O$

SAME AS CYTOSTATIC

$C_9H_{13}N_3O_5$
$C_9H_{12}N_3O_5.HCL$

Health & Safety Hazards/US Department of Transportation (DOT)/US Environmental Protection Agency (EPA)—Sources

Mutagen—University of Maryland at College Park, Toxic—Material Safety Data Sheet, National Fire Protection Association Health 2, Flammability (0) Instability/Reactivity (0)—Material Safety Data Sheet, Hazardous Materials Identification System (R) and/or US Department of Defense System Health (2) Fire Hazard (0) Reactivity (0) Personal Protection Code (-)—Material Safety Data Sheet. Pregnancy (D)—US Food and Drug Administration and US Navy, NA—US California Proposition 65, National Fire Protection Association Health (2) Flammability (1) Instability/Reactivity (0)—Material Safety Data Sheet, Hazardous Materials Identification System (R) and/or US Department of Defense System Health (2) Fire Hazard (1) Reactivity (0) Personal Protection Code (E) (Safety Glasses, Chemical Gloves, Dust Respirator)—Material Safety Data Sheet.

CYTOSINE can cause fetal harm; breastfeeding should be discontinued because of potential for reproductive and developmental hazards. (*A Guide for Occupational Health Professionals Technical Manual*, Navy Environmental Health Center [NEHC-TM-OEM 6260.01a].

CYTOSINE is a white solid.

First Aid/Medical Information/ Occupational Exposure Limits

First Aid Measures to include: Use general first aid measures except for the following:

Ingestion: Do not induce vomiting. If conscious and alert, rinse mouth out and drink 2–4 cups of milk or water. Seek medical assistance.

Medical Information:

Caution and Warning Statements: Toxic—CYTOSINE ARABINOSIDE exposure may cause skin irritation and allergic skin reaction. May cause adverse reproductive effects based upon animal studies and may cause congenital malformation in the fetus. May cause harm to the unborn child. This drug is harmful by inhalation, in contact with skin, and if swallowed.

CYTOSINE ARABINOSIDE may cause sensitization by skin contact. Cytosine is irritating to eyes, respiratory system, and skin. It is listed as a possible mutagen. Laboratory experiments have shown mutagenic effects. If ingested, may cause digestive tract irritation. Exposure may cause sensitization by skin contact.

Target Organs/Systems: Bone marrow, immune system, reproductive systems, central nervous system (nerves), GI, respiratory tracts, skin (dermal), and eyes

Medical Conditions Generally Aggravated by Exposure:

▪ Pregnancy and preexisting skin condition.

Specific Medical Surveillance Information: Reproductive and pregnancy counseling.

Occupational Exposure Level/Limit (OEL) & Sampling Methods: Not otherwise specified

Environmental Sentinel Contamination Action Level (ESCAL): Not otherwise specified

Supplemental Response Information

Extinguishing Media: Use extinguishing agent which is the most appropriate to extinguish surrounding fire (carbon dioxide, foam, dry chemical or water fog as extinguishing media).

Solubility: CYTOSINE ARABINOSIDE is slightly water soluble.

Chemical Degradation/Neutralization Method: Not otherwise specified

Note: If a specific degradation or neutralization method is not provided on this table and you do not have other specific information that will guide you on how to clean up the specific material spilled, then follow the general spill procedure found at the introduction section of this table.

Incompatibility: CYTOSINE ARABINOSIDE is incompatible with oxidizing agents.

CYTOXAN ANHYDROUS FORM

CYCLOPHOSPHAMIDE HYDRATE/MONO-HYDRATE (1)
CYCOLOPHOSPHAMIDE (*sye-kloe-FAHS-fah-mide*)
CTX
PROCYTOX®37

Chemical Abstract Service (CAS) Registry
Numbers: 50-18-0, 6055-19-2, 60007-96-7,
60030-72-0, 6007-95-6 (mixture)
RTECS: RP6157750
RTECS: RP5950000

NSC 26271
$C_7-H_{15}-C_{12}-N_2-0_2-P.H_{20}$
$C_7H_{15}Cl_2N_2O_2P$
(Two Degradation Methods)

Health & Safety Hazards/US Department of Transportation (DOT)/US Environmental Protection Agency (EPA)—Sources

Carcinogen G1—International Agency for Research on Cancer, Carcinogen N1—US National Toxicology Program and Material Safety Data Sheet, Carcinogen—Berkeley University Hazardous Chemical List, Carcinogen—University of Maryland at College Park, Carcinogen Material Safety Data Sheet, Mutagen—Material Safety Data Sheet, Teratogen—University of Maryland at College Park, Teratogen—Material Safety Data Sheet, Reproductive Effector—Centre College, Embryotoxic—Material Safety Data Sheet, Acutely Toxic—Material Safety Data Sheet, Pregnancy Category (D)—US Food and Drug Administration, Carcinogen and Developmental Male and Female—US California Proposition 65, Cytotoxic—Material Safety Data Sheet, Cytotoxic—British Columbia Cancer Agency Canada, Ototoxic—T. C. Hain, Non-vesicant—British Columbia Cancer Agency Canada, National Fire Protection Association Health (2) Flammability (0) Instability/Reactivity (0)—Material Safety Data Sheet, National Fire Protection Association Health (3) Flammability (l) Instability/Reactivity (1)—Material Safety Data Sheet, National Fire Protection Association Health (2) Flammability (1) Instability/Reactivity (0)—Material Safety Data Sheet; Hazardous Materials Identification System (R) and/or US Department of Defense System Health (2) Fire Hazard (1) Reactivity (0) Personal Protection Code (E) (Safety Glasses, Chemical Gloves, Dust Respirator)—Material Data Safety Sheet, Hazardous Materials Identification System (R) and/or US Department of Defense System (2★) with additional chronic hazard present Fire Hazard (0) Reactivity (0) Personal Protection Code (-) (None stated)—Material Safety Data Sheet, U058; UN 2811, CLASS 6.1, GROUP III; MIDI: HW01—(http://usaphcapps.amedd.army.mil/midi/), US California Environmental Protection Agency Listed.

CYCLOPHOSPHAMIDE is available as an injection and as tablets.

CYCLOPHOSPHAMIDE: Breastfeeding is contraindicated because of possible immune suppression, association with carcinogenesis, and neutropenia. This drug is distributed into breast milk and may cause reproductive and developmental harm (*A Guide for Occupational Health Professionals Technical Manual*, Navy Environmental Health Center [NEHC-TM-OEM 6260.01a]).

CYCLOPHOSPHAMIDE is a colorless fluid from powder and 50 mg pink or 50 mg white tablets.

CYCLOPHOSPHAMIDE is supplied in 25 mg tablets (light blue) and 50 mg tablets (light blue).

First Aid/Medical Information/ Occupational Exposure Limits

First Aid Measures to include: Use the general first aid measures except for the following:

Dermal contact: Skin should not be rinsed with organic solvent or scanned with UV light. Avoid rubbing skin or increasing its temperature. Irritated skin can be covered with emollient. Seek medical attention.

Ingestion: Drink milk or water and induce vomiting only if conscious and alert. Seek medical assistance.

Physicians Note (A): In case of accidental exposure, treat symptomatically and supportively.

Physician's note (B): Overdose treatment—since there is no known antidote for CYCLOPHOSPHA-MIDE overdose, treatment should be supportive, and including appropriate treatment for any concurrent infection, myelosuppression, or cardiac toxicity should it occur. Liberal fluid intake and frequent urination are advised to reduce the risk of cystitis, but care must be taken to avoid water retention and intoxication.

Medical Information:

Caution and Warning Statements: CYCLOPHOSP-AMIDE monohydrate is a human carcinogen. Acutely toxic if swallowed. Exposure may cause heritable genetic damage and may cause harm to the unborn child. Exposure may cause skin irritation (permeator) and severe eye irritation. Material may be irritating to mucous membranes and upper respiratory tract. Male and female reproductive toxicity has been documented. CYTOXAN ANHYDROUS may be a cardiotoxic substance. CYTOXAN may cause delayed bone marrow suppression and possibly cardiotoxicity substance. RTECS lists CYTOXAN as a suspected cardiovascular or blood toxicant; as a gastrointestinal or liver toxicant; as a kidney toxicant and as a neurotoxicant.

Exposure may cause nausea, vomiting, anorexia, headache, dizziness, rash, conjunctivitis, GI effects, cystitis, genito-urinary, kidney damage, alopecia, pulmonary fibrosis, changes in metabolism, and permanent sterility.

Caution: Females and males planning to have a child, pregnant women, and nursing mothers should exercise caution regarding potential occupational exposure to this cytotoxic drug. No information or not enough information exists or was provided concerning occupational exposure that may potentially occur while handling this drug and its affects on reproductive systems, the fetus, and/or if it is secreted along with breast milk, which may harm nursing infants. Staff members should consult with the occupational health physician monitoring workers' health in your facility to be apprised of potential hazards and should be advised to avoid becoming pregnant and/or breastfeeding or should be transferred in accordance with policy/procedures to other duties that do not involve preparation, handling, and administering this drug.

Target Organs/Systems: Eyes, bone marrow, bladder, upper respiratory tract, skin, reproductive, and cardiovascular system

Medical Conditions Generally Aggravated by Exposure:

- Low platelet, leukocyte counts, coagulation disorders, renal, pulmonary, cardiac diseases, recent radiation, chemotherapy, and reproductive and pregnancy issues.

Specific Medical Surveillance Information: Reproductive and pregnancy counseling.
Bladder cancer

- Nmp22@bladderchek (nuclear matrix protein) to detect elevated levels of tumor markers in the urine (reported to be more accurate than below)
- Urinalysis to detect microscopic heamaturia
- Urine cytology
- Urine culture to rule out urinary tract infection

Occupational Exposure Level/Limit (OEL) & Sampling Methods:

Environmental Sentinel Contamination Action Level (ESCAL): Air, surface

Supplemental Response Information

Extinguishing Media: Use extinguishing agent which is the most appropriate to extinguish surrounding fire (carbon dioxide, foam, dry chemical or water fog as extinguishing media).

Solubility: CYTOXAN ANHYDROUS is water solubility (40 g/l water). It is freely soluble in alcohol (1% solution has a pH of 4.5).

Chemical Degradation/Neutralization Method: There are two recommended methods (bleach [sodium hypochlorite] solution method and potassium hydroxide in methanol solution method) for CYCLOPHOSPHA-MIDE (see below and above).

A manufacturer's Material Safety Data Sheet (MSDS) recommends treating CYCOPHOSPHAMIDE spill surfaces with a 0.2n solution of potassium hydroxide in methanol after absorbing liquids with inert absorbent pads or removing any powder present: allow solution to stand for up to one hour, and then thoroughly wash spilled surfaces with soap and water; sample to determine if surface contamination is still present (if sampling method is available). If drug is still present, repeat above steps; dispose of wastes in accordance with your local procedures, state, and federal regulations.

Incompatibility: CYTOXAN ANHYDROUS is incompatible with strong bases, strong acids, alkalis, and strong oxidizing agents. Benzyl alcohol preserved diluents. Avoid exposure to heat.

D

DACARBAZINE (*da-CAR-ba-zeen*)

DTIC-DOME®35
DTIC®38

　CAS Registry Number: 4342-03-4
　C_6-H_{10}-N_6O

DACARBAZINE

　CAS Registry Number: 64038-56-8

DACARBINE CUTRATE

　Chemical Abstract Service (CAS) Registry
　　Number: 55390-090-10 (injection solution),
　　37626-23-6
　RTECS: NI3950000

Health & Safety Hazards/US Department of Transportation (DOT)/US Environmental Protection Agency (EPA)—Sources

Carcinogen G2B—International Agency for Research on Cancer, Carcinogen—US National Toxicology Program and Material Safety Data Sheet, Carcinogen C2—US National Toxicology Program, Carcinogen—Berkeley University Hazardous Chemical List, Carcinogen—University of Maryland at College Park, Carcinogen—Material Safety Data Sheet, Teratogen—Material Safety Data Sheet, Cytotoxic—Material Safety Data Sheet, Cytotoxic—British Columbia Cancer Agency Canada, Toxic—Material Safety Data Sheet, Mutagen—Material Safety Data Sheet, Photosensitizer—Material Safety Data Sheet, Irritant—British Columbia Cancer Agency Canada, Lactation-Avoid Breastfeeding (World Health Organization), Pregnancy Category (C)—US Food and Drug Administration, arcinogen and Developmental—US California Proposition 65, Toxic—US State of Florida, Carcinogen—US State of Minnesota, Hazardous Materials Identification System (R) and/or US Department of Defense System Health (3) Fire Hazard (1) Reactivity (0) Personal Protection Code (X) (ask supervisor), National Fire Protection Association Health (2) Flammability (1) Instability/Reactivity (0), National Fire Protection Association Health (2) Flammability (0), Instability/Reactivity (0)—Material Safety Data Sheet, US California Environmental Protection Agency Listed.

　DACARBAZINE (DTIC) is a colorless to pale yellow liquid from powder (200 mg for injection).

　DACARBAZINE: Breastfeeding is contraindicated (US Navy).

　Reduction of DACARBAZINE with nickel-aluminum alloy in dilute base appears to be a good method for the destruction of this drug (Reference MSDS) (no supportive research).

　DACARBAZINE for injection is a sterile parenteral dosage form for reconstitution. When reconstituted each ml of the solution in the 200 milligram vial contains DACARBAZINE, citric acid two milligrams and mannitol 3.75 milligrams with a pH in the range of 3.0 to 4.0.

First Aid/Medical Information/Occupational Exposure Limits

First Aid Measures to include: Use general first aid measures except for the following:

Ingestion: Do not induce vomiting. If conscious and alert, rinse mouth and drink 2–4 cups of milk or water. Seek medical attention.

Physician's note: Physician may induce vomiting and should monitor blood count and liver count during post-exposure period. Treat symptomatically and supportively.

Medical Information:

Caution and Warning Statements: Contain a carcinogen. DACARBAZINE is a cytotoxic agent. All work practices must be designed to reduce human exposure to the lowest level.

DACARBAZINE is a toxic substance that may cause cancer and may cause heritable genetic damage. Cancers of the lining of the heart and bladder were observed in animal studies. Animal studies have indicated that it may be a possible teratogen. May cause nausea, vomiting, decreased appetite, diarrhea, rash, muscle/joint aches, decreased white and/or red blood cells. DACARBAZINE can produce variety of health effects to the respiratory, blood-forming, digestive, and reproductive systems. DACARBAZINE may cause irritation to the eyes, skin photo-sensitizer, and respiratory tract irritant because of being corrosive. Exposure to DACARBAZINE may cause nausea, vomiting, decreased appetite, diarrhea, rash, muscle/joint aches, decreased white/red cells, hair loss, and liver damage. RTECS classifies and lists DACARBAZINE as a suspected neurotoxicant. BC Cancer Agency lists DARBAZINE as an irritant.

May produce immunosuppression in individuals occupationally exposed to this material (drug).

Caution: Females and males planning to have a child, pregnant women, and nursing mothers should exercise caution regarding potential occupational exposure to this cytotoxic drug. No information or not enough information exists or was provided concerning occupational exposure that may potentially occur while handling this drug and its affects on reproductive systems, the fetus, and/or if it is secreted along with breast milk, which may harm nursing infants. Staff members should consult with the occupational health physician monitoring workers' health in your facility to be apprised of potential hazards and should be advised to avoid becoming pregnant and/or breastfeeding or should be transferred in accordance with policy/procedures to other duties that do not involve preparation, handling, and administering this drug.

Therapeutic Levels: There are no adequate and well-controlled studies in pregnant women. It is not known whether this drug is excreted in human milk. DACARBAZINE has been assigned to Food and Drug Administration Pregnancy Category (C). Animal studies have revealed evidence of teratogenicity.

Target Organs/Systems: Skin, eyes, blood, bone marrow, kidneys, GI system, liver, cancer, possibly reproductive system, and fetus

Medical Conditions Generally Aggravated by Exposure:

- Citric acid may cause sensitization of the skin after prolonged or repeated overexposure.
- Persons with sensitivity to DACARBAZINE or those who have conditions with depressed white and/or red blood cells. Furthermore, individuals

with liver, kidney, and skin conditions should be evaluated prior to working in areas where exposure could occur.
- Reproductive and pregnancy issues.

Specific Medical Surveillance Information: Reproductive and pregnancy counseling.

Monitor blood count and liver count during post-exposure period.

Occupational Exposure Level/Limit (OEL) & Sampling Methods:

> *Environmental Sentinel Contamination Action Level (ESCAL)*: Not otherwise specified
> California no significant risk level: Chemical Abstract Service (CAS) Registry Number: 4342-03-4: 0.01 ÆG/day NSRL
> (Method not listed or specified)

Supplemental Response Information

Extinguishing Media: Use extinguishing agent which is the most appropriate to extinguish surrounding fire (carbon dioxide, foam, dry chemical or water fog as extinguishing media).

Solubility: DACARBAZINE (DTIC-DOME®35) is slightly water soluble to water soluble (1 mg/ml at room temp) in the pH range of 3–4 when reconstituted with water (Bedford Laboratories MSDS). This drug is slightly soluble in alcohol.

Chemical Degradation/Neutralization Method: Not otherwise specified

Note: If a specific degradation or neutralization method is not provided on this table and you do not have other specific information that will guide you on how to clean up the specific material spilled, then follow the general spill procedure found at the introduction section of this table.

Incompatibility: DACARBAZINE is incompatible with strong oxidizing agents. Avoid light and heat.

DACTINOMYCIN (*DAK-tin-o-MY-sin*)
ACTINOMYCIN D®39
COSMEGEN LYOVAC®40

> Chemical Abstract Service (CAS) Registry Number: 50-76-0 (may be a mixture or single substance)
> RTECS: AU1575000
> $C_{62}H_{86}N_{12}O_{16}$

Health & Safety Hazards/US Department of Transportation (DOT)/US Environmental Protection Agency (EPA)—Sources

Carcinogen G3—International Agency for Research on Cancer, Reproductive Effector—US National Institute of Environmental Health Sciences (NIEHS), Developmental Toxic—Centre College, Mutagen—University of Maryland at College Park, Teratogen—University of Maryland at College Park, Tumorigenic—Material Safety Data Sheet, Carcinogen—University of Maryland at College Park, Carcinogen—Berkeley University Hazardous Chemical List, Highly Toxic—Material Safety Data Sheet, Sensitizer—Material Safety Data Sheet, Corrosive—Material Safety Data Sheet, Cytotoxic—British Columbia Cancer Agency Canada, Vesicant—British Columbia Cancer Agency Canada, Lactation—Avoid Breastfeeding (World Health Organization) Pregnancy Category (D) US Food and Drug Administration—British Columbia Cancer Agency Canada, Pregnancy Category (C) US Food and Drug Administration—US Navy, Carcinogen and Developmental—US California Proposition 65, National Fire Protection Association Health (3) Flammability (0) Instability/Reactivity (0)—Material Safety Data Sheet, National Fire Protection Association Health (3) Flammability (1) Instability/Reactivity (0)—Material Safety Data Sheet; National Fire Protection Association Health (4) Flammability (1) Instability/Reactivity (0)—Material Safety Data Sheet, National Fire Protection Association Health (3) Flammability (2) Instability/Reactivity (1), Hazardous Materials Identification System (R) and/or US Department of Defense System (4★) with additional chronic hazard present Fire Hazard (1) Reactivity (0) Personal Protection Code (A) (Safety Glasses)—Material Safety Data Sheet, Hazardous Materials Identification System (R) and/or US Department of Defense System (3★) with additional chronic hazard present Fire Hazard (0) Reactivity (0) Personal Protection Code (-) (None stated), Hazardous Materials Identification System (R) and/or US Department of Defense System (3★) with additional chronic hazard present Fire Hazard (2) Reactivity (1) Personal Protection code (-) (None stated)—Material Safety Data Sheet, UN 2811, Class 6.1, or UN 3462, Class 6.1, Group II, or NA 1993, Comb Liquid, Group III.

DACTINOMYCIN (COSMEGEN LYOVAC) is a yellow fluid prepared from a powder.

DACTINOMYCIN is a bright red, somewhat hygroscopic, crystalline powder.

DACTINOMYCIN can cause malformations and embryotoxicity in animals; breastfeeding should be discontinued because of potential for reproductive and developmental harm (*A Guide for Occupational Health Professionals Technical Manual*, Navy Environmental Health Center [NEHC-TM-OEM 6260.01a]).

DACTINOMYCIN is an antineoplastic antibiotic produced by Streptomyces Parvulus and other species of Streptomyces.

First Aid/Medical Information/ Occupational Exposure Limits

First Aid Measures to include: Use general first aid measures except for the following:

Ingestion: Do no induce vomiting unless told to do so by a physician. Only if conscious and alert, give water. Avoid alcoholic beverages. Be alert to early indication of allergic reactions or hypersensitivity. Seek medical assistance.

Physician's note: There is no known specific antidote. Gastric lavage may be effective if indicated for ingestion. Activated carbon may provide detoxification activity. Blood pathologies may include agranulocytosis, leucopenia, thrombopenia, reticulocytopenia, and pancytopenia. Small systemic doses may cause a minor health hazard although individual sensitivity may vary. Observe for 24 hours. Monitor hepatic function, white blood cell (leukocyte) count and/or morphology, and platelet count. Be alert to early indications of allergic reactions or hypersensitivity. Be prepared for emergency hypersensitivity reaction intervention. Anaphylactoid reactions may require emergency epinephrine administration. Hypersensitivity reactions may require oxygen, intravenous steroids, and airway management including intubation as indicated.

Medical Information:

Caution and Warning Statements:

Danger! DACTINOMYCIN (COSMEGEN) is classified as a poison, highly toxic, and may be fatal if swallowed. Exposure may cause birth defects and may cause heritable genetic damage. Limited evidence of a carcinogenic effect, listed by IARC as a Group 3 Carcinogen. Exposure to DACTINOMYCIN (COSMEGEN) may cause severe eye irritation, may cause blindness. This drug is a possible sensitizer. Extremely corrosive to skin and allergic skin reaction. Inhalation may be irritating to mucous membranes or respiratory tract. Animal study shows that COSMEGEN is highly toxic by ingestion. DACTINOMYCIN (COSMEGEN) may damage the developing fetus. RTECS lists DACTI-NOMYCN (ACTINOMYCIN D®39) as a suspected cardiovascular or blood toxicant and as a gastrointestinal or liver toxicant. BC Cancer Agency lists DACTINO-MYCIN as a vesicant.

Caution: Females and males planning to have a child, pregnant women, and nursing mothers should exercise caution regarding potential occupational exposure to this cytotoxic drug. No information or not enough information exists or was provided concerning occupational exposure that may potentially occur while handling this drug and its affects on reproductive systems, the fetus, and/or if it is secreted along with breast milk, which may harm nursing infants. Staff members should consult with the occupational health physician monitoring workers' health in your facility to be apprised of potential hazards and should be advised to avoid becoming pregnant and/or breastfeeding or should be transferred in accordance with policy/procedures to other duties that do not involve preparation, handling, and administering this drug.

Target Organs/Systems: Hypersensitization, bone marrow, liver, kidneys, eyes, skin, respiratory, GI tracts, muscle tissue, testes, developing fetus, and cancer

Medical Conditions Generally Aggravated by Exposure: Exposure to ACTINOMYCIN D®39 at therapeutic levels may aggravate pregnancy. Exposure to ACTINOMYCIN D®39 may cause congenital malformation in the fetus. Medical Conditions Generally Aggravated by exposure: allergy or hypersensitivity to antibiotics aminoglycoside antibiotics (e.g., KANAMYCIN, STREPTOMYCIN).

It has been reported that COSMEGEN treatments should not be given at or about the time of infection with chickenpox or herpes zoster because of the risk of severe generalized disease, which may result in death.

DACTINOMYCIN exposure—hypersensitivity to material, chicken pox (including recent exposure), herpes zoster, bone marrow depression, impaired liver function, infection, and previous cytotoxic drug or radiation therapy. Repeated exposure to a highly toxic material may produce general deterioration of health by an accumulation in one or more human organs.

Specific Medical Surveillance Information: Reproductive and pregnancy counseling.

Occupational Exposure Level/Limit (OEL) & Sampling Methods:

Environmental Sentinel Contamination Action Level (ESCAL): Surface

DACTINOMYCIN Occupational Exposure Level (OEL): Merck, Sharp & Dohme
DACTINOMYCIN zero exposure★
Merck exposure control limit (ECL); ★zero exposure is an internally derived exposure control limit based on the carcinogenic potential of the compound.
(Method not listed or specified)

Supplemental Response Information

Extinguishing Media: Use extinguishing agent which is the most appropriate to extinguish surrounding fire (carbon dioxide, foam, dry chemical or water fog as extinguishing media).

Solubility: DACTINOMYCIN has been reported in various MSDSs to be water soluble to almost insoluble.

Chemical Degradation/Neutralization Method: A DACTINOMYCIN Material Safety Data Sheet (MSDS) recommends a neutralizing agent of 5% trisodium phosphate for at least 15 to 30 minutes, and then cleaned with soap and water.

Incompatibility: DACTINOMYCIN is incompatible with strong oxidizing agents, acid chlorides, phosphorus halides, strong reducing agents, acids, or bases (alkalis).

DAUNORUBICIN HYDROCHLORIDE (HCL) (1)
(*DAWN-o-ROU-bi-sin*)
DAUNORUBICIN FREE BASE
CERUBIDINE®41
DAUNOXOME®42
LIPOSOMA
DAUNOMYCIN

Chemical Abstract Service (CAS) Registry Number: 23541-50-6
C_{27}-H_{29}-NO_{10}.HCL
C_{27}-H_{29}-$N0_{10}$
$C_{27}H_{30}ClNO_{10}$

DAUNORUBICIN HYDROCHLORIDE

CAS Registry Number: 20830-81-3

DAUNORUBICIN

RTECS: HB7878000
NSC 82151
(Three Degradation Methods)

Health & Safety Hazards/US Department of Transportation (DOT)/US Environmental Protection Agency (EPA)—Sources

Ca G2B—International Agency for Research on Cancer, Reproductive Effector—Centre College, Carcinogen—US National Institute of Health (NIH) and Material Safety Data Sheet, Mutagen—US National Institute of Health (NIH) and Material Safety Data Sheet, Teratogen—US National Institute of Health (NIH) and Material Safety Data Sheet, Highly Toxic—Material Safety Data Sheet, Mutagen—Material Safety Data Sheet, Cytotoxic—British Columbia Cancer Agency Canada, Corrosive—British Columbia Cancer Agency Canada, Vesicant—British Columbia Cancer Agency Canada, Irritant—Material Safety Data Sheet, Lactation—Avoid Breastfeeding (World Health Organization) Pregnancy Category (D)—US Food and Drug Administration, Developmental—US California Proposition 65 and Material Safety Data Sheet, Developmental—Material Safety Data Sheet, National Fire Protection Association Health (1) Flammability (0) Instability/Reactivity (0)—Material Safety Data Sheet, National Fire Protection Association Health (2) Flammability (1) Instability/Reactivity (0)—Material Safety Data Sheet, National Fire Protection Association Health (2) Flammability (0) Instability/Reactivity (0)—Material Safety Data Sheet, National Fire Protection Association Health (3) Flammability (0) Instability/Reactivity (0)—Material Safety Data Sheet, Hazardous Materials Identification System (R) and/or US Department of Defense System Health (2*) with additional chronic hazard present Fire Hazard (1) Reactivity (0) Personal Protection Code (A) (Safety Glasses); Hazardous Materials Identification System (R) and/or US Department of Defense System Health (3*) with additional chronic hazard present Fire Hazard (0) Reactivity (0) Personal Protection Code (-) (None stated)—Material Safety Data Sheet, MIDI: HW01—(http://usaphcapps .amedd.army.mil/midi/), ORAL RAT 290 MG/KG, ORAL MOUSE 205 MG/KG, US California Environmental Protection Agency Listed, U059, UN 2811, UN 2810.

DAUNORUBICIN is a red fluid from powder for injection.

DAUNORUBICIN is an orange-red, hygroscopic, crystalline powder.

DAUNORUBICIN is available as an injection.

DAUNORUBICIN—May cause fetal harm; breastfeeding should be discontinue because of potential for reproductive and developmental harm (*A Guide for Occupational Health Professionals Technical Manual,* Navy Environmental Health Center [NEHC-TM-OEM 6260.01a]).

First Aid/Medical Information/ Occupational Exposure Limits

First Aid Measures to include: Use general first aid measures except for the following:

Note: Medical attention should be sought immediately after the initiating first aid measures.

Ingestion: If the product is swallowed, call physician or poison control center for most current information. If professional advice is not available, do not induce vomiting. Victim should drink milk, egg whites, or large quantities of water. Never induce vomiting or give diluents (milk or water) to someone who is unconscious, having convulsions, or who cannot swallow.

Physician's note (A): Due to its action, DAUNORUBICIN should be treated as potentially carcinogenic and may be mutagenic, teratogenic, or allergenic. If respiratory distress occurs after inhalation of airborne droplets, administer emergency airway support and 100% humidified supplemental oxygen with assisted ventilation if needed. If coughing or difficulty in breathing develops, evacuating for respiratory tract irritation, bronchitis, or pneumonitis. Medical attention should be sought immediately after the initiating first aid measures.

Physician's note (B): Treatment of anthracycline antineoplastic overdose should be symptomatic and supportive and may include the following:

1. Filgrastim may be useful in treating severe granulocytopenia. For fever or infection, take cultures and administer appropriate antibiotics.
2. Treat bleeding from bone marrow suppression with transfusions of packed red blood cells and platelets.
3. Cardiac monitoring is recommended.
4. DEXRAZOXANE may prevent cardiomyopathy.
5. Treatment of cardiomyopathy consists of vigorous management of congestive heart failure with digitalis preparations, diuretics, and after-load reducers such as ace inhibitors.
6. Hemodialysis is not likely to be effective, however, hemoperfusion initiated within minutes of overdose may reduce serum levels.

Medical Information:

Caution and Warning Statements: DAUNORUBICIN HCL is a cytotoxic agent. All work practices must be designed to eliminate or greatly reduce human exposure. Exposure to DAUNORUBICIN HCL may cause birth defect hazard, cancer, heritable genetic damage, and male and female reproductive toxicity. DAUNORUBICIN HCL may cause sensitization by inhalation and skin contact. May cause skin and eye irritation. Exposure to DAUNORUBICIN HCL has been known to cause kidney damage.

Exposure to DAUNORUBICIN HCL can cause nausea, vomiting, gastrointestinal disturbances, poor appetite, and abdominal pain. High exposure can cause irregular heart rhythm and may lead to permanent damage of the heart muscle. BC Cancer Agency lists DAUNORUBICIN as a vesicant.

Caution: Females and males planning to have a child, pregnant women, and nursing mothers should exercise caution regarding potential occupational exposure to this cytotoxic drug. No information or not enough information exists or was provided concerning occupational exposure that may potentially occur while handling this drug and its affects on reproductive systems, the fetus, and/or if it is secreted along with breast milk, which may harm nursing infants. Staff members should consult with the occupational health physician monitoring workers' health in your facility to be apprised of potential hazards and should be advised to avoid becoming pregnant and/or breastfeeding or should be transferred in accordance with policy/procedures to other duties that do not involve preparation, handling, and administering this drug.

Target Organs/Systems: Reproductive systems (embryotoxic), liver, kidneys, cardiovascular system (heart), CNS, bone marrow, blood, and skin; a mutagen and a possible human carcinogen

Medical Conditions Generally Aggravated by Exposure:

- It is recommended that personnel with preexisting dermatitis, cardiovascular symptoms, bone marrow suppression, kidney and liver disorders, and blood system disorders, as well as women during the first three months of pregnancy should not be exposed to DAUNORUBICIN HCL. Breastfeeding is not recommended due to the potential for the drug to be secreted into breast milk.
- Persons sensitive to other anthracyclines may be sensitive to this material.

Specific Medical Surveillance Information: Reproductive and pregnancy counseling.

Medical Surveillance may consist of liver and kidney functions tests, hematological (complete blood count) work up, EKG, and cardiovascular examination.

Occupational Exposure Level/Limit (OEL) & Sampling Methods: Not otherwise specified

Environmental Sentinel Contamination Action Level (ESCAL): Not otherwise specified

Supplemental Response Information

Extinguishing Media: Use extinguishing agent which is the most appropriate to extinguish surrounding fire (carbon dioxide, foam, dry chemical or water fog as extinguishing media).

Solubility: DAUNORUBICIN HCL is easily to freely soluble in cold water. DAUNORUBICIN pH range is 5.5–8.8 (reconstituted solution). Another notation: pH 4.5–6.5 reference standard (0.5%) aqueous solution; soluble in methanol/aqueous alcohols.

Chemical Degradation/Neutralization Method: There are three recommended methods (sodium hydroxide method, bleach [sodium hypochlorite] method and sulphuric acid/potassium permanganate method) for DAUNORUBICIN HCL. See below for procedures.

A manufacturer's Material Safety Data Sheet (MSDS) recommends treating spill surfaces with a ~2 mol/liter (~8 g/100 ml), aqueous caustic soda (sodium hydroxide) solution after absorbing liquids with inert absorbent pads or removing any powder present: allow solution to stand for up to one hour, and then thoroughly wash spilled surfaces with soap and water; sample to determine if surface contamination is still present (if sampling method is available). If drug is still present, repeat above steps; dispose of wastes in accordance with your local procedures, state, and federal regulations.

Incompatibility: DAUNORUBICIN HCL is incompatible with strong oxidizing agents. Water reactivates acids, caustics, and aluminum. Avoid exposure to light, heat, and moisture.

DAUNORUBICIN HCL (2)

DAUNORUBICIN FREE BASE (*DAWN-o-ROU-bi-sin*)
CERUBIDINE®41
DAUNOXOME®42
LIPOSOMA

Chemical Abstract Service (CAS) Registry Number: 23541-50-6
C_{27}-H_{29}-NO_{10}·HCL
C_{27}-H_{29}-NO_{10}

DAUNORUBICIN HYDROCHLORIDE)

CAS Registry Number: 20830-81-3

DAUNORUBICIN

RTECS: HB7878000
NSC 82151
(Three Degradation Methods)

Health & Safety Hazards/US Department of Transportation (DOT)/US Environmental Protection Agency (EPA)—Sources

Carcinogen G2B—International Agency for Research on Cancer, Reproductive Effector—Centre College, Carcinogen—US National Institute of Health (NIH) and Material Safety Data Sheet, Mutagen—US National Institute of Health (NIH) and Material Safety Data Sheet, Teratogen—US National Institute of Health (NIH) and Material Safety Data Sheet, Highly Toxic—Material Safety Data Sheet, Mutagen—Material Safety Data Sheet, Cytotoxic—British Columbia Cancer Agency Canada, Corrosive—British Columbia Cancer Agency Canada, Vesicant—British Columbia Cancer Agency Canada, Irritant—Material Safety Data Sheet, Lactation Avoid Breastfeeding (World Health Organization) Pregnancy Category (D)—US Food and Drug Administration, Carcinogen and Development—US California Proposition 65, National Fire Protection Association Health (1) Flammability (0) Instability/Reactivity (0)—Material Safety Data Sheet, National Fire Protection Association Health (2) Flammability (1) Instability/Reactivity (0)—Material Safety Data Sheet, National Fire Protection Association Health (2) Flammability (0) Instability/Reactivity (0)—Material Safety Data Sheet, National Fire Protection Association Health (3) Flammability (0) Instability/Reactivity (0)—Material Safety Data Sheet, Hazardous Materials Identification System (R) and/or US Department of Defense System (2★) with additional chronic hazard present Fire Hazard (1) Reactivity (0) Personal Protection Code (A) (Safety Glasses); (3★) with additional chronic hazard present Fire Hazard (0) Reactivity (0) Personal Protection Code (-) (None stated)—Material Safety Data Sheet, Hazardous Materials Identification System (R) and/or US Department of Defense System Health (3) Fire hazard (0) Reactivity (0) Personal Protection Code (X) (Ask Supervisor)—Material Safety Data Sheet, MIDI:HW01—(http://usaphcapps.amedd.army.mil/midi/), U059, UN 2811ORAL RAT 290 MG/KG, ORAL MOUSE 205 MG/KG, US California Environmental Protection Agency Listed.

DAUNORUBICIN is a red fluid from powder for injection.

DAUNORUBICIN is an orange-red, hygroscopic, crystalline powder.

DAUNORUBICIN is available as an injection.

DAUNORUBICIN may cause fetal harm; breast-feeding should be discontinued because of potential for reproductive and developmental harm (*A Guide for Occupational Health Professionals Technical Manual*, Navy Environmental Health Center [NEHC-TM-OEM 6260.01a]).

First Aid/Medical Information/ Occupational Exposure Limits

First Aid Measures to include: Use general first aid measures except for the following:

Ingestion: If the product is swallowed, call physician or poison control center for most current information. If professional advice is not available, do not induce vomiting. Victim should drink milk, egg whites, or large quantities of water. Never induce vomiting or give diluents (milk or water) to someone who is unconscious, having convulsions, or who cannot swallow.

Physician's note (A): Due to its action, DAUNORUBICIN should be treated as potentially carcinogenic, and may be mutagenic, teratogenic, or allergenic. If respiratory distress occurs after inhalation of airborne droplets, administer emergency airway support and 100% humidified supplemental oxygen with assisted ventilation if needed. If coughing or difficulty in breathing develops, evacuating for respiratory tract irritation, bronchitis, or pneumonitis. Because of the potentially hazardous nature of DAUNORUBICIN, if the solution is swallowed, in eyes or in contact with the skin, medical attention should be sought immediately after the preceding first aid measures are taken.

Physician's note (B): Treatment of anthracycline antineoplastic overdose should be symptomatic and supportive and may include the following:

1. Filgrastim may be useful in treating severe granulocytopenia. For fever or infection, take cultures and administer appropriate antibiotics.
2. Treat bleeding from bone marrow suppression with transfusions of packed red blood cells and platelets.
3. Cardiac monitoring is recommended.
4. DEXRAZOXANE may prevent cardiomyopathy.
5. Treatment of cardiomyopathy consists of vigorous management of congestive heart

failure with digitalis preparations, diuretics, and after-load reducers such as ace inhibitors.

Hemodialysis is not likely to be effective, however, hemoperfusion initiated within minutes of overdose may reduce serum levels

Medical Information:

Caution and Warning Statements: DAUNORUBI-CIN HCL is a cytotoxic agent. All work practices must be designed to eliminate or greatly reduce human exposure. Exposure to DAUNORUBICIN HCL may cause birth defect hazard, cancer, heritable genetic damage, and male and female reproductive toxicity. DAUNORUBICIN HCL may cause sensitization by inhalation and skin contact. May cause skin and eye irritation. Exposure to DAUNORUBICIN HCL has been known to cause kidney damage.

Exposure to DAUNORUBICIN HCL can cause nausea, vomiting, gastrointestinal disturbances, poor appetite, and abdominal pain. High exposure can cause irregular heart rhythm and may lead to permanent damage of the heart muscle.

Caution: Females and males planning to have a child, pregnant women, and nursing mothers should exercise caution regarding potential occupational exposure to this cytotoxic drug. No information or not enough information exists or was provided concerning occupational exposure that may potentially occur while handling this drug and its affects on reproductive systems, the fetus, and/or if it is secreted along with breast milk, which may harm nursing infants. Staff members should consult with the occupational health physician monitoring workers' health in your facility to be apprised of potential hazards and should be advised to avoid becoming pregnant and/or breastfeeding or should be transferred in accordance with policy/procedures to other duties that do not involve preparation, handling, and administering this drug.

Therapeutic Levels: It is recommended that during the first three months of pregnancy should not be exposed to DAUNORUBICIN HCL. Breastfeeding is not recommended due to the potential for the drug to be secreted into breast milk.

Target Organs/Systems: Reproductive systems (embryotoxic), liver, kidneys, cardiovascular system, CNS, bone marrow, blood, skin, a mutagen, and a possible human carcinogen

Medical Conditions Generally Aggravated by Exposure:

- It is recommended that personnel with preexisting hypersensitivity, dermatitis, cardiovascular symptoms, kidney and liver disorders, and blood system disorders, as well as women during the first three months of pregnancy, should not be exposed to DAUNORUBICIN HCL. Breastfeeding is not recommended due to the potential for the drug to be secreted into breast milk.

- Persons sensitive to other anthracyclines may be sensitive to this material.

Specific Medical Surveillance Information: Reproductive and pregnancy counseling.

Medical Surveillance may consist of liver and kidney functions tests, hematological (complete blood count) work up, EKG, and cardiovascular examination.

Occupational Exposure Level/Limit (OEL) & Sampling Methods: Not otherwise specified

Environmental Sentinel Contamination Action Level (ESCAL): Not otherwise specified

Supplemental Response Information

Extinguishing Media: Use extinguishing agent which is the most appropriate to extinguish surrounding fire (carbon dioxide, foam, dry chemical or water fog as extinguishing media).

Solubility: DAUNORUBICIN HCL is easily to freely soluble in cold water. DAUNORUBICIN pH range is 5.5–8.8 (reconstituted solution). Another reference: pH 4.5–6.5 reference standard (0.5%) aqueous solution.

DAUNORUBICIN is soluble in methanol/aqueous alcohols.

Chemical Degradation/Neutralization Method: There are three recommended methods (sodium hydroxide method, bleach [sodium hypochlorite] method and sulphuric acid/potassium permanganate method) for DAUNORUBICIN HCL. See below and above for procedures.

The International Agency for Research on Cancer (IARC) recommended degradation method for DAUNORUBICIN HCL:

The IARC recommends treating spill surfaces with a 5.25% sodium hypochlorite (bleach) solution after absorbing liquids with inert absorbent pads or removing any powder present: allow solution to stand for up to one hour, and then thoroughly wash spilled surfaces with soap and water; sample to determine if surface contamination is still present (if sampling method is available). If drug is still present, repeat above steps; dispose of wastes in accordance with your local procedures, state, and federal regulations.

Incompatibility: DAUNORUBICIN HCL is incompatible with strong oxidizing agents, acids, caustics, and aluminum. Avoid exposure to light, heat, and moisture.

DAUNORUBICIN HCL (3)
DAUNORUBICIN FREE BASE
CERUBIDINE®41
DAUNOXOME®42
LIPOSOMA

Chemical Abstract Service (CAS) Registry
    Number: 23541-50-6
C_{27}-H_{29}-$N0_{10}$.HCL
C_{27}-H_{29}-$N0_{10}$

DAUNORUBICIN HYDROCHLORIDE

Chemical Abstract Service (CAS) Registry
    Number: 20830-81-3

DAUNORUBICIN)

RTECS: HB7878000
NSC 82151
(Three Degradation Methods)

Health & Safety Hazards/Department of Transportation (DOT)/US Environmental Protection Agency (EPA)—Sources

Carcinogen G2B—International Agency for Research on Cancer, Reproductive Effector—Centre College, Carcinogen—US National Institute of Health (NIH) and Material Safety Data Sheet, Mutagen—US National Institute of Health (NIH) and Material Safety Data Sheet, Teratogen—US National Institute of Health (NIH) and Material Safety Data Sheet, Highly Toxic—Material Safety Data Sheet, Mutagen—Material Safety Data Sheet, Cytotoxic—British Columbia Cancer Agency Canada, Corrosive—British Columbia Cancer Agency Canada, Vesicant—British Columbia Cancer Agency Canada, Irritant—Material Safety Data Sheet, Lactation—Avoid Breastfeeding (World Health Organization) Pregnancy Category (D)—US Food and Drug Administration, Carcinogen and Developmental—US California Proposition 65, National Fire Protection Association Health (1) Flammability (0) Instability/Reactivity (0)—Material Safety Data Sheet, National Fire Protection Association Health (2) Flammability (1) Instability/Reactivity (0)—Material Safety Data Sheet, National Fire Protection Association Health (2) Flammability (0) Instability/Reactivity (0)—Material Safety Data Sheet, National Fire Protection Association Health (3) Flammability (0) Instability/Reactivity (0)—Material Safety Data Sheet, Hazardous Materials Identification System (R) and/or US Department of Defense System (2★) with additional chronic hazard present Health (1) Fire hazard (0) Personal Protection (A) (Safety Glasses)—Material Safety Data Sheet, Hazardous Materials Identification System (R) and/or US Department of Defense System Health (3★) with additional chronic hazard present Fire Hazard (0) Reactivity (0) Personal Protection Code (-)(None stated), Hazardous Materials Identification System (R) and/or US Department of Defense System Health (3) Fire Hazard (0) Reactivity (0) Personal Protection Code (X) (ask supervisor), MIDI: HW01—(http://usaphcapps.amedd.army.mil/midi/), U059, UN 2811, UN 2810, US California Environmental Protection Agency Listed.

DAUNORUBICIN is a red fluid from powder for injection.

DAUNORUBICIN is an orange-red, hygroscopic, crystalline powder.

DAUNORUBICIN is available as an injection.

DAUNORUBICIN may cause fetal harm; breastfeeding should be discontinued because of potential for reproductive and developmental harm (*A Guide for Occupational Health Professionals Technical Manual*, Navy Environmental Health Center [NEHC-TM-OEM 6260.01a]).

First Aid/Medical Information/Occupational Exposure Limits

First Aid Measures to include: Use general first aid measures except for the following:

Note: Medical attention should be sought immediately after the initiating first aid measures.

Ingestion: If the product is swallowed, call physician or poison control center for most current information. If professional advice is not available, do not induce vomiting. Victim should drink milk, egg whites, or large quantities of water. Never induce vomiting or give diluents (milk or water) to someone who is unconscious, having convulsions, or who cannot swallow.

Physician's note (A): Due to its action, DAUNORUBICIN should be treated as potentially carcinogenic, and may be mutagenic, teratogenic, or allergenic. If respiratory distress occurs after inhalation of airborne droplets, administer emergency airway support and 100% humidified supplemental oxygen with assisted ventilation if needed. If coughing or difficulty in breathing develops, evacuating for respiratory tract irritation, bronchitis, or pneumonitis.

Medical attention should be sought immediately after the initiating first aid measures.

Physician's note (B): Treatment of anthracycline antineoplastic overdose should be symptomatic and supportive and may include the following:

1. Filgrastim may be useful in treating severe granulocytopenia. For fever or infection, take cultures and administer appropriate antibiotics.
2. Treat bleeding from bone marrow suppression with transfusions of packed red blood cells and platelets.
3. Cardiac monitoring is recommended.
4. Dexrazoxane may prevent cardiomyopathy.
5. Treatment of cardiomyopathy consists of vigorous management of congestive heart failure with digitalis preparations, diuretics, and after-load reducers such as ace inhibitors.
6. Hemodialysis is not likely to be effective, however, hemoperfusion initiated within minutes of overdose may reduce serum levels.

Medical Information:

Caution and Warning Statements: DAUNORUBICIN HCL is a cytotoxic agent. All work practices must be designed to eliminate or greatly reduce human exposure. Exposure to DAUNORUBICIN HCL may cause birth defect hazard, cancer, heritable genetic damage, and male and female reproductive toxicity. DAUNORUBICIN HCL may cause sensitization by inhalation and skin contact. May cause skin and eye irritation. Exposure to DAUNORUBICIN HCL has been known to cause kidney damage.

Exposure to DAUNORUBICIN HCL can cause nausea, vomiting, gastrointestinal disturbances, poor appetite, and abdominal pain. High exposure can cause irregular heart rhythm and may lead to permanent damage of the heart muscle. BC Cancer Agency lists DAUNORUBICIN as a vesicant.

Caution: Females and males planning to have a child, pregnant women, and nursing mothers should exercise caution regarding potential occupational exposure to this cytotoxic drug. No information or not enough information exists or was provided concerning occupational exposure that may potentially occur while handling this drug and its affects on reproductive systems, the fetus, and/or if it is secreted along with breast milk, which may harm nursing infants. Staff members should consult with the occupational health physician monitoring workers' health in your facility to be apprised of potential hazards and should be advised

to avoid becoming pregnant and/or breastfeeding or should be transferred in accordance with policy/procedures to other duties that do not involve preparation, handling, and administering this drug.

Therapeutic Levels: It is recommended that during the first three months of pregnancy personnel are not to be exposed to DAUNORUBICIN HCL. Breastfeeding is not recommended due to the potential for the drug to be secreted into breast milk.

Target Organs/Systems: Reproductive systems (embryotoxic), liver, kidneys, cardiovascular system (heart), CNS, bone marrow, blood, skin; a mutagen and a possible human carcinogen

Medical Conditions Generally Aggravated by Exposure:

- It is recommended that personnel with preexisting dermatitis, cardiovascular symptoms, bone marrow suppression, kidney and liver disorders, and blood system disorders, as well as women during the first three months of pregnancy not to be exposed to DAUNORUBICIN HCL. Breastfeeding is not recommended due to the potential for the drug to be secreted into breast milk.
- Persons sensitive to other anthracyclines may be sensitive to this material.

Specific Medical Surveillance Information: Reproductive and pregnancy counseling.

Medical surveillance may consist of liver and kidney functions tests, hematological (complete blood count) work up, EKG, and cardiovascular examination.

Occupational Exposure Level/Limit (OEL) & Sampling Methods: Not otherwise specified

Environmental Sentinel Contamination Action Level (ESCAL): Not otherwise specified

Supplemental Response Information

Extinguishing Media: Use extinguishing agent which is the most appropriate to extinguish surrounding fire (carbon dioxide, foam, dry chemical or water fog as extinguishing media).

Solubility: DAUNORUBICIN HCL is easily soluble in cold water. This drug pH range is 5.5–8.8 (reconstituted solution) and a pH 4.5–6.5 reference standard (0.5%) aqueous solution.

DAUNORUBICIN is soluble in methanol/aqueous alcohols.

Chemical Degradation/Neutralization Method: There are three recommended methods (sodium hydroxide method, bleach [sodium hypochlorite] method and sulphuric acid/potassium permanganate method) for DAUNORUBICIN HCL. See below and above for procedures.

A manufacturer's Material Safety Data Sheet (MSDS) recommends treating spill surfaces with spills may be treated with 3 m sulphuric acid and 0.3 m potassium permanganate (2:1) solution. After absorbing liquids with inert absorbent pads or removing any powder present: allow solution to stand for up to one hour, and then thoroughly wash spilled surfaces with soap and water; sample to determine if surface contamination is still present (if sampling method is available at your facility). If still present, repeat above steps; dispose of wastes in accordance with your local procedures, state, and federal regulations.

Incompatibility: DAUNORUBICIN HCL is incompatible with strong oxidizing agents, water reactive chemicals, acids, caustics, and aluminum. Avoid exposure to light, heat, and moisture.

DIAMINOCYCLOHEXANE (OXALATOPLATINUM)

C_8-H_{14}-N_2-O_4-Pt

(+)-(S,S)-1,2-DIAMINOCYCLOHEXANE)

Chemical Abstract Service (CAS) Registry
    Number: 21436-03-3
$C_8H_{12}N_2O_4Pt$

OXALIPLATIN
ELOXATIN®88

Chemical Abstract Service (CAS) Registry
    Number: 61825-94-3
RTECS: TP2275850

Health & Safety Hazards/US Department of Transportation (DOT)/US Environmental Protection Agency (EPA)—Sources

Corrosive—Material Safety Data Sheet, Pregnancy Category (D)—US Food and Drug Administration, National Fire Protection Association Health (3) Flammability (0) Instability/Reactivity (0), Hazardous Materials Identification System (R) and/or US Department of Defense System Health (3★) with additional chronic hazard present Fire Hazard (0) Reactivity (0) Personal Protection Code (-) (None stated), Hazardous Materials Identification System (R) and/or US Department of Defense System Health (2) Fire Hazard (1) Reactivity

(1) Personal Protection Code (-) (None stated)—Material Safety Data Sheet, UN 3259, Class 8.

OXALIPLATIN is available as an injection.

First Aid/Medical Information/ Occupational Exposure Limits

First Aid Measures to include: Use general first aid measures.

Medical Information:

Caution and Warning Statements: The acute and chronic toxicity of DIAMINOCYCLOHEXANE OXALATOPLATINUM is not fully known. It has a corrosive effect on skin and mucous membranes. Furthermore, it has a strong corrosive effect on the eye. It is an irritant to skin and mucous membranes.

Exposure to DIAMINOCYCLOHEXANE OXALATOPLATINUM may cause respiratory tract, eyes, skin, and digestive tract damage from the material's corrosive characteristics. Eye contact may result in permanent damage and complete vision loss. Inhalation may result in respiratory effects such as inflammation, edema, and chemical pneumonitis. This drug may cause coughing, wheezing, laryngitis, shortness of breath, headache, nausea, and vomiting. Ingestion may cause damage to the mouth, throat, and esophagus. Contact may cause skin burns or irritation depending in the severity of exposure. Swallowing will lead to a strong corrosive effect on mouth and throat and to the danger of perforation of esophagus and stomach.

Caution: Females and males planning to have a child, pregnant women, and nursing mothers should exercise caution regarding potential occupational exposure to this cytotoxic drug. No information or not enough information exists or was provided concerning occupational exposure that may potentially occur while handling this drug and its affects on reproductive systems, the fetus, and/or if it is secreted along with breast milk, which may harm nursing infants. Staff members should consult with the occupational health physician monitoring workers' health in your facility to be apprised of potential hazards and should be advised to avoid becoming pregnant and/or breastfeeding or should be transferred in accordance with policy/procedures to other duties that do not involve preparation, handling, and administering this drug.

Therapeutic Levels: ELOXATIN®88 may cause fetal harm when administered to a pregnant woman. Pregnant rats were administered 1 mg/kg/day OXALIPLATIN (less than one-tenth the recommended human dose based on body surface area) during gestation days 1–5 (pre-implantation), 6–10, or 11–16 (during organogenesis). OXALIPLATIN caused developmental mortality (increased early resorption) when administered on days 6–10 and 11–16 and adversely affected fetal growth (decreased fetal weight, delayed ossification) when administered on days 6–10. Nursing mothers—it is not known whether ELOXATIN®88 or its derivatives are excreted in human milk.

Target Organs/Systems: Skin, mucous membranes, respiratory tract, digestive tract, eyes, and possibly fetus (**Note**: Acute or chronic toxicity is not fully unknown.)

Medical Conditions Generally Aggravated by Exposure:

- Preexisting respiratory condition.
- Reproductive and pregnancy issues.

Specific Medical Surveillance Information: Reproductive and pregnancy counseling.

Occupational Exposure Level/Limit (OEL) & Sampling Methods: Not otherwise specified

Environmental Sentinel Contamination Action Level (ESCAL): Not otherwise specified

Supplemental Response Information

Extinguishing Media: Use extinguishing agent which is the most appropriate to extinguish surrounding fire (carbon dioxide, foam, dry chemical or water fog as extinguishing media).

Solubility: DIAMINOCYCLOHEXANE OXALATOPLATINUM is water soluble (7.9 mg/ml) (Merck).

Chemical Degradation/Neutralization Method: Not otherwise specified

Note: If a specific degradation or neutralization method is not provided on this table and you do not have other specific information that will advise you on how to clean up the specific material spilled, then follow the general spill procedure found at the introduction section of this table.

Incompatibility: DIAMINOCYCLOHEXANE OXALATOPLATINUM is incompatible with oxidizing agents, acids, and carbon dioxide.

DIANHYDROGALACTITOL
DAD
DAG
DULCITOLDIEPOXIDE

Chemical Abstract Service (CAS) Registry
Number: 23261-20-3
RTECS: LW5320000
NSC-132313
$C_6-H_{10}-O_4$

Health & Safety Hazards/US Department of Transportation (DOT)/US Environmental Protection Agency (EPA)—Sources

Toxic—Sax's "Dangerous Properties of Industrial Materials," Mutagen—University of Maryland at College Park, Mutagen Tendencies—ToxReport.

First Aid/Medical Information/ Occupational Exposure Limits

First Aid Measures to include: Use general first aid measures.

Medical Information:

Caution and Warning Statements: One of the cytotoxic dihalohexitols that may have alkylating antineoplastic activity. It causes bone marrow toxicity.

Target Organs/Systems: Bone marrow

Medical Conditions Generally Aggravated by Exposure:

- Preexisting conditions that affect bone marrow.

Specific Medical Surveillance Information: Not otherwise specified

Occupational Exposure Level/Limit (OEL) & Sampling Methods: Not otherwise specified

Environmental Sentinel Contamination Action Level (ESCAL): Not otherwise specified

Supplemental Response Information

Extinguishing Media: Use extinguishing agent which is the most appropriate to extinguish surrounding fire (carbon dioxide, foam, dry chemical or water fog as extinguishing media).

Solubility: DIANHYDROGALACTITOL: Not otherwise specified

Chemical Degradation/Neutralization Method: Not otherwise specified

Note: If a specific degradation or neutralization method is not provided on this table and you do not have other specific information that will guide you on how to clean up the specific material spilled, then follow the general spill procedure found at the introduction section of this table.

Incompatibility: Not otherwise specified

DIAZIQUONEB
AZQ

Chemical Abstract Service (CAS) Registry
Number: 57998-68-2
RTECS: EY8794000
NSC 182986
$C_{16}-H_{20}-N_4-O_6$

Health & Safety Hazards/US Department of Transportation (DOT)/US Environmental Protection Agency (EPA)—Sources

Carcinogen—Material Safety Data Sheet, Mutagen—Material Safety Data Sheet, Sensitizer—Material Safety Data Sheet, Pregnancy Category (None)—Food and Drug Administration.

First Aid/Medical Information/ Occupational Exposure Limits

First Aid Measures to include: Use general first aid measures.

Medical Information:

Caution and Warning Statements:

Harmful: There is limited evidence of a carcinogenic effect. This drug may be a possible mutagen and possible sensitizer. Sensitization may occur if prolonged or repeated exposure; may cause allergic reactions in certain sensitive individuals. There is a possible risk of irreversible effects.

Target Organs/Systems: Bone marrow, sensitization: prolonged or repeated exposure may cause allergic reactions in certain sensitive individuals

Medical Conditions Generally Aggravated by Exposure:

- Sensitization: Prolonged or repeated exposure may cause allergic reactions in certain sensitive individuals.

Specific Medical Surveillance Information: Not otherwise specified

Occupational Exposure Level/Limit (OEL) & Sampling Methods: Not otherwise specified

Environmental Sentinel Contamination Action Level (ESCAL): Not otherwise specified

Supplemental Response Information

Extinguishing Media: Use extinguishing agent which is the most appropriate to extinguish surrounding fire (carbon dioxide, foam, dry chemical or water fog as extinguishing media).

Solubility: DIAZIQUONE is water soluble (0.72 mg/ml) or 0.5 mg/ml (Merck).

Chemical Degradation/Neutralization Method: Not otherwise specified

Note: If a specific degradation or neutralization method is not provided on this table and you do not have other specific information that will guide you on how to clean up the specific material spilled, then follow the general spill procedure found at the introduction section of this table.

Incompatibility: DIAZIQUONE is incompatible with strong oxidizing agents.

DICHLOROMETHOTREXATE
NCI-CO 4875
DCM

Chemical Abstract Service (CAS) Registry Number: 528-74-5
NSC 29630
$C_{20}-H_{20}-CL_2-N_8-O_5$

DICHLOROMETHOTREXATE

Chemical Abstract Service (CAS) Registry Number: 88442-77-7

OTHER—DICHLOROMETHOTREXATE

Chemical Abstract Service (CAS) Registry Number: 88442-77-7 (NTP listing)
RTECS: MA1250000

Health & Safety Hazards/US Department of Transportation (DOT)/US Environmental Protection Agency (EPA)—Sources

Moderate Toxic—US National Institute of Health (NIH) and Material Safety Data Sheet, Mutagen—Chemdplus (US National Library of Medicine), Reproductive—Chemdplus (US National Library of Medicine), Carcinogen—US National Institute of Health (NIH) and Material Safety Data Sheet, Ototoxic—Butterworth-Heinman.

DICHLOROMETHOTREXATE is a yellow-orange crystalline compound in pure form.

(Fluorescent: exc = 420 nm; em = 480 nm (similar to those of Methotrexate)

First Aid/Medical Information/ Occupational Exposure Limits

First Aid Measures to include: Use general first aid measures except for the following:

Ingestion: If victim is conscious and alert, drink plenty of water or milk. Induce vomiting. Seek medical attention. Refer for gastric lavage.

Dermal contact: Avoid washing with solvents. Avoid rubbing of skin or increasing its temperature. For skin exposure, remove contaminated clothing and wash skin with soap and water.

Eye contact: For eyes exposure, irrigate immediately with sodium bicarbonate solution, followed by copious quantities of running water for at least 15 minutes. Obtain ophthalmological evaluation.

Medical Information:

Caution and Warning Statements: There is little information concerning chemical, physical and biological properties of DICHLOROMETHOTREXATE.

DICHLOROMETHOTREXATE is readily absorbed through the skin, respiratory, and intestinal tracts. (Folic acid antagonists—pharm action.)

DICHLOROMETHOTREXATE is about one-tenth as toxic as methotrexate; there are no data concerning mutagenicity, teratogenicity, and embryotoxicity, and its carcinogenicity is slight. (NIH MSDS)

Target Organs/Systems: Permanent cochleovestibular toxicity

Medical Conditions Generally Aggravated by Exposure: Not otherwise specified

Specific Medical Surveillance Information: Not otherwise specified

Occupational Exposure Level/Limit (OEL) & Sampling Methods:

Environmental Sentinel Contamination Action Level (ESCAL): Not otherwise specified

Supplemental Response Information

Extinguishing Media: Use extinguishing agent which is the most appropriate to extinguish surrounding fire (carbon dioxide, foam, dry chemical or water fog as extinguishing media).

Solubility: DICHLOROMETHOTREXATE is reported as being water soluble to practically water insoluble (as <0.1 g/100 ml at 22 deg. C) with a higher solubility in dilute alkali, hydroxide, or carbonate. Stated to be ten times more lipid soluble than METHOTREXATE.

Chemical Degradation/Neutralization Method: The international agency for research on cancer (IARC) recommended a removal method for DICHLOROMETHOTRETATE:

Caution: Not a complete deactivation method.

The IARC recommends treating spill surfaces with a 3 mol/liter sulfuric acid and take up the rinse with inert absorbent pads or removing any powder present: allow solution to stand for several minutes and then thoroughly wash spilled surfaces with soap and water; sample to determine if surface contamination is still present (if sampling method is available). If drug is still present, repeat above steps; dispose of wastes in accordance with your local procedures, state, and federal regulations.

Incompatibility: Conditions contributing to instability are acid, alkali, elevated temperatures, and prolonged exposure to ultraviolet light.

DIETHYLSTILBESTROL TOZOCIN
ZANOSAR®44
STN
STRZ
STREPTOZOCIN

$C_8H_{15}N_3O_7$
Chemical Abstract Service (CAS) Registry
    Number: 18883-66-4

STREPTOZOCIN

Chemical Abstract Service (CAS) Registry
    Numbers: 66395-18-4, 66395-17-3

DES
STILPHOSTROL
RTECS: LZ5775000

Health & Safety Hazards/US Department of Transportation (DOT)/US Environmental Protection Agency (EPA)—Sources

Carcinogen G2B—International Agency for Research on Cancer, Carcinogen C2—US National Toxicology Program, Carcinogen—US National Institute of Health (NIH) and Material Safety Data Sheet, Teratogen—US National Institute of Health (NIH) and Material Safety Data Sheet, Mutagen—US National Institute of Health (NIH) and Material Safety Data Sheet, Mutagen—Material Safety Data Sheet, Tumorigenic and Toxic—Materials Safety Data Sheet, Reproductive Toxic—Material Safety Data Sheet, Vesicant—British Columbia Cancer Agency Canada, Cytotoxic—British Columbia Cancer Agency Canada, Pregnancy Category (D)—US Food and Drug Administration, Carcinogen and Developmental Male and Female, US California Proposition 65, National Fire Protection Association Health (2) Flammability (1) Instability/Reactivity (0)—Material Safety Data Sheet, Hazardous Materials Identification System (R) and/or US Department of Defense System Health (2) Fire Hazard (1) Reactivity (0) Personal Protection Code (E) (Safety Glasses, Chemical Gloves, Dust Respirator)—Material Safety Data Sheet, Hazardous Materials Identification System (R) and/or US Department of Defense System Health (0★) with additional chronic hazards present Fire Hazard (0) Reactivity (0)—Material Safety Data Sheet, National

Fire Protection Association Health (3) Flammability (0) Instability/Reactivity (0), U206.

STREPTOZOCIN is a colorless odorless fluid from powder.

STREPTOZOCIN: breastfeeding should be discontinued because of potential for reproductive and developmental harm (*A Guide for Occupational Health Professionals Technical Manual*, Navy Environmental Health Center [NEHC-TM-OEM 6260.01a]).

First Aid/Medical Information/ Occupational Exposure Limits

First aid measure to include: Use general first aid measures except for the following:

Dermal contact: Follow general first aid measures first, may cover the irritated skin with an emollient (antibacterial cream). Seek medical attention.

Medical Information:

Caution and Warning Statements: Exposure to DIETHYLSTILBESTROL TOZOCIN (STREPTOZOCIN) may cause cancer and is a possible teratogen/reproductive effector (males/females). Exposure may cause skin, eyes, and mucous membranes and upper respiratory tract irritation. Exposure may be harmful if absorbed through the skin. May be harmful if ingested; may cause systemic effects include renal dysfunction (kidneys) and impaired liver function. DIETHYLSTILBESTROL TOZOCIN is readily absorbed by various body tissues through the intestinal tract and transplacentally, skin and eye irritant. This drug exerts a specific toxic effect on the b cells of the pancreas. Exposure may affect glucose metabolism. This drug may cause male and female reproductive toxicity. May cause harm to the unborn child.

Exposure to DIETHYLSTILBESTROL TOZOCIN (STREPTOZOCIN) may cause drowsiness, nausea, and irritation to the eyes, skin, and upper respiratory tract. High and repeated exposures may cause anemia, leukopenia, thrombocytopenia, and diabetes. BC Cancer Agency lists STREPTOZOCIN has a vesicant.

Caution: Females and males planning to have a child, pregnant women, and nursing mothers should exercise caution regarding potential occupational exposure to this cytotoxic drug. No information or not enough information exists or was provided concerning occupational exposure that may potentially occur while handling this drug and its affects on reproductive systems, the fetus, and/or if it is secreted along with breast milk, which may harm nursing infants. Staff members should consult with the occupational health physician monitoring workers' health in your facility to be apprised of potential hazards and should be advised to avoid becoming pregnant and/or breastfeeding or should be transferred in accordance with policy/procedures to other duties that do not involve preparation, handling, and administering this drug.

Target Organs/Systems: Kidney, liver, reproductive and cardiovascular systems, pancreas, blood, bone marrow, skin, and eyes

Medical Conditions Generally Aggravated by Exposure:

- Medical surveillance may consist of a complete blood count, liver and kidney function tests. Animal studies have shown that exposure may induce diabetes. Refer to caution and warning statement section above. Repeated or prolonged exposure to the substance can produce target organ(s) damage and aggravate pregnancy.

Specific Medical Surveillance Information: Reproductive and pregnancy counseling.

Medical surveillance may consist of a complete blood count, liver and kidney function tests. Refer to the caution and warning statement section above for more medical surveillance information.

Occupational Exposure Level/Limit (OEL) & Sampling Methods: Not otherwise specified

Environmental Sentinel Contamination Action Level (ESCAL): Not otherwise specified

Supplemental Response Information

Extinguishing Media: Use extinguishing agent which is the most appropriate to extinguish surrounding fire (carbon dioxide, foam, dry chemical or water fog as extinguishing media).

Solubility: DIETHYLSTILBESTROL TOZOCIN is water soluble (cold and hot water) and soluble in lower alcohols and ketones. However, is insoluble in non-polar organic solvents.

Chemical Degradation/Neutralization Method: A DIETHYSTIBESTROL TOZOCIN (STREPTOZOCIN) Material Safety Data Sheet (MSDS) recommends that deactivation of small qualities of DIETHYLSTILBESTROL TOZOCIN (STREPTOZOCIN) use sulfamic acid at a ratio of 0.5 gm sulfamic acid/3 ml water.

Incompatibility: DIETHYLSTILBESTROL TOZOCIN (STREPTOZOCIN) is incompatible with strong acids, bases, and oxidizers. Avoid heat.

E

EPIRUBICIN (1) (*eh-pih-ROO-bih-cin*)
ELLENCE®46
EPIRUBICN HCL
PHARMORUBICIN®45

Chemical Abstract Service (CAS) Registry
Number: 56420-45-2
NSC-256942 (IMI-28)

EPIRUBICIN

Chemical Abstract Service (CAS) Registry
Number: 56390-90-1

EPIRUBICIN HCL

RTECS: QI9295750
$C_{27}-H_{29}-NO_{11}$.HCL
(Two Degradation Methods)

Health & Safety Hazards/US Department of Transportation (DOT)/US Environmental Protection Agency (EPA)—Sources

Mutagen—Material Safety Data Sheet, Mutagen—British Columbia Cancer Agency Canada, Reproductive Effector British Columbia Cancer Agency Canada, Carcinogen—British Columbia Cancer Agency Canada, CARDIOTOXIC, Pregnancy Category (D)—US Food and Drug Administration, National Fire Protection Administration Health (1) Flammability (1) Instability/Reactivity (0), Hazardous Materials Identification System (R) and/or US Department of Defense System Health (1) Fire Hazard (1) Reactivity (0) Personal Protection Code (E) (Safety Glasses, Chemical Gloves, Dust Respirator).

EPIRUBICIN is available as an injection.

EPIRUBICIN is a red fluid.

EPIRUBICIN HYDROCHLORIDE is a yellow to orange to red solid or powder.

First Aid/Medical Information/ Occupational Exposure Limits

First Aid Measures to include: Use general first aid measures.

Medical Information:

Caution and Warning Statements: EPIRUBICIN (ELLENCE®46) is classified as a possible human mutagen. It is hazardous in case of inhalation, ingestion, and skin contact (permeator). May cause heritable genetic effects based on animal data. There is a possible risk of irreversible effects with exposure to EPIRUBICIN (ELLENCE®46).

Caution: The toxicological properties of most cytotoxic drugs have not been fully investigated, particularly as it pertains to occupational exposure. EPIRUBICIN (ELLENCE®46) is one of the drugs that has little occupational hazards information available. Therefore, therapeutic dose information was extrapolated below to assist in determining occupational toxicity, and signs and symptoms of overexposure. Therefore, it is prudent to minimize occupational exposure to EPIRUBICIN (ELLENCE®46).

Exposure to EPIRUBICIN (ELLENCE®46) may cause nausea, vomiting, diarrhea, mouth sores, dehydration, fever, infection, symptoms of congestive heart failure (swelling of ankles, shortness of breath, etc.), hair loss, low red blood counts (anemia), temporary or permanent loss of menstrual cycle in women, feeling tired, hot flashes, and rash/itch. Besides gastrointestinal symptoms, it is may present neutropenic complications. Ellence®46 has a hematological toxicity and is a cardiotoxic drug.

Caution: Females and males planning to have a child, pregnant women, and nursing mothers should exercise caution regarding potential occupational exposure to this cytotoxic drug. No information or not enough information exists or was provided concerning occupational exposure that may potentially occur while handling this drug and its affects on reproductive systems, the fetus, and/or if it is secreted along with breast milk, which may harm nursing infants. Staff members should consult with the occupational health physician monitoring workers' health in your facility to be apprised of potential hazards and should be advised to avoid becoming pregnant and/or breastfeeding or should be transferred in accordance with policy/procedures to other duties that do not involve preparation, handling, and administering this drug.

Target Organs/Systems: Heart, blood, bone marrow, liver, possibly reproductive system, and fetus

Medical Conditions Generally Aggravated by Exposure:

- EPIRUBICIN—Hypersensitivity to EPIRUBICIN, to anthracyclines (DAUNORUBICIN, DOXORUBICIN), and to anthracenediones (MITOXANTRONE, MITOMYCIN); severe hepatic impairment, severe myocardial infarction, severe arrhythmias, history of severe cardiac disease.

- Repeated exposure to highly toxic materials may produce general deterioration of health by an accumulation in one or more human organs.
- Reproductive and pregnancy issues.

Specific Medical Surveillance Information: Reproductive and pregnancy counseling.

Occupational Exposure Level/Limit (OEL) & Sampling Methods: Not otherwise specified

Environmental Sentinel Contamination Action Level (ESCAL): Not otherwise specified

Supplemental Response Information

Extinguishing Media: Use extinguishing agent which is the most appropriate to extinguish surrounding fire (carbon dioxide, foam, dry chemical or water fog as extinguishing media).

Solubility: EPIRUBICIN (ELLENCE®46) is easily soluble in cold water and is soluble in methyl alcohol and slightly soluble in dehydrated alcohol.

Chemical Degradation/Neutralization Method: There are two or more recommended methods for ERIRU-BICIN. See below or above for optional method.

The International Agency for Research on Cancer (IARC) recommended degradation method for EPI-RUDICIN:

The IARC recommends treating spill surfaces with a 5.25% sodium hypochlorite (bleach) solution after absorbing liquids with inert absorbent pads or removing any powder present: allow solution to stand for up to one hour, and then thoroughly wash spilled surfaces with soap and water; sample to determine if surface contamination is still present (if sampling method is available). If drug is still present, repeat above steps; dispose of wastes in accordance with your local procedures, state, and federal regulations.

Incompatibility: Not otherwise specified

EPIRUBICIN (2) (*eh-pih-ROO-bih-cin*)

ELLENCE®46
EPIRUBICIN HCL
PHARMORUBICIN® 45

Chemical Abstract Service (CAS) Registry
Number: 56420-45-2
NSC-256942 (IMI-28)

EPIRUBICIN

Chemical Abstract Service (CAS) Registry
Number: 56390-09-1

EPIRUBICIN HCL

RTECS: QI9295840
C_{27}-H_{29}-N-O_{11}.CL-H
(Two Degradation Methods)

Health & Safety Hazards/US Department of Transportation (DOT)/US Environmental Protection Agency (EPA)—Sources

Mutagen—Material Safety Data Sheet, Mutagen—British Columbia Cancer Agency Canada, Reproductive Effector—British Columbia Cancer Agency Canada, Carcinogen—British Columbia Cancer Agency Canada, Cardiotoxic—British Columbia Cancer Agency Canada, Cytotoxic—British Columbia Cancer Agency Canada, Vesicant—British Columbia Cancer Agency Canada, Pregnancy Category (D)—US Food and Drug Administration, National Fire Protection Administration Health (1) Flammability (1) Instability/Reactivity (0)—Material Safety Data Sheet.

EPIRUBICIN is available as an injection.

EPIRUBICIN is a red fluid.

EPIRUBICIN HYDROCHLORIDE is an orange-red powder.

First Aid/Medical Information/Occupational Exposure Limits

First Aid Measures to include: Use general first aid measures.

Medical Information:

Caution and Warning Statements: EPIRUBICIN (ELLENCE®46) is classified as a possible human mutagen. It is hazardous in case of inhalation, ingestion, and skin contact (permeator). May cause heritable genetic effects based on animal data. This is a possible risk of irreversible effects with exposure to EPIRUBICIN (ELLENCE®46).

Caution: The toxicological properties of most cytotoxic drugs have not been fully investigated, particularly as it pertains to occupational exposure. EPIRUBICIN (ELLENCE®46) is one of the drugs that has little occupational hazards information available. Therefore, therapeutic dose information was extrapolated below to assist in determining occupational toxicity, and signs and symptoms of overexposure. Therefore, it is prudent to minimize occupational exposure to EPIRUBICIN (ELLENCE®46).

Exposure to EPIRUBICIN (ELLENCE®46) may cause nausea, vomiting, diarrhea, mouth sores, dehydration, fever, infection, symptoms of congestive heart failure (swelling of ankles, shortness of breath, etc.), hair loss, low red blood counts (anemia), temporary or permanent loss of menstrual cycle in women, feeling tired, hot flashes, and rash/itch. Besides gastrointestinal symptoms, it is may present neutropenic complications. (ELLENCE®46) has a hematological toxicity and is a cardiotoxic drug. BC Cancer Agency lists EPIRUBICIN as a vesicant.

Caution: Females and males planning to have a child, pregnant women, and nursing mothers should exercise caution regarding potential occupational exposure to this cytotoxic drug. No information or not enough information exists or was provided concerning occupational exposure that may potentially occur while handling this drug and its affects on reproductive systems, the fetus, and/or if it is secreted along with breast milk, which may harm nursing infants. Staff members should consult with the occupational health physician monitoring workers' health in your facility to be apprised of potential hazards and should be advised to avoid becoming pregnant and/or breastfeeding or should be transferred in accordance with policy/procedures to other duties that do not involve preparation, handling, and administering this drug.

Target Organs/Systems: Heart, blood, bone marrow, liver, and possibly reproductive systems and fetus

Medical Conditions Generally Aggravated by Exposure:

- EPIRUBICIN—Hypersensitivity to EPIRUBICIN, to anthracyclines (DAUNORUBICIN, DOXORUBICIN), and to anthracenediones (MITOXANTRONE, MITOMYCIN); severe hepatic impairment, severe myocardial infarction, severe arrhythmias, history of severe cardiac disease.
- Repeated exposure to highly toxic materials may produce general deterioration of health by an accumulation in one or more human organs.
- Reproductive and pregnancy issues.

Specific Medical Surveillance Information: Reproductive and pregnancy counseling.

Occupational Exposure Level/Limit (OEL) & Sampling Methods: Not otherwise specified

Environmental Sentinel Contamination Action Level (ESCAL): Not otherwise specified

Supplemental Response Information

Extinguishing Media: Use extinguishing agent which is the most appropriate to extinguish surrounding fire (carbon dioxide, foam, dry chemical or water fog as extinguishing media).

Solubility: EPIRUBICIN (ELLENCE®46) is easily soluble in cold water and is soluble in methyl alcohol and slightly soluble in dehydrated alcohol.

Chemical Degradation/Neutralization Method: There are two or more recommended procedures for EPIRUBICIN. See below for optional method.

A manufacturer's Material Safety Data Sheet (MSDS) recommends treating spill surfaces with a ~2 mol/liter (~8 g/100 ml), aqueous caustic soda (sodium hydroxide) solution after absorbing liquids with inert absorbent pads or removing any powder present: allow solution to stand for up to one hour, and then thoroughly wash spilled surfaces with soap and water; sample to determine if surface contamination is still present (if sampling method is available). If drug is still present, repeat above steps; dispose of wastes in accordance with your local procedures, state, and federal regulations.

Incompatibility: ELLENCE®46 is incompatible with HEPARIN AND FLUORACIL resulting in a chemical reaction and possible precipitation of materials.

ERBITUX®47
CETUXIMAB (*se-TUK-see-mab*)

> Chemical Abstract Service (CAS) Registry Number: 205923-56-4
> $C_{6484}H_{10042}N_{1732}O_{2023}S_{36}$

Health & Safety Hazards/US Department of Transportation (DOT)/US Environmental Protection Agency (EPA)—Sources

Cytotoxic—British Columbia Cancer Agency Canada, Nonvesicant—British Columbia Cancer Agency Canada, Pregnancy Category (C)—US Food and Drug Administration.

ERBITUX®47 (CETUXIMAB) is available as an injection (50 ml vial).

First Aid/Medical Information/ Occupational Exposure Limits

First Aid Measures to include: Use general first aid measures except for the following:

Ingestion: Induction of vomiting should be considered for significant ingestions if person is conscious and not experiencing convulsions. Seek medical attention.

Inhalation: **Warning**—it may be hazardous to the person providing aid to give mouth-to-mouth resuscitation when the inhaled material is toxic.

Medical Information:

Caution and Warning Statements:

Caution: CETUXIMAB is not fully tested; handle material with appropriate care to minimize exposure. Avoid inhalation, ingestion, and skin and eye contact. Exposure may cause acne-like rash and hypersensitivity or acute allergic reactions (throat closing, swelling of lips, hives, and low blood pressure) and difficulty breathing. A Material Safety Data Sheet (MSDS) stated that the material was a non-infectious biologic fluid in solution.

Caution: Females and males planning to have a child, pregnant women, and nursing mothers should exercise caution regarding potential occupational exposure to this cytotoxic drug. No information or not enough information exists or was provided concerning occupational exposure that may potentially occur while handling this drug and its affects on reproductive systems, the fetus, and/or if it is secreted along with breast milk, which may harm nursing infants. Staff members should consult with the occupational health physician monitoring workers' health in your facility to be apprised of potential hazards and should be advised to avoid becoming pregnant and/or breastfeeding or should be transferred in accordance with policy/procedures to other duties that do not involve preparation, handling, and administering this drug.

Therapeutic Levels: CETUXIMAB binds to the placenta and the potential for harm is unknown, therefore, pregnant women should avoid exposure. Nursing mothers should avoid exposure to CETUXIMAB because of the possibility of passing to child.

Target Organs/Systems: Skin, lungs, fetus, and eyes

Medical Conditions Generally Aggravated by Exposure:

- If preexisting allergy to ERBITUX®47 or mouse protein and other allergens (prescription or over-the-counter drug).
- Reproductive and pregnancy issues.
- Avoid prolonged exposure to sunlight or artificial UV lights during treatment or after being exposure/overexposed to CETUXIMAB.

Specific Medical Surveillance Information: Reproductive and pregnancy counseling.

Occupational Exposure Level/Limit (OEL) & Sampling Methods:

Environmental Sentinel Contamination Action Level (ESCAL): Not otherwise specified

Occupational Exposure Level (OEL): Bristol-Myers Squibb Company

0.01 mg/m3

(Method not listed or specified)

Supplemental Response Information

Extinguishing Media: Use extinguishing agent which is the most appropriate to extinguish surrounding fire (carbon dioxide, foam, dry chemical or water fog as extinguishing media).

Solubility: ERBITUX®47 (CETUXIMAB): Not otherwise specified

ERBITUX®47 has a pH range of 7.0–7.4.

Chemical Degradation/Neutralization Method: A manufacturer's Material Safety Data Sheet (MSDS) recommends using alkaline soap/detergent and water to clean spill surfaces after absorbing liquids with inert absorbent pads or removing any powder present: repeat using soap and water; sample to determine if surface contamination is still present (if sampling method is available). If drug is still present, repeat above steps; dispose of wastes in accordance with your local procedures, state, and federal regulations.

Incompatibility: Not otherwise specified

ESORUBICIN
$C_{27}H_{29}N\text{-}O_{10}$

4'-DEOXYADRIAMYCIN

Chemical Abstract Service (CAS) Registry Number: 63521–85–7
NSC267469

ESORUBICIN

Chemical Abstract Service (CAS) Registry Number: 63950–06–1

DEXYDOXORUBICIN HYDROCLORIDE

RTECS: QI9443000
$C_{27}H_{29}NO_{10}\cdot ClH$

Health & Safety Hazards/US Department of Transportation (DOT)/US Environmental Protection Agency (EPA)—Sources

Pregnancy Category (None)—Food and Drug Administration, Cardiotoxic—Material Safety Data Sheet.

First Aid/Medical Information/ Occupational Exposure Limits

First Aid Measures to include: Use general first aid measures.

Medical Information:

Caution and Warning Statements: ESORUBICIN this drug is a non-infectious biologic fluid in solution. ESORUBICIN may be cardiotoxicity.

Caution: Females and males planning to have a child, pregnant women, and nursing mothers should exercise caution regarding potential occupational exposure to this cytotoxic drug. No information or not enough information exists or was provided concerning occupational exposure that may potentially occur while handling this drug and its affects on reproductive systems, the fetus, and/or if it is secreted along with breast milk, which may harm nursing infants. Staff members should consult with the occupational health physician monitoring workers' health in your facility to be apprised of potential hazards and should be advised to avoid becoming pregnant and/or breastfeeding or should be transferred in accordance with policy/procedures to other duties that do not involve preparation, handling, and administering this drug.

Target Organs/Systems: Skin

Medical Conditions Generally Aggravated by Exposure:

- Preexisting cardiopulmonary disease.
- Reproductive and pregnancy issues.

Specific Medical Surveillance Information: Reproductive and pregnancy counseling.

Occupational Exposure Level/Limit (OEL) & Sampling Methods: Not otherwise specified

Environmental Sentinel Contamination Action Level (ESCAL): Not otherwise specified

Supplemental Response Information

Extinguishing Media: Use extinguishing agent which is the most appropriate to extinguish surrounding fire (carbon dioxide, foam, dry chemical or water fog as extinguishing media).

Solubility: ESORUBICIN: Not otherwise specified ESORUBICIN has a pH range of 7.0—7.4.

Chemical Degradation/Neutralization Method: Not otherwise specified

Note: If a specific degradation or neutralization method is not provided on this table and you do not have other specific information that will guide you on how to clean up the specific material spilled, then follow the general spill procedure found at the introduction section of this table.

Incompatibility: Not otherwise specified

ESTRAMUSTINE PHOSPHATE
(es-tra-MUS-teen)
ESTRAMUSTINE SODIUM PHOSPHATE
ESTRAMUSTINE
GUEMCYT
EMCYT®48 (LEO 275)

Chemical Abstract Service (CAS) Registry Number: 2998-57-4
RO 21-8837
NSC89201

ESTRAMUSTINE

Chemical Abstract Service (CAS) Registry Number: 52205-73-9
$C_{23}H_{31}Cl_2NO_3$

ESTRAMUSTINE SODIUM PHOSPHATE

Chemical Abstract Service (CAS) Registry Number: 4891-15-0

ESTRAMUSTINE PHOSPHATE

RTECS: KG7355000, RTECS: KG4250000

ESTRADIOL

(Mixture)

Health & Safety Hazards/US Department of Transportation (DOT)/US Environmental Protection Agency (EPA)—Sources

Carcinogen—British Columbia Cancer Agency Canada, Mutagen—British Columbia Cancer Agency Canada, Reproductive Effector—Material Safety Data Sheet, Cardiotoxic and Material Safety Data Sheet, Pregnancy Category (None)—US Food and Drug Administration, Carcinogen—US California Proposition 65.

EMCYT® 48 (ESTRAMUSTINE) is available as a capsule.

ESTAMUSTINE SODIUM PHOSPHATE is a white or almost white powder.

First Aid/Medical Information/ Occupational Exposure Limits

First Aid Measures to include: Use general first aid measures.

Medical Information:

Caution and Warning Statements:

Caution: The toxicological properties of most cytotoxic drugs have not been fully investigated, particularly as it pertains to occupational exposure. ESTRAMUSTINE PHOSPHATE (EMCYT®48) is one of the drugs that has little occupational hazard information available. Therefore, therapeutic dose information was extrapolated below to assist in determining occupational toxicity, and signs and symptoms of overexposure. Furthermore, it is prudent to minimize occupational exposure to ESTRAMUSTINE PHOSPHATE (EMCYT®48).

ESTRAMUSTINE is potentially mutagenic and carcinogenic.

ESTRAMUSTINE PHOSPHATE (EMCYT®48) may cause nausea, vomiting, diarrhea, impotence or decreased sex drive, elevated liver function tests, low WBC (myelosuppression), skin rash, breast swelling or tenderness (gynecomastia).

Caution: Females and males planning to have a child, pregnant women, and nursing mothers should exercise caution regarding potential occupational exposure to this cytotoxic drug. No information or not enough information exists or was provided concerning occupational exposure that may potentially occur while handling this drug and its affects on reproductive systems, the fetus, and/or if it is secreted along with breast milk, which may harm nursing infants. Staff members should consult with the occupational health physician monitoring workers' health in your facility to be apprised of potential hazards and should be advised to avoid becoming pregnant and/ or breastfeeding or should be transferred in accordance with policy/procedures to other duties that do not involve preparation, handling, and administering this drug.

Therapeutic Levels: Patient should be advised to use birth control if their partner is of childbearing age. Breastfeeding is not recommended due to the potential secretion into breast milk and because it interferes with milk volume and content.

Target Organs/Systems: Kidneys, liver, blood, immune, reproductive, and cardiovascular systems

Medical Conditions Generally Aggravated by Exposure:

The following information was taken from therapeutic dose information.

- ESTRAMUSTINE PHOSPHATE (EMCYT®48) is contraindicated in patients with severe hepatic or cardiac disease, or active thrombophlebitis or thromboembolic disorders and known hypersensitivity to either Estradiol or MECHLORETHAMINE.
- Reproductive and pregnancy issues.

Specific Medical Surveillance Information: Reproductive and pregnancy counseling.

Therapeutic lab monitoring are CBC, liver function tests, and kidney function tests.

Occupational Exposure Level/Limit (OEL) & Sampling Methods: Not otherwise specified

Environmental Sentinel Contamination Action Level (ESCAL): Not otherwise specified

Supplemental Response Information

Extinguishing Media: Use extinguishing agent which is the most appropriate to extinguish surrounding fire (carbon dioxide, foam, dry chemical or water fog as extinguishing media).

Solubility: ESTRAMUSTINE PHOSPHATE SODIUM (EMCYT®48) is readily water soluble and methyl alcohol slightly soluble in dehydrated alcohol and in chloroform (pH of 8.5 to 10.0 in a 0.5% solution of water).

Chemical Degradation/Neutralization Method: Not otherwise specified

Note: If a specific degradation or neutralization method is not provided on this table and you do not have other specific information that will advise you on how to clean up the specific material spilled, then follow the general spill procedure found at the introduction section of this table.

Incompatibility: Not otherwise specified

ETOPOSIDE (1) (*e-TOE-poe-side*)
VEPESID®49 INJECTION (VP-16)
VESPESID®49

Chemical Abstract Service (CAS) Registry
Numbers: 33419-42-0, 33419-42-9 (NTP MSDS) (mixture)
RTECS: KC0190000
NSC 141540
$C_{29}-H_{32}-O_{13}$
(Four Degradation Methods)

Health & Safety Hazards/US Department of Transportation (DOT)/US Environmental Protection Agency (EPA)—Sources

Carcinogen G2A—International Agency for Research on Cancer, Carcinogen—US National Toxicology Program, Mutagen—Material Safety Data Sheet, Mutagen—University of Maryland at College Park, Teratogen—Material Safety Data Sheet, Teratogen—University of Maryland at College Park, Toxic—Material Safety Data Sheet, Cytotoxic—Material Safety Data Sheet, Cytotoxic—British Columbia Cancer Agency Canada, US California Environmental Protection Agency Listed, Irritant—British Columbia Cancer Agency Canada, Lactation Avoid Breastfeeding (World Health Organization) Pregnancy (D)—US Food and Drug Administration, Developmental—US California Proposition 65, Flammable—Material Safety Data Sheet, National Fire Protection Association Health (0) Flammability (1) Instability/Reactivity (0)—Material Safety Data Sheet, National Fire Protection Association Health (1) Flammability (1) Instability/Reactivity (0)—Material Safety Data Sheet, National Fire Protection Association Health (1) Flammability (0) Instability/Reactivity (0)—Material Safety Data Sheet, Hazardous Materials Identification System (R) and/or US Department of Defense System Health (0★) with additional chronic hazard present Fire Hazard (1) Reactivity (0) Personal Protection Code (A) (Safety Glasses)—Material Safety Data Sheet, Hazardous Materials Identification System (R) and/or US Department of Defense System Health (1★) with additional chronic hazard present Fire hazard (0) Reactivity (0) Personal Protective Code (-) (None stated)—Material Safety Data Sheet, D001 DOT FLAMMABLE LIQUIDS, N.O.S, UN 1993, CLASS 3, GROUP II.

ETOPOSIDE is a white or almost white crystalline powder.

ETOPOSIDE is a colorless fluid or pale pink capsule 50 mg and 100 mg.

ETOPOSIDE Breastfeeding is contraindicated and should be avoided because of possible reproductive and developmental harm (*A Guide for Occupational Health Professionals Technical Manual*, Navy Environmental Health Center [NEHC-TM-OEM 6260.01a]).

First Aid/Medical Information/ Occupational Exposure Limits

First Aid Measures to include: Use general first aid measures except for the following:

Physician's note (A): Overdose treatment: there is no proven antidote for ETOPOSIDE overdose. Treatment is supportive and includes the following:

1. Hypotension is managed by the administration of fluids.
2. Anaphylaxis is treated by administering pressor agents, adrenocorticoids, antihistamines, or volume expanders.

Physician's note (B): Due to its action, ETOPOSIDE should be treated as potentially carcinogenic and may be mutagenic, teratogenic, or allergenic. If respiratory distress occurs after inhalation of airborne droplets, administer emergency airway support and 100% humidified supplemental oxygen with assisted ventilation if needed. If coughing or difficulty in breathing develops, evacuating for respiratory tract irritation, bronchitis, or pneumonitis. Because of the potentially hazardous nature of ETOPOSIDE, if the solution is swallowed, gets in eyes or in contact with the skin, medical attention should be sought immediately after the preceding first aid measures are taken.

Medical Information:

Caution and Warning Statements: ETOPOSIDE is toxic by inhalation, in contact with skin, and if swallowed. This material may cause cancer and causes heritable genetic damage. ETOPOSIDE may cause harm to the unborn child. RTECS lists ETOPOSIDE as a suspected cardiovascular or blood toxicant; as an endocrine toxicant; and as a gastrointestinal or liver toxicant. This drug has possible hypersensitization and cancer tendencies. BC Cancer Agency lists ETOPOSIDE has an irritant.

Caution: Females and males planning to have a child, pregnant women, and nursing mothers should exercise caution regarding potential occupational exposure to this cytotoxic drug. No information or not enough information exists or was provided concerning occupational exposure that may potentially occur while handling this drug and its affects on reproductive systems, the fetus, and/or if it is secreted along with breast milk, which may harm nursing infants. Staff members should consult with the occupational health physician monitoring workers' health in your facility to be apprised of potential hazards and should be advised to avoid becoming pregnant and/or breastfeeding or should be transferred in accordance with policy/procedures to other duties that do not involve preparation, handling, and administering this drug.

Target Organs/Systems: Blood, bone marrow, lungs, reproductive systems (male and female), heart, peripheral nervous system, gastrointestinal tract, cardiovascular system, respiratory tract, skin, ears, muscle tissue, eyes (lens or cornea), and throat

Medical Condition Generally Aggravated by Exposure:

- Anemia, other forms of bone marrow suppression, and birth defect hazard. Pre-existing skin and respiratory conditions. Repeated exposure to a highly toxic material may produce general deterioration of health by an accumulation in one or more human organs. Hypersensitivity to the material, bone marrow depression, chickenpox (including recent exposure), herpes zoster, and infection.
- Reproductive and pregnancy issues.

Specific Medical Surveillance Information: Reproductive and pregnancy counseling.

A pre-placement physical examination and history for employees with potential exposure to ETOPOSIDE is recommended. A complete blood count with differential, blood test for renal and liver function, and a urine analysis may be taken to provide a baseline. Based on opportunity for exposure and duration of exposure a periodic follow-up examination may be considered. This exam is overseen by a physician thoroughly knowledgeable about both the toxicity of ETOPOSIDE and the extent of workplace exposure.

Occupational Exposure Level/Limit (OEL) & Sampling Methods:

Environmental Sentinel Contamination Action Level (ESCAL): Air, surface

Pharmacia & Upjohn exposure limit for ETOPOSIDE occupational exposure

TWA: the exposure limit will be at the no detection (ND) limit.

Occupational Exposure Level (OEL): Bristol Myers Squibb

VEPESID®49—0.000014 mg/m3 TWA 8-hr (dust control)★

★Adherence to this target level should protect most employees who handle this drug from experiencing adverse effects from this substance, however, exposure to this substance should be maintained as low as reasonably possible.

(Methods not listed or specified)

Supplemental Response Information

Extinguishing Media: Use extinguishing agent which is the most appropriate to extinguish surrounding fire (carbon dioxide, foam, dry chemical or water fog as extinguishing media).

Solubility: ETOPOSIDE is very soluble in methanol and in chloroform slightly soluble in ethanol and alcohol, while being sparingly to slightly water soluble (<1 mg/ml with a ph range of 3.0 to 4.0).

Chemical Degradation/Neutralization Method: There are four recommended procedures for ETOPOSIDE (VEPESID®49). See below for optional methods.

A manufacturer's Material Safety Data Sheet (MSDS) recommends treating spill surfaces with a ~2 mol/liter (~8 g/100 ml) (5.25%), aqueous caustic soda (sodium hydroxide) solution after absorbing liquids with inert absorbent pads or removing any powder present: allow solution to stand for up to one hour, and then thoroughly wash spilled surfaces with soap and water; sample to determine if surface contamination is still present (if sampling method is available). If drug is still present, repeat above steps; dispose of wastes in accordance with your local procedures, state, and federal regulations.

Incompatibility: ETOPOSIDE: Slightly reactive with oxidizing agents and reducing agents.

ETOPOSIDE is a mixture. Mixed with ethyl alcohol and benzyl alcohol both substances have many incompatibilities. Review other literature before deactivation and cleanup.

ETOPOSIDE (2) (*e-TOE-poe-side*)
VEPESID®49 INJECTION) (VP-16)
VESPESID®49

Chemical Abstract Service (CAS) Registry Number: 33419-42-0, 33419-42-9 (NTP) (mixture)
RTECS: KCO190000
NSC 141540
C_{29}-H_{32}-O_{13}
(Four Degradation Methods)

Health & Safety Hazards/US Department of Transportation (DOT)/US Environmental Protection Agency (EPA)—Sources

Carcinogen G2A—International Agency for Research on Cancer, Carcinogen—US National Toxicology Program, Mutagen—Material Safety Data Sheet,

Mutagen—University of Maryland at College Park, Teratogen—Material Safety Data Sheet, Teratogen—University of Maryland at College Park, Toxic—Material Safety Data Sheet, Cytotoxic—Material Safety Data Sheet, Cytotoxic—British Columbia Cancer Agency Canada, US California Environmental Protection Agency Listed, Irritant—British Columbia Cancer Agency Canada, Pregnancy Category (D)—US Food and Drug Administration, Developmental US California Proposition 65, Flammable—Material Safety Data Sheet, National Fire Protection Association Health (0 Flammability (1) Instability/Reactivity (0)—Material Safety Data Sheet; National Fire Protection Association Health (1) Flammability (1) Instability/Reactivity (0)—Material Safety Data Sheet, National Fire Protection Association Health (1) Flammability (0) Instability/Reactivity (0)—Material Safety Data Sheet, Hazardous Materials Identification System (R) and/or US Department of Defense System Health (0★) with additional chronic hazard present Fire Hazard (1) Reactivity (0) Personal Protection Code (A) (Safety Glasses)—Material Safety Data Sheet; Hazardous Materials Identification System (R) and/or US Department of Defense System Health (1★) with additional chronic hazard present Fire Hazard (0) Reactivity (0) Personal Protection Code (-) (None stated), D001, DOT, FLAMMABLE LIQUIDS, N.O.S, UN 1993, CLASS 3, GROUP II.

ETOPOSIDE is a white or almost white crystalline powder.

ETOPOSIDE is a colorless fluid or pale pink capsule 50 mg and 100 mg.

ETOPOSIDE Breastfeeding (contraindicated) should be avoided because of potential for reproductive and developmental harm (*A Guide for Occupational Health Professionals Technical Manual*, Navy Environmental Health Center [NEHC-TM-OEM 6260.01a]).

First Aid/Medical Information/Occupational Exposure Limits

First Aid Measures to include: Use general first aid measures except for the following:

Physician's note (A): Overdose treatment: there is no proven antidote for ETOPOSIDE overdose. Treatment is supportive and includes the following:

1. Hypotension is managed by the administration of fluids.
2. Anaphylaxis is treated by administering pressor agents, adrenocorticoids, antihistamines, or volume expanders.

Physician's Note (B): Due to its action, ETOPOSIDE should be treated as potentially carcinogenic and may be mutagenic, teratogenic, or allergenic. If respiratory distress occurs after inhalation of airborne droplets, administer emergency airway support and 100% humidified supplemental oxygen with assisted ventilation if needed. If coughing or difficulty in breathing develops, evacuating for respiratory tract irritation, bronchitis or pneumonitis. Because of the potentially hazardous nature of ETOPOSIDE, if the solution is swallowed, gets in eyes or in contact with the skin, medical attention should be sought immediately after the preceding first aid measures are taken.

Medical Information:

Caution and Warning Statements: ETOPOSIDE is toxic by inhalation, in contact with skin, and if swallowed. This material may cause cancer and causes heritable genetic damage. ETOPOSIDE may cause harm to the unborn child. RTECS lists ETOPOSIDE as a suspected cardiovascular or blood toxicant; as an endocrine toxicant; and as a gastrointestinal or liver toxicant. This drug has possible hypersensitization and cancer tendencies. BC Cancer Agency lists ETOPOSIDE has an irritant.

Caution: Females and males planning to have a child, pregnant women, and nursing mothers should exercise caution regarding potential occupational exposure to this cytotoxic drug. No information or not enough information exists or was provided concerning occupational exposure that may potentially occur while handling this drug and its affects on reproductive systems, the fetus, and/or if it is secreted along with breast milk, which may harm nursing infants. Staff members should consult with the occupational health physician monitoring workers' health in your facility to be apprised of potential hazards and should be advised to avoid becoming pregnant and/or breastfeeding or should be transferred in accordance with policy/procedures to other duties that do not involve preparation, handling, and administering this drug.

Target Organs/Systems: Blood, bone marrow, lungs, reproductive systems (male and female), heart, peripheral nervous system, gastrointestinal tract, cardiovascular system, respiratory tract, skin, ears, muscle tissue, eyes (lens or cornea), and throat

Medical Condition Generally Aggravated by Exposure:

- Medical condition aggravated by exposure is anemia, other forms of bone marrow suppression, and birth defect hazard. Preexisting skin and respiratory conditions.

Repeated exposure to a highly toxic material may produce general deterioration of health by an accumulation in one or more human organs. Hypersensitivity to the material, bone marrow depression, chickenpox (including recent exposure), herpes zoster, and infection.

- Reproductive and pregnancy issues.

Specific Medical Surveillance Information: Reproductive and pregnancy counseling.

A pre-placement physical examination and history for employees with potential exposure to ETOPO-SIDE is recommended. A complete blood count with differential, blood test for renal and liver function, and a urine analysis may be taken to provide a base-line. Based on opportunity for exposure and duration of exposure, a periodic follow-up examination may be considered. This exam is overseen by a physician thoroughly knowledgeable about both the toxicity of ETOPOSIDE and the extent of workplace exposure.

Occupational Exposure Level/Limit (OEL) & Sampling Methods:

Environmental Sentinel Contamination Action Level (ESCAL): Air, surface
Pharmacia & Upjohn exposure limit for ETOPOSIDE occupational exposure
TWA: The exposure limit will be at the no detection (ND) limit.

Occupational Exposure Limit (OEL): Bristol Myers Squibb
VEPESID®49—0.000014 mg/m3 TWA 8-hr (dust control)*

*Adherence to this target level should protect most employees who handle this drug from experiencing adverse effects from this material, however, exposure to this substance should be maintained as low as reasonably possible.
(Method not listed or specified)

Supplemental Response Information

Extinguishing Media: Use extinguishing agent which is the most appropriate to extinguish surrounding fire (carbon dioxide, foam, dry chemical or water fog as extinguishing media).

Solubility: ETOPOSIDE is very soluble in methanol and in chloroform slightly soluble in ethanol, while being sparingly to slightly water soluble (<1 mg/ml with a pH range of 3.0 to 4.0).

Chemical Degradation/Neutralization Method: There are four recommended procedures for ETOPOSIDE (VEPESID®49). See below and above for optional methods.

A manufacturer's Material Safety Data Sheet (MSDS) recommends treating spill surfaces with a 9 fold molar excess of potassium permanganate ($KMNO_4$) solution after absorbing liquids with inert absorbent pads or removing any powder present: allow solution to stand for up to one hour, and then thoroughly wash spilled surfaces with soap and water; sample to determine if surface contamination is still present (if sampling method is available). If drug is still present, repeat above steps; dispose of wastes in accordance with your local procedures, state, and federal regulations.

Incompatibility: ETOPOSIDE: Slightly reactive with oxidizing agents and reducing agents.

ETOPOSIDE is a mixture. Mixed with ethyl alcohol and benzyl alcohol, both substances have many incompatibilities. Review other literature before deactivation and cleanup.

ETOPOSIDE (3) (*e-TOE-poe-side*)
VEPESID®49 INJECTION (VP-16)
VESPESID®49

Chemical Abstract Service (CAS) Registry Numbers: 33419-42-0, 33419-42-9 (NTP) (mixture)
RTECS: KC0190000
NSC 141540
$C_{29}H_{32}O_{13}$
(Four Degradation Methods)

Health & Safety Hazards/US Department of Transportation (DOT)/US Environmental Protection Agency (EPA)—Sources

Carcinogen G2A—International Agency for Research on Cancer, Carcinogen—US National Toxicology Program, Mutagen—Material Safety Data Sheet, Mutagen—University of Maryland at College Park, Teratogen—Material Safety Data Sheet, Teratogen—University of Maryland at College Parks, Toxic—Material Safety Data Sheet, Cytotoxic—Material Safety Data Sheet, US California Environmental Protection Agency Listed, Pregnancy Category (D)—US Food and Drug Administration, Developmental—US California Proposition 65, Flammable—Material Safety Data Sheet, National Fire Protection Association Health (0) Flammability (1) Instability/Reactivity (0)—Material Safety Data Sheet, National Fire Protection Association Health (1) Flammability (1) Instability/Reactivity (0)—Material

Safety Data Sheet, National Fire Protection Association Health (1) Flammability (0) Instability/Reactivity (0)—Material Safety Data Sheet, Hazardous Materials Identification System (R) and/or US Department of Defense System Health (0★) with additional chronic hazard present Fire Hazard (1) Reactivity (0) Personal Protection Code (A) (Safety Glasses)—Material Safety Data Sheet, Hazardous Materials Identification System (R) and/or US Department of Defense System (1★) with additional chronic hazard present Fire Hazard (0) Reactivity (0) Personal Protection Code (-) (None state), D001, DOT, FLAMMABLE LIQUIDS, N.O.S, UN 1993, CLASS 3, GROUP II.

ETOPOSIDE is a white or almost white crystalline powder.

ETOPOSIDE is a colorless fluid or pale pink 50 mg and 100 mg capsules.

ETOPOSIDE: Breastfeeding is contraindicated because of potential for reproductive and developmental harm (*A Guide for Occupational Health Professionals Technical Manual*, Navy Environmental Health Center [NEHC-TM-OEM 6260.01a]).

First Aid/Medical Information/ Occupational Exposure Limits

First Aid Measures to include: Use general first aid measures except for the following:

Physician's note (A): Overdose treatment: there is no proven antidote for ETOPOSIDE overdose. Treatment is supportive and includes the following:

1. Hypotension is managed by the administration of fluids.
2. Anaphylaxis is treated by administering pressor agents, adrenocorticoids, antihistamines, or volume expanders.

Physician's note (B): Due to its action, ETOPOSIDE should be treated as potentially carcinogenic and may be mutagenic, teratogenic, or allergenic. If respiratory distress occurs after inhalation of airborne droplets, administer emergency airway support and 100% humidified supplemental oxygen with assisted ventilation if needed. If coughing or difficulty in breathing develops, evacuating for respiratory tract irritation, bronchitis, or pneumonitis. Because of the potentially hazardous nature of ETOPOSIDE, if the solution is swallowed, gets in eyes or in contact with the skin, medical attention should be sought immediately after the preceding first aid measures are taken.

Medical Information:

Caution and Warning Statements: ETOPOSIDE is toxic by inhalation, in contact with skin, and if swallowed. This material may cause cancer and causes heritable genetic damage. ETOPOSIDE may cause harm to the unborn child. RTECS lists ETOPOSIDE as a suspected cardiovascular or blood toxicant; as an endocrine toxicant; and as a gastrointestinal or liver toxicant. This drug has possible hypersensitization and cancer tendencies.

Caution: Females and males planning to have a child, pregnant women, and nursing mothers should exercise caution regarding potential occupational exposure to this cytotoxic drug. No information or not enough information exists or was provided concerning occupational exposure that may potentially occur while handling this drug and its affects on reproductive systems, the fetus, and/or if it is secreted along with breast milk, which may harm nursing infants. Staff members should consult with the occupational health physician monitoring workers' health in your facility to be apprised of potential hazards and should be advised to avoid becoming pregnant and/or breastfeeding or should be transferred in accordance with policy/procedures to other duties that do not involve preparation, handling, and administering this drug.

Target Organs/Systems: Blood, bone marrow, lungs, reproductive systems, heart, peripheral nervous system, gastrointestinal tract, cardiovascular system, respiratory tract, skin, ears, muscle tissue, eyes (lens or cornea), and throat

Medical Condition Generally Aggravated By Exposure:

- Anemia, other forms of bone marrow suppression, and birth defect hazard. Pre-existing skin and respiratory conditions.
- Repeated exposure to a highly toxic material may produce general deterioration of health by an accumulation in one or more human organs. Hypersensitivity to the material, bone marrow depression, chickenpox (including recent exposure), herpes zoster, and infection.
- Reproductive and pregnancy issues.

Specific Medical Surveillance Information: Reproductive and pregnancy counseling.

A pre-placement physical examination and history for employees with potential exposure to ETOPOSIDE is recommended. A complete blood count with differential, blood test for renal and liver function, and a urine analysis may be taken to provide a baseline. Based on opportunity for exposure and duration of exposure, a periodic follow-up examination may be considered. This exam is overseen by a physician thoroughly knowledgeable about both the toxicity of ETOPOSIDE and the extent of workplace exposure.

Occupational Exposure Level/Limit (OEL) & Sampling Methods:

> *Environmental Sentinel Contamination Action Level (ESCAL)*: Air, surface
> Pharmacia & Upjohn exposure limit for ETOPOSIDE occupational exposure
> TWA: The exposure limit will be at the no detection (ND) limit.
> (Method not listed or specified)

Supplemental Response Information

Extinguishing Media: Use extinguishing agent which is the most appropriate to extinguish surrounding fire (carbon dioxide, foam, dry chemical or water fog as extinguishing media).

Solubility: ETOPOSIDE is very soluble in methanol and in chloroform slightly soluble in ethanol & alcohol, while being sparingly to slightly water soluble (<1 mg/ml with a pH range of 3.0 to 4.0).

Chemical Degradation/Neutralization Method: There are four recommended procedures for ETOPOSIDE (VEPESID®49). See below and above for optional methods.

A manufacturer's Material Safety Data Sheet (MSDS) recommends treating spill surfaces with a 7.5 fold molar.

Excess of 5.25% bleach (sodium hypochlorite) solution after absorbing liquids with inert absorbent pads or removing any powder present: allow solution to stand for up to one hour, and then thoroughly wash spilled surfaces with soap and water; sample to determine if surface contamination is still present (if sampling method is available at your facility). If still present, repeat above steps; dispose of wastes in accordance with your local procedures, state, and federal regulations.

Incompatibility: ETOPOSIDE: Slightly reactive with oxidizing agents and reducing agents.

ETOPOSIDE is a mixture. Mixed with ethyl alcohol and benzyl alcohol both substances have many incompatibilities. Review other literature before deactivation and cleanup.

ETOPOSIDE (4) (*e-TOE-poe-side*)
VEPESID®49 INJECTION (VP-16)
VESPESID®49

> Chemical Abstract Service (CAS) Registry
>   Numbers: 33419-42-0, 33419-42-9 (NTP)
>   (mixture)
> RTECS: KC0190000
> NSC 141540
> $C_{29}H_{32}O_{13}$
> (Four Degradation Methods)

Health & Safety Hazards/US Department of Transportation (DOT)/US Environmental Protection Agency (EPA)—Sources

Carcinogen G2A—International Agency for Research on Cancer, Carcinogen—US National Toxicology Program, Mutagen—Material Safety Data Sheet, Mutagen—University of Maryland at College Park, Teratogen—Material Safety Data Sheet, Teratogen—University of Maryland at College Park, Toxic—Material Safety Data Sheet, Cytotoxic—Material Safety Data Sheet, US California Environmental Protection Agency Listed, Pregnancy Category (D)—US Food and Drug Administration, Developmental—US California Proposition 65, Flammable—Material Safety Data Sheet, National Fire Protection Association Health (0) Flammability (1) Instability/Reactivity (0)—Material Safety Data Sheet, National Fire Protection Association Health (1) Flammability (1) Instability/Reactivity (0)—Material Safety Data Sheet, National Fire Protection Association Health (1) Flammability (0) Instability/Reactivity (0)—Material Safety Data Sheet, Hazardous Materials Identification System (R) and/or US Department of Defense System Health (0*) with additional chronic hazard present Fire Hazard (1) Reactivity (0) Personal Protection Code (A) (Safety Glasses)—Material Safety Data Sheet, Hazardous Materials Identification System (R) and/or US Department of Defense System Health (1*) with additional chronic hazard present Fire Hazard (0) Reactivity (0) Personal Protection Code (–) (None stated)—Material Safety Data Sheet, D001, DOT, FLAMMABLE LIQUIDS, N.O.S, UN 1993, CLASS 3, GROUP II.

ETOPOSIDE is a white or almost white crystalline powder.

ETOPOSIDE is a colorless fluid or pale pink 50 mg and 100 mg capsules.

ETOPOSIDE: Breastfeeding is contraindicated because of potential for reproductive and developmental harm (*A Guide for Occupational Health Professionals Technical Manual*, Navy Environmental Health Center [NEHC-TM-OEM 6260.01a]).

First Aid/Medical Information/ Occupational Exposure Limits

First Aid Measures to include: Use general first aid measures except for the following:

Physician's note (A): Overdose treatment: there is no proven antidote for ETOPOSIDE overdose. Treatment is supportive and includes the following:

1. Hypotension is managed by the administration of fluids.
2. Anaphylaxis is treated by administering pressor agents, adrenocorticoids, antihistamines, or volume expanders.

Physician's note (B): Due to its action, ETOPOSIDE should be treated as potentially carcinogenic, and may be mutagenic, teratogenic, or allergenic. If respiratory distress occurs after inhalation of airborne droplets, administer emergency airway support and 100% humidified supplemental oxygen with assisted ventilation if needed. If coughing or difficulty in breathing develops, evacuating for respiratory tract irritation, bronchitis, or pneumonitis. Because of the potentially hazardous nature of ETOPOSIDE, if the solution is swallowed, gets in eyes or in contact with the skin, medical attention should be sought immediately after the preceding first aid measures are taken.

Medical Information:

Caution and Warning Statements: ETOPOSIDE is toxic by inhalation, in contact with skin, and if swallowed. This material may cause cancer and causes heritable genetic damage. ETOPOSIDE may cause harm to the unborn child. RTECS lists ETOPOSIDE as a suspected cardiovascular or blood toxicant; as an endocrine toxicant; and as a gastrointestinal or liver toxicant. This drug has possible hypersensitization and cancer tendencies.

Caution: Females and males planning to have a child, pregnant women, and nursing mothers should exercise caution regarding potential occupational exposure to this cytotoxic drug. No information or not enough information exists or was provided concerning occupational exposure that may potentially occur while handling this drug and its affects on reproductive systems, the fetus, and/or if it is secreted along with breast milk, which may harm nursing infants. Staff members should consult with the occupational health physician monitoring workers' health in your facility to be apprised of potential hazards and should be advised to avoid becoming pregnant and/or breastfeeding or should be transferred in accordance with policy/procedures to other duties that do not involve preparation, handling, and administering this drug.

Target Organs/Systems: Blood, bone marrow, lungs, reproductive systems, heart, peripheral nervous system, gastrointestinal tract, cardiovascular system, respiratory tract, skin, ears, muscle tissue, eyes (lens or cornea), and throat

Medical Condition Generally Aggravated by Exposure:

- Anemia, other forms of bone marrow suppression, and birth defect hazard. Preexisting skin and respiratory conditions.
- Repeated exposure to a highly toxic material may produce general deterioration of health by an accumulation in one or more human organs. Hypersensitivity to the material, bone marrow depression, chickenpox (including recent exposure), herpes zoster, and infection.
- Reproductive and pregnancy issues.

Specific Medical Surveillance Information: Reproductive and pregnancy counseling.

A pre-placement physical examination and history for employees with potential exposure to ETOPOSIDE is recommended. A complete blood count with differential, blood test for renal and liver function, and a urine analysis may be taken to provide a baseline. Based on opportunity for exposure and duration of exposure, a periodic follow-up examination may be considered. This exam is overseen by a physician thoroughly knowledgeable about both the toxicity of ETOPOSIDE and the extent of workplace exposure.

Occupational Exposure Level/Limit (OEL) & Sampling Methods:

Environmental Sentinel Contamination Action Level (ESCAL): Air, surface
Pharmacia & Upjohn exposure limit for ETOPOSIDE occupational exposure
TWA: The exposure limit will be at the no detection (ND) limit. (Method not listed or specified)

Supplemental Response Information

Extinguishing Media: Use extinguishing agent which is the most appropriate to extinguish surrounding fire (carbon dioxide, foam, dry chemical or water fog as extinguishing media).

Solubility: ETOPOSIDE is very soluble in methanol and in chloroform slightly soluble in ethanol, while being sparingly to slightly water soluble (<1 mg/ml with a pH range of 3.0 to 4.0).

Chemical Degradation/Neutralization Method: There are four recommended procedures for ETOPOSIDE (VEPESID®49). See below and above for optional methods.

A manufacturer's Material Safety Data Sheet (MSDS) recommends treating spill surfaces with a 9 fold molar excess of potassium permanganate (KMNO4) solution after absorbing liquids with inert absorbent pads or removing any powder present: al-low solution to stand for up to one hour, and then thoroughly wash spilled surfaces with soap and water; sample to determine if surface contamination is still present (if sampling method is available at your facility). If still present, repeat above steps; dispose of wastes in accordance with your local procedures, state, and federal regulations.

Incompatibility: ETOPOSIDE: Slightly reactive with oxidizing agents and reducing agents.

ETOPOSIDE is a mixture. Mixed with ethyl alcohol and benzyl alcohol both substances have many incompatibilities. Review other literature before deactivation and cleanup.

F

FINASTERIDE (*fih-NAH-steh-ride*)
PROSCAR®50

$C_{23}H_{36}N_2O_2$

PROPECIA®51

Chemical Abstract Service (CAS) Registry
Number: 98319-26-7
RTECS: CL5245000

Health & Safety Hazards/US Department of Transportation (DOT)/US Environmental Protection Agency (EPA)—Sources

Toxic—Material Safety Data Sheet, Reproductive Effector Male—Material Safety Data Sheet, Teratogen—Material Safety Data Sheet, US California Proposition 65 (Na), Pregnancy Category (X) US Food and Drug Administration—Material Safety Data Sheet.

FINASTERIDE (PROSCAR®50) (PROPECIA®51) is available as tablets (1 mg and 5 mg).

FINASTERIDE—Risk to male fetus; women should not handle crushed or broken tablets when pregnant or may potentially be pregnant; breastfeeding: this drug is not indicated for use in women; not known if excreted in breast milk (facts and comparisons), is contraindicated because of potential for reproductive and developmental harm (*A Guide for Occupational Health Professionals Technical Manual*, Navy Environmental Health Center [NEHC-TM-OEM 6260.01a]).

FINASTERIDE is a white to off-white crystalline powder.

First Aid/Medical Information/ Occupational Exposure Limits

First Aid Measures to include: Use general first aid measures.

Medical Information:
Caution and Warning Statements:

Caution: The toxicological properties of most cytotoxic drugs have not been fully investigated, particularly as it pertains to occupational exposure. FINASTERIDE (PROSCAR®50) is one of the drugs that has little occupational hazards information available. Therefore, therapeutic dose information was extrapolated below to assist in determining occupational toxicity, and signs and symptoms of overexposure. Furthermore, it is prudent to minimize occupational exposure to FINASTERIDE (PROSCAR®50).

Pregnant women should avoid exposure to FINASTERIDE (PROSCAR®50) because it may cause abnormalities of the external genitalia of a male fetus. Furthermore, it is not known whether FINASTERIDE is excreted in human milk.

Caution: Women should not handle crushed or broken tablets when they are or may potentially be pregnant.

Caution: Females and males planning to have a child, pregnant women, and nursing mothers should exercise caution regarding potential occupational exposure to this cytotoxic drug. No information or not enough information exists or was provided concerning occupational exposure that may potentially occur while handling this drug and its affects on reproductive systems, the fetus, and/or if it is secreted along with breast milk, which may harm nursing infants. Staff members should consult with the occupational health physician monitoring workers' health in your facility to be apprised of potential hazards and should be advised to avoid becoming pregnant and/or breastfeeding or should be transferred in accordance with policy/procedures to other duties that do not involve preparation, handling, and administering this drug.

Target Organs/Systems: Fetus and reproductive systems (male)

Medical Conditions Generally Aggravated by Exposure:

- Refer to the caution and warning statements section above.

Specific Medical Surveillance Information: Reproductive and pregnancy counseling.

Occupational Exposure Level/Limit (OEL) & Sampling Methods: Not otherwise specified

Environmental Sentinel Contamination Action Level (ESCAL): Not otherwise specified

Supplemental Response Information

Extinguishing Media: Use extinguishing agent which is the most appropriate to extinguish surrounding fire (carbon dioxide, foam, dry chemical or water fog as extinguishing media).

Solubility: FINASTERIDE is practically water insoluble (0.05 mg/ml at 25 C) to very slightly soluble. It is freely soluble in chloroform and in lower alcohol solvents.

Chemical Degradation/Neutralization Method: Not otherwise specified

Note: If a specific degradation or neutralization method is not provided on this table and you do not have other specific information that will advise you on how to clean up the specific material spilled, then follow the general spill procedure found at the introduction section of this table.

Incompatibility: FINASTERIDE is incompatible with strong oxidizing agents.

FLOXURIDINE (*floks-YOOR-ih-deen*)
FUDR, 5-FLUORODEOXYURIDINE
FUDR®52
5-FUDR

NSC27640

2'-DEOXY-5-FLUOROURIDINE

Chemical Abstract Service (CAS) Registry
Number: 50-91-9
RTECS: YU7525000
$C_9-H_{11}-FN_2-0_5$

Health & Safety Hazards/US Department of Transportation (DOT)/US Environmental Protection Agency (EPA)—Sources

Carcinogen—Material Safety Data Sheet, Toxic—Material Safety Data Sheet, Experimental Terato-gen—Material Safety Data Sheet, Experimental Mutagen—Material Safety Data Sheet, Experimental Fetotoxic—Material Safety Data Sheet, Lactation Harmful—Material Safety Data Sheet, Cytotoxic—Material Safety Data Sheet, Pregnancy Category (D)—US Food and Drug Administration, National Fire Protection Association Health (2) Flammability (0) Instability/Reactivity (0)—Material Safety Data Sheet, Hazardous Materials Identification System (R) and/or US Department of Defense System (2★) with additional chronic hazard present Fire Hazard (0) Reactivity (0) Personal Protection Code (-) (None stated)—Material Safety Data Sheet, UN 3249.

FLOXURIDINE available as an injection.

First Aid/Medical Information/ Occupational Exposure Limits

First Aid Measures to include: Use general first aid measures except for the following:

Ingestion: If victim is conscious and alert, give 2–4 cups of milk or water. Seek medical attention.

Medical Information:

Caution and Warning Statements: FLOXURIDINE is a suspect carcinogen.

FLOXURIDINE exposure may irritate eyes, skin, and/or respiratory tract. Exposure may cause allergic reaction. FLOXURIDINE has shown to be teratogenic, mutagenic, and fetotoxic in animal studies, FLOXURIDINE is a suspected cancer causing agent. This material poses possible risks for irreversible effects from exposure to FLOXURIDINE.

If ingested, may cause gastrointestinal irritations with nausea, vomiting, and diarrhea occuring. Stomatitis (inflammation of the mucous membranes in the mouth) is a common sign of toxicity. Chronic exposure may cause hair loss, nail changes, dermatitis, and increased pigmentation of the skin.

Caution: Females and males planning to have a child, pregnant women, and nursing mothers should exercise caution regarding potential occupational exposure to this cytotoxic drug. No information or not enough information exists or was provided concerning occupational exposure that may potentially occur while handling this drug and its affects on reproductive systems, the fetus, and/or if it is secreted along with breast milk, which may harm nursing infants. Staff members should consult with the occupational health physician monitoring workers' health in your facility to be apprised of potential hazards and should be advised to avoid becoming pregnant and/or breastfeeding or should be transferred in accordance with policy/procedures to other duties that do not involve preparation, handling, and administering this drug.

Therapeutic Levels: FUDR®52 may cause fetal harm when administered to a pregnant woman. It has been shown to be teratogenic in the chick embryo, mouse (at doses of 2.5 to 100 mg/kg), and rat (at doses of 75 to 150 mg/kg). Malformations included cleft palates; skeletal defects; and deformed appendages, paws, and tails. The dosages that were teratogenic in animals are 4.2 to 125 times the recommended human therapeutic dose. There are no adequate and well-controlled studies with FUDR®52 in pregnant women.

Target Organs/Systems: Gastrointestinal system, central nervous system, blood forming systems, kidneys, vascular system, immune system, liver, eyes, heart, fetus, and skin

Medical Conditions Generally Aggravated by Exposure:

- Digestive and respiratory disorders and previously existing cardiovascular, liver, kidney, blood disorders, serious infections and nutritional deficiency, individuals in poor nutritional state, with depressed bone marrow function, or those with potentially serious infections. Furthermore, reproductive and pregnancy issues.

Specific Medical Surveillance Information: Reproductive and pregnancy counseling.

Occupational Exposure Level/Limit (OEL) & Sampling Methods:

Environmental Sentinel Contamination Action Level (ESCAL): Not otherwise specified
Occupational Exposure Level (OEL): Bedford Lab 10 μ/m3
(Method not listed or specified)

Supplemental Response Information

Extinguishing Media: Use extinguishing agent which is the most appropriate to extinguish surrounding fire (carbon dioxide, foam, dry chemical or water fog as extinguishing media).

Solubility: FLOXURIDINE is freely water soluble with a pH range of 4.0–5.5. Solubility: other diethyl acetamide and propylene glycol. FLOXURIDINE is soluble in acetone and in alcohol; insoluble in chloroform, in ether, and in benzene.

Chemical Degradation/Neutralization Method: A manufacturer's Material Safety Data Sheet (MSDS) recommends treating spill surfaces with a ~2 mol/liter (~8 g/100 ml), aqueous caustic soda (sodium hydroxide) solution after absorbing liquids with inert absorbent pads or removing any powder present: allow solution to stand for up to one hour, and then thoroughly wash spilled surfaces with soap and water; sample to determine if surface contamination is still present (if sampling method is available). If drug is still present, repeat above steps; dispose of wastes in accordance with your local procedures, state, and federal regulations.

Incompatibility: FLOXURIDINE is incompatible with strong oxidizing agents and strong bases.

FLUOROURACIL (1)
(flure-oh-YOOR-a-sil)
5-FLUOROURACIL
5-FU (FU)
ADRUCIL®53

Chemical Abstract Service (CAS) Registry Number: 51-21-8
RTECS: YR0350000
NSC 19893
$C_4H_3FN_2O_2$
(Two Degradation Methods)

Health & Safety Hazards/US Department of Transportation (DOT)/US Environmental Protection Agency (EPA)—Sources

Suspect Human Carcinogenic—Material Safety Data Sheet, Carcinogen G3—International Agency for Research on Cancer, Experimental Mutagen—Material Safety Data Sheet, Teratogen—US National Institute of Health (NIH)—Material Safety Data Sheet, Reproductive Effector—Material Safety Data Sheet, Moderate Toxic—US National Institute of Health (NIH) and Material Safety Data Sheet, Photosensitizer—Material Safety Data Sheet, Corrosive—Material Safety Data Sheet, Cytotoxic—British Columbia Cancer Agency Canada, Nonvesicant—British Columbia Cancer Agency Canada, Lactation—Avoid Breastfeeding (World Health Organization), Pregnancy Category (D) US Food and Drug Administration—Box Warning, Pregnancy Category (X) US Food and Drug Administration—Product Information, and US Navy, Carcinogen and Developmental—US California Proposition 65, National Fire Protection Association Health (2) Flammability (0) Instability/Reactivity (0)—Material Safety Data Sheet, National Fire Protection Association Health (2) Flammability (1) Instability/Reactivity (0)—Material Safety Data Sheet, National Fire Protection Association Health (2) Flammability (1) Instability/Reactivity (1), National Fire Protection Association Health (3) Flammability (1) Instability/

Reactivity (0)—Material Safety Data Sheet, National Fire Protection Association Health (3) Flammability (0) Instability/Reactivity (0)—Material Safety Data Sheet, Hazardous Materials Identification System (R) and/or US Department of Defense System Health (2) Fire Hazard (1) Reactivity (0) Personal Protection Code (E) (Safety Glasses, Chemical Gloves, Dust Respirator)—Material Safety Data Sheet, Hazardous Materials Identification System (R) and/or US Department of Defense System Health (3) Fire Hazard (1) Reactivity (0) Personal Protection Code (E) (Safety Glasses, Chemical Gloves, Dust Respirator)—Material Safety Data Sheet, Hazardous Materials Identification System (R) and/or US Department of Defense System Health (3★) with additional chronic hazards present Fire Hazard (0) Reactivity (0) Personal Protection Code (-) (None stated)—Material Safety Data Sheet, US Environmental Protection Agency (EPA) SARA 302, US Environmental Protection Agency (EPA) SARA 313, UN 3249, UN 2811, CLASS 6.1.

FLUOROURACIL is a white or almost white crystalline powder.

FLUOROURACIL is a clear, colorless liquid and is odorless.

FLUOROURACIL   (5-FLUOROURACIL) Breastfeeding is contraindicated because of potential for reproductive and developmental harm (*A Guide for Occupational Health Professionals Technical Manual*, Navy Environmental Health Center [NEHC-TM-OEM 6260.01a]).

First Aid/Medical Information/ Occupational Exposure Limits

First Aid Measures to include: Use general first aid measures except for the following:

Ingestion: If victim is conscious and alert, rinse mouth out and drink plenty of sodium bicarbonate solution, water, or milk.

Physician's note: Physician should treat symptomatically and supportively. Refer for gastric lavage. Note: examine the lips and mouth to ascertain whether the tissues are damaged, a possible indication that the toxic material was ingested; the absence of such signs, however, is not conclusive.

Dermal contact: Avoid rubbing of skin or increasing its temperature; will increase absorption. Avoid exposure to UV light.

Medical Information:

Caution and Warning Statements: FLUOROURACIL is a cytotoxic agent and a corrosive. All work practices must be designed to reduce human exposure to the lowest level.

Warning: 5-FLUOROURACIL is harmful if swallowed. Severe overexposure can result in death. This drug may cause adverse reproductive effects, birth defects, and irritate the skin, eyes, and respiratory system. Material is harmful if swallowed, inhaled, and/or with skin contact. Exposure to 5-FLUOROURACIL may cause heritable genetic damage. May cause harm to the unborn child. This drug may cause photosensitivity.

5-FLUOROURACIL is listed by RTECS as a cardiovascular or blood toxicant and as a gastrointestinal or liver toxicant.

Exposure to 5-FLUOROURACIL can cause nausea, vomiting, diarrhea, headache, fatigue, dizziness, mental confusion, and abdominal pain. Repeated contact may cause hair loss, nail changes, atrophy and a change in skin color. This drug is considered to be toxic to blood. Repeated or prolonged exposure to this substance can produce target organs damage. Repeated exposure to a highly toxic material may produce general deterioration of health by an accumulation in one or more human organs. 5-FLUOROURACIL acute and chronic toxicity is not fully known. This drug is a photosensitizer.

Caution: Females and males planning to have a child, pregnant women, and nursing mothers should exercise caution regarding potential occupational exposure to this cytotoxic drug. No information or not enough information exists or was provided concerning occupational exposure that may potentially occur while handling this drug and its affects on reproductive systems, the fetus, and/or if it is secreted along with breast milk, which may harm nursing infants. Staff members should consult with the occupational health physician monitoring workers' health in your facility to be apprised of potential hazards and should be advised to avoid becoming pregnant and/or breastfeeding or should be transferred in accordance with policy/procedures to other duties that do not involve preparation, handling, and administering this drug.

Target Organs/Systems: Heart (cardiovascular), bone marrow, blood, central nervous system, immune and reproductive systems, skin, and eyes

Medical Conditions Generally Aggravated by Exposure:

- Preexisting cardiovascular, central nervous, and immune system disorders.
- Reproductive and pregnancy issues.
- Impaired hepatic or renal function and/or previous chemotherapy. Repeated or prolonged

exposure to the substance can produce target organs damage. Repeated exposure to a highly toxic material may produce general deterioration or health by an accumulation in one or more human organs.

Specific Medical Surveillance Information: 5-FLUO-ROURACIL absorbed by various body tissues, skin, respiratory, and intestinal and transplacentally.

Reproductive and pregnancy counseling is recommended.

Recommendation for a complete blood count is performed prior to employment, administering 5-FLUOROURACIL and at regular times afterwards. If symptoms develop or/and overexposure is suspected, the following are recommended: EKG and evaluation by a qualified allergist to help diagnoses skin allergy.

Occupational Exposure Level/Limit (OEL) & Sampling Methods:

Environmental Sentinel Contamination Action Level (ESCAL): Surface
US American Conference of Governmental Industrial Hygienist (ACGIH):
TLV 2.5 mg/m3 (2.0 mg/m3)
(Method not listed or specified)

Supplemental Response Information

Extinguishing Media: Use extinguishing agent which is the most appropriate to extinguish surrounding fire (carbon dioxide, foam, dry chemical or water fog as extinguishing media).

Solubility: 5-FLUOROURACIL is slightly, sparingly, or partially soluble in cold water and methanol. Furthermore this material is insoluble in diethyl ether (pH ~ 9.2), and in a 1% solution in water it has a pH of 4.5 to 5.0.

Chemical Degradation/Neutralization Method: There are two or more recommended procedures (alkaline soap/detergent method and bleach [sodium hypochlorite] solution) method) for 5-FLUOROURACIL (ADRUCIL®53). See below for optional method.

A manufacturer's Material Safety Data Sheet (MSDS) recommends using a 5.25% bleach (sodium hypochlorite) solution) and water to clean spill surfaces after absorbing liquids with inert absorbent pads or removing any powder present. After applying the bleach solution, leave solution on spill for at least 15 minutes. After removing the bleach solution, rinse with soap and water. Sample to determine if surface contamination is still present (if sampling method is available at your

facility). If contamination is still present, repeat above steps; dispose of wastes in accordance with your local procedures, state, and federal regulations.

Incompatibility: 5-FLUOROURACIL is incompatible with strong oxidizing agents, strong bases, and strong acids.

FLUOROURACIL (2)
(*flure-oh-YOOR-a-sil*)
5-FLUOROURACIL
5-FU FU
ADRUCIL®53

Chemical Abstract Service (CAS) Registry Number: 51-21-8
RTECS: YR0350000
NSC 19893
$C_4H_3FN_2O_2$
(Two Degradation Methods)

Health & Safety Hazards/US Department of Transportation (DOT)/US Environmental Protection Agency (EPA)—Sources

Suspected Human Carcinogen—Material Safety Data Sheet, Carcinogen G3—International Agency for Research on Cancer, Experimental Mutagen—Material Safety Data Sheet, Teratogen—US National Institute of Health (NIH) and Material Safety Data Sheet, Reproductive Effector—Material Safety Data Sheet, Moderate Toxic—US National Institute of Health (NIH) and Material Safety Data Sheet, Photosensitizer—Material Safety Data Sheet, Corrosive—Material Safety Data Sheet, Cytotoxic—British Columbia Cancer Agency Canada, Nonvesicant—British Columbia Cancer Agency Canada, Lactation Avoid Breastfeeding (World Health Organization), Pregnancy Category (D)—US Food and Drug Administration, Pregnancy Category (X) US Food and Drug Administration—Product Information and US Navy, Carcinogen and Developmental US California Proposition 65, National Fire Protection Association Health (2) Flammability (0) Instability/Reactivity (0)—Material Safety Data Sheet, National Fire Protection Association Health (2) Flammability (1) Instability/Reactivity (0)—Material Safety Data Sheet, National Fire Protection Association Health (2) Flammability (1) Instability/Reactivity (1)—Material Safety Data Sheet, National Fire Protection Association Health (3) Flammability (1) Instability/Reactivity (0)—Material Safety Data Sheet, National Fire Protection Association Health (3) Flammability (0) Instability/Reactivity (0)—Material Safety Data Sheet,

Hazardous Materials Identification System (R) and/ or US Department of Defense System Health (2) Fire Hazard (1) Reactivity (0) Personal Protection Code (E) (Safety Glasses, Chemical Gloves, Dust Respirator)—Material Safety Data Sheet, Hazardous Materials Identification System (R) and/or US Department of Defense System Health (3) Fire Hazard (1) Reactivity (0) Personal Protection Code (E) (Safety Glasses, Chemical Gloves, Dust Respirator)—Material Safety Data Sheet, Hazardous Materials Identification System (R) and/or US Department of Defense System Health (3★) with additional chronic hazards present Fire Hazard (0) Reactivity (0) Personal Protection Code (-) (None stated)—Material Safety Data Sheet, US Environmental Protection Agency (EPA) SARA 302, US Environmental Protection Agency (EPA) SARA 313, UN 3249, UN 2811, CLASS 6.1.

FLUOROURACIL is a white or almost white crystalline powder.

FLUOROURACIL is clear, colorless liquid; odorless.

FLUOROURACIL (5-FLUOROURACIL) Breastfeeding is contraindicated because of potential for reproductive and developmental harm (*A Guide for Occupational Health Professionals Technical Manual*, Navy Environmental Health Center [NEHC-TM-OEM 6260.01a]).

First Aid/Medical Information/ Occupational Exposure Limits

First Aid Measures to include: Use general first aid measures except for the following:

Ingestion: If victim is conscious and alert, rinse mouth out and drink plenty of sodium bicarbonate solution, water, or milk.

Physician's note: Physician should treat symptomatically and supportively. Refer for gastric lavage. Note: examine the lips and mouth to ascertain whether the tissues are damaged, a possible indication that the toxic material was ingested; the absence of such signs, however, is not conclusive.

Dermal contact: Avoid rubbing of skin or increasing its temperature; will increase absorption. Avoid exposure to UV light.

Medical Information:

Caution and Warning Statements: Fluorouracil is a cytotoxic agent and a corrosive. All work practices must be designed to reduce human exposure to the lowest level.

Warning: 5-FLUOROURACIL is harmful if swallowed. Severe overexposure can result in death. This drug may cause adverse reproductive effects. and birth detects. Irritate the skin, eyes, and respiratory system. Material is harmful if swallowed, inhaled and/or with skin contact. Exposure to 5-FLUOROURACIL may cause heritable genetic damage. May cause harm to the unborn child. This drug may cause photosensitivity.

5-FLUOROURACIL is listed by RTECS as a cardiovascular or blood toxicant and as a gastrointestinal or liver toxicant.

Exposure to 5-FLUOROURACIL can cause nausea, vomiting, diarrhea, headache, fatigue, dizziness, mental confusion, and abdominal pain. Repeated contact may cause hair loss, nail changes, atrophy, and a change in skin color. This drug is considered to be toxic to blood. Repeated or prolonged exposure to this substance can produce target organs damage. Repeated exposure to a highly toxic material may produce general deterioration of health by an accumulation in one or more human organs. 5-FLUOROURACIL acute and chronic toxicity is not fully known. This drug is a photosensitizer.

Caution: Females and males planning to have a child, pregnant women, and nursing mothers should exercise caution regarding potential occupational exposure to this cytotoxic drug. No information or not enough information exists or was provided concerning occupational exposure that may potentially occur while handling this drug and its affects on reproductive systems, the fetus, and/or if it is secreted along with breast milk, which may harm nursing infants. Staff members should consult with the occupational health physician monitoring workers' health in your facility to be apprised of potential hazards and should be advised to avoid becoming pregnant and/or breastfeeding or should be transferred in accordance with policy/procedures to other duties that do not involve preparation, handling, and administering this drug.

Target Organs/Systems: Heart (cardiovascular), bone marrow, blood, central nervous system, immune, reproductive systems, skin, and eyes

Medical Conditions Generally Aggravated by Exposure:

- Preexisting cardiovascular, central nervous, and immune system disorders. May be aggravated by Exposure to 5-FLUOROURACIL.
- Reproductive and pregnancy issues.
- Impaired hepatic or renal function and/or previous chemotherapy; if nutritional deficiencies and protein depletion may have a reduced tolerance to 5-FLUOROURACIL (Gilman 1985, p. 1270). Repeated or prolonged exposure

to the substance can produce target organs damage. Repeated exposure to a highly toxic material may produce general deterioration or health by an accumulation in one or more human organs.

Specific Medical Surveillance Information: 5-FLUOROURACIL absorbed by various body tissues, skin, respiratory and intestinal, and transplacentally.

Reproductive and pregnancy counseling is recommended.

Therapeutic Levels: Recommendation for a complete blood count is performed prior to employment, administering 5-FLUOROURACIL and at regular times afterwards. If symptoms develop or/and overexposure is suspected, the following are recommended: EKG and evaluation by a qualified allergist to help diagnoses skin allergy.

Occupational Exposure Level/Limit (OEL) & Sampling Methods:

Environmental Sentinel Contamination Action Level (ESCAL): Surface
US American Conference of Governmental Industrial Hygienists (ACGIH):
TLV 2.5 mg/m3 (2.0 mg/m3)
(Method not listed or specified)

Supplemental Response Information

Extinguishing Media: Use extinguishing agent which is the most appropriate to extinguish surrounding fire (carbon dioxide, foam, dry chemical or water fog as extinguishing media). (Do not use water jet.)

Solubility: 5-FLUOROURACIL is slightly water soluble partially soluble in cold water and methanol. Furthermore this material is insoluble in diethyl ether (pH ~ 9.2) (a 1% solution in water has a pH of 4.5 to 5.0).

Chemical Degradation/Neutralization Method: There are two or more recommended procedures (alkaline soap/detergent and bleach [sodium hypochlorite] solution) for 5-FLUOROURACIL (ADRUCIL®53). See below for optional method.

A manufacturer's Material Safety Data Sheet (MSDS) recommends using alkaline soap/detergent and water to clean spill surfaces after absorbing liquids with inert absorbent pads or removing any powder present: repeat using soap and water; sample to determine if surface contamination is still present (if sampling method is available). If drug is still present, repeat above steps; dispose of wastes in accordance with your local procedures, state, and federal regulations.

Incompatibility: 5-FLUOROURACIL is incompatible with strong oxidizing agents, strong bases, and strong acids.

FLUOXYMESTERONE (*floo-oks-ih-MESS-te-rone*)
HALOTESTIN®54

$C_{20}H_{29}FO_3$

ANDROFLUORENE

Chemical Abstract Service (CAS) Registry Number: 76-43-7 (mixture)
RTECS: BV8390000

Health & Safety Hazards/US Department of Transportation (DOT)/US Environmental Protection Agency (EPA)—Sources

Carcinogen G2A—International Agency For Research on Cancer, Teratogen—University of Maryland at College Park, Carcinogen—Material Safety Data Sheet, Reproductive Effector—Material Safety Data Sheet, Reproductive Effector—Registry of Toxic Effects of Chemical Substances (RTECS), Photosensitive—Material Safety Data Sheet, Mutagen—Registry of Toxic Effects of Chemical Substances (RTECS), Pregnancy Category (X) US Food and Drug Administration—US Navy, Developmental Male and Female US California Proposition 65, National Fire Protection Association Health (1) Flammability (1) Instability/Reactivity (0)—Material Safety Data Sheet, Hazardous Materials Identification System (R) and/or US Department of Defense System Health (1) Fire Hazard (1) Reactivity (0) Personal Protection Code (E) (Safety Glasses, Chemical Gloves, Dust Respirator)—Material Safety Data Sheet, Hazardous Materials Identification System (R) and/or US Department of Defense System Health (1★) with additional chronic hazards present Fire Hazard (3) Reactivity (3) Personal Protection Code (-) (None stated)—Material Safety Data Sheet, National Fire Protection Association Health (1) Flammability (3) Instability/Reactivity (3)—Material Safety Data Sheet, National Fire Protection Association Health (0) Flammability (0) Instability/Reactivity (0)—Material Safety Data Sheet, Hazardous Materials Identification System (R) and/or US Department of Defense System Health (0★) with additional chronic hazards present Fire Hazard (0) Reactivity (0) Personal Protection Code (-) (None stated)—Material Safety Data Sheet, Flammable—Material Safety Data Sheet,

Peroxide Former—Material Safety Data Sheet, US California Environmental Protection Agency Listed.

FLUOXYMESTERONE—Male: fertility effects (may be dose dependent; genotoxic effects). Breast-feeding should be discontinued because of potential for reproductive and developmental harm (*A Guide for Occupational Health Professionals Technical Manual*, Navy Environmental Health Center [NEHC-TM-OEM 6260.01a]).

First Aid/Medical Information/ Occupational Exposure Limits

First Aid Measures to include: Use general first aid measures except for the following.

Physician's note: Acute overexposure to FLUOXYMESTERONE requires supportive care and is the only treatment necessary or appropriate for acute intoxication.

Medical Information:

Caution and Warning Statements: Exposure to FLUOXYMESTERONE may impair fertility and pose a possible risk of harm to the unborn child. Anabolic steroid abuse has been known to cause cancer after long-term use. FLUOXYMESTERONE is classified as suspect developmental toxic (female and male).

Acute: Contact (dermal and/or inhalation) with drug may cause skin, eye, and respiratory tract irritation. Ingestion may cause upset stomach, vomiting, diarrhea, bad breath odor, thirst, weight gain, tenderness of the abdomen, abdominal or stomach pain, purple or red spots on the body or inside the mouth or nose, frequent need to pass urine, changes in skin color, edema or fluid retention, itching, hives, changes in sexual desire, and other signs of liver problems. It may also affect behavior/central nervous system. For females: deepening of the voice, clitoral growth, scalp hair loss, acne, absence or changes in menstrual periods, or growth of facial hair. For males: frequent or persistent erections, decrease sperm production, and inhibition of testicular function, difficulty urinating, or acne.

Chronic: Ingestion/inhalation: prolonged or repeated exposure may cause hypersensitivity, with skin manifestations (dermatitis) and anaphylactoid reactions. Prolonged exposure may affect the liver, endocrine system, blood, and may cause adverse reproductive effects and birth defects.

Caution: Females and males planning to have a child, pregnant women, and nursing mothers should exercise caution regarding potential occupational exposure to this cytotoxic drug. No information or not enough information exists or was provided concerning occupational exposure that may potentially occur while handling this drug and its affects on reproductive systems, the fetus, and/or if it is secreted along with breast milk, which may harm nursing infants. Staff members should consult with the occupational health physician monitoring workers' health in your facility to be apprised of potential hazards and should be advised to avoid becoming pregnant and/or breastfeeding or should be transferred in accordance with policy/procedures to other duties that do not involve preparation, handling, and administering this drug.

Therapeutic Levels: Contraindicated during pregnancy due to possible masculinization of the fetus. Breastfeeding is not recommended due to the potential secreted into breast milk.

Human studies have shown that androgens administered during pregnancy cause masculinization of the external genitalia of the female fetus; the degree of masculinization is dose related.

RTECS lists FLUOXYMESTERONE (HALO-TESTIN®54) as a suspected respiratory toxicant and as a skin or sense organ toxicant.

Target Organs/Systems: Liver, kidneys, CNS, endocrine system, blood, male and female reproductive effects (to include impotence in men), virilization in women, premature cardiovascular disease, testicular atrophy, azoospermia, and prostatic hypertrophy in men, and fetus

Medical Conditions Generally Aggravated by Exposure:

- Clinical/Therapeutic Levels: Contraindicated in males with cancer of the prostate. Known hypersensitivity to FLUOXYMESTERONE. If on WARFARIN (COUMADIN) medication, which will cause significant interaction. Males with breast or prostate cancer; hypocalcaemia due to metastatic breast cancer; preexisting liver, kidney, heart problems, and enlarged prostate gland.
- Diabetes, heart disorders, kidney and liver disorders.
- Reproductive and pregnancy issues.

Specific Medical Surveillance Information: Reproductive and pregnancy counseling.

Clinical/Therapeutic: The following tests can be relevant in the investigation of chronic anabolic steroid abuse: full blood count (CBC), electrolytes and renal function tests, hepatic function tests, testosterone, luteinizing hormone, prostatic acid phosphatase or prostate related antigen, blood glucose concentration, calcium, and cholesterol concentration.

Toxicological analysis: Urinary analysis for anabolic steroids and their metabolites.

Occupational Exposure Level/Limit (OEL) & Sampling Methods: Not otherwise specified

Environmental Sentinel Contamination Action Level (ESCAL): Not otherwise specified

Supplemental Response Information

Extinguishing Media: Use extinguishing agent which is the most appropriate to extinguish surrounding fire (carbon dioxide, foam, dry chemical).

Note: Water may be effective for cooling, but may not effect extinguishment.

Solubility: FLUOXYMESTERONE is insoluble in cold water but sparingly (slightly) soluble in alcohol.

Chemical Degradation/Neutralization Method: Short term products of biodegradation are not likely. However, long term degradation products may arise. The products of degradation are more toxic than the product itself.

Incompatibility: FLUOXYMESTERONE is incompatible with oxidizing agents; avoid exposure to light.

FLUTAMIDE (*FLEW-tuh-mide*)
EULEXIN®55
FLUTAMIDE-3H(G)

Chemical Abstract Service (CAS) Registry
   Number: 13311-84-7
RTECS: UG5700000
$C_{11}H_{11}F_3N_2O_3$
(Mixture)

Health & Safety Hazards/US Department of Transportation (DOT)/US Environmental Protection Agency (EPA)—Sources

FLUTAMIDE: Mutagen—University of Maryland at College Park, Teratogen—University of Maryland at College Park, Pregnancy Category (D)—US Food and Drug Administration, Carcinogen—Material Safety Data Sheet, Developmental—US California Proposition 65, US California Environmental Protection Agency Listed, National Fire Protection Association Health (1) Flammability (1) Instability/Reactivity (0)—Material Safety Data Sheet, Flutamide-3h(G): Developmental US California Proposition 65—Material Safety Data Sheet, Neurotoxicant—Scorecard,

Mutagen—University of Maryland at College Park, Teratogen—University of Maryland at College Park, Hazardous Materials Identification System (R) and/or US Department of Defense System Health (2★) with additional chronic hazards present Fire Hazard (3) Reactivity (0) Personal Protection Code (None)—Material Safety Data Sheet, National Fire Protection Association Health (2) Flammability (3) Instability/Reactivity (0)—Material Safety Data Sheet.

EULEXIN®55 (FLUTAMIDE) are available in capsules 125 mg.

FLUTAMIDE is a pale yellow crystalline powder.

FLUTAMIDE causes reduced sperm counts and spermatogenesis in males. Breastfeeding: this drug is only indicated for use in males because of reproductive and developmental harm (*A Guide for Occupational Health Professionals Technical Manual*, Navy Environmental Health Center [NEHC-TM-OEM 6260.01a]).

First Aid/Medical Information/Occupational Exposure Limits

First Aid Measures to include: Use general first aid measures except for the following:

Ingestion: Give copious amounts of water and induce vomiting, if conscious and alert. Obtain medical attention.

Physician's Note: Treatment for overdose should be symptomatic and supportive and may include the following:

1. Administer activated charcoal as a slurry;
2. Consider gastric lavage if it can be performed soon after ingestion unless contraindicated. Control seizures prior to initiation and protect airway;
3. For mild or moderate hypertension, sedation with benzodiazepines may be helpful; for severe hypertension, administer nitroprusside, labetalol, nitroglycerin, or phentolamine;
4. For methemoglobinemia, administer methylene blue intravenously;
5. Monitor liver and kidney function tests and ECG;
6. Hemodialysis is not likely to be effective.

Medical Information:
Caution and Warning Statements:
Warning: Possible carcinogen, antiandrogen inhibits, neutralizes effects of male sex hormones (male reproductive hazard).

Exposure to EULEXIN®55 (FLUTAMIDE/FLU-TAMIDE-3H (G) may cause eyes, skin, and upper respiratory irritation. Exposure may cause sensitization and/or allergic reactions to the skin. Ingestion of large amounts may result in dizziness, nausea, vomiting, hot flashes, impotence, loss of libido, diarrhea, anemia, jaundice, adverse liver effects, and gynecomastia (breast enlargement). EULEXIN®55 capsules contain FLU-TAMIDE which has been shown to suppress sperm production in animal studies. FLUTAMIDE exposure to pregnant women may cause fetal harm. Exposure may produce hot flashes, impotence, loss of libido, diarrhea, nausea, vomiting, and gynecomastia (breast enlargement). In some individuals FLUTAMIDE has caused anemia, jaundice, and adverse live effects. RTECS classified and lists FLUTAMIDE as a suspected neurotoxicant.

Therapeutic Levels: FLUTAMIDE exposure to pregnant women may cause fetal harm. FLUTAMIDE therapy results in reduced sperm count in men. Pregnancy studies in rats found a decrease in the survival of offspring, feminization of male offspring, and other developmental variations in the fetus. Studies in rabbits found a decrease in offspring survival. The antiadrogenic effects of FLUTAMIDE could cause femination of a male fetus in humans. This drug is listed by the Food and Drug Administration as a Pregnancy Category (D).

Food and Drug Administration Pregnancy Category (D): Use in women: EULEXIN®55 capsules are for use only in men. This product has no indication for women, and should not be used in this population, particularly for non-serious or non-life threatening conditions. Fetal toxicity: FLUTAMIDE may cause fetal harm when administered to a pregnant woman.

FLUTAMIDE-3H(G) is highly flammable because of ethyl alcohol mixture.

Target Organs/Systems: FLUTAMIDE: Fetus, male reproductive systems, breast, blood, bladder (cancer), eyes, skin, liver, kidney, and upper respiratory system FLUTAMIDE-3H(G): Nerves, heart, and liver.

Medical Conditions Generally Aggravated by Exposure:

- Hypersensitivity to material impaired liver function, and conditions predisposing to aniline toxicity, such as G6PD deficiency, hemoglobin M disease, or tobacco smoking.
- Reproductive and pregnancy issues.

Specific Medical Surveillance Information: Reproductive and pregnancy counseling.

Occupational Exposure Level/Limit (OEL) & Sampling Methods:

Environmental Sentinel Contamination Action Level (ESCAL): Air, surface

Supplemental Response Information

Extinguishing Media: Use extinguishing agent which is the most appropriate to extinguish surrounding fire (carbon dioxide, foam, dry chemical or water fog as extinguishing media).

Solubility: FLUTAMIDE (EULEXIN®55) is listed as insoluble in water to slightly soluble. FLUTAMIDE is freely soluble in acetone, in ethyl acetate, methanol, and in methyl alcohol; soluble in chloroform and in ether.

Chemical Degradation/Neutralization Method: A manufacturer's Material Safety Data Sheet (MSDS) recommends using alkaline soap (detergent) and water to clean spill surfaces after absorbing liquids with inert absorbent pads or removing any powder present: repeat using soap and water; sample to determine if surface contamination is still present (if sampling method is available). If drug is still present, repeat above steps; dispose of wastes in accordance with your local procedures, state, and federal regulations.

Incompatibility: FLUTAMIDE is incompatible with oxidizers, strong acids, and bases. Avoid contact with moisture.

FLUTAMIDE-3H (G) is incompatible with alkali metals, ammonia, oxidizing, peroxides, acid anhydrides, acid chlorides, and acids. Avoid contact with moisture.

G

GANCICLOVIR (*gan-SYE-kloe-veer*)
VITRASERT®57
VALCYTE®58
CYTOVENE®56

RS21592

DHPG

Chemical Abstract Service (CAS) Registry
     Number: 82410-32-0
RTECS: MF8407000
$C_9\text{-}H_{13}\text{-}N_5\text{-}O_4$

GANCICLOVIR SODIUM
CYTOVENE®56

C_9-H_{13}-N_5-O_4NA

CYMEVENE®59

Chemical Abstract Service (CAS) Registry
Number: 84245-13-6
RTECS: MF8407000
BW759U
RS21592-030

Health & Safety Hazards/US Department of Transportation (DOT)/US Environmental Protection Agency (EPA)—Sources

Potential Carcinogen—Material Safety Data Sheet, Reproductive Effector—Material Safety Data Sheet, Teratogen—Material Safety Data Sheet, Mutagen—Material Safety Data Sheet, Mutagen Toxic—Material Safety Data Sheet, Pregnancy Category (C)—US Food and Drug Administration (US) and US Navy, Pregnancy Category (D)—US Food and Drug Administration (AU), Toxic—Material Safety Data Sheet, Carcinogen and Developmental Male US California Proposition 65, Vesicant—Material Safety Data Sheet, Hazardous Materials Identification System (R) and/or US Department of Defense System Health (4) Fire hazard (0) Reactivity (1) Personal Protection Code (-) (None stated)—Material Safety Data Sheet; Hazardous Materials Identification System (R) and/or US Department of Defense System Health (2) Fire Hazard (0) Reactivity (1) Personal Protection Code (X) (ask supervisor)—Material Safety Data Sheet, Hazardous Materials Identification System (R) and/or US Department of Defense System Health (1★) with additional chronic hazards present Fire Hazard (1) Reactivity (0) Personal Protective Code (A) (Safety Glasses)—Material Safety Data Sheet; National Fire Protection Association Health (2) Flammability (1) Instability/Reactivity (0)—Material Safety Data Sheet; National Fire Protection Association Health (4) Flammability (0) Instability/Reactivity (1)—Material Safety Data Sheet; National Fire Protection Association Health (1) Flammability (1) Instability/Reactivity (0)—Material Safety Data Sheet, US California Environmental Protection Agency Listed.

GANCICLOVIR is available in capsules, injection, IV, and intravitreal implant.

GANCICLOVIR is an odorless solid white crystalline powder.

GANCICLOVIR may be teratogenic or embryotoxic; breastfeeding should be discontinued because of potential for reproductive and developmental harm (*A Guide for Occupational Health Professionals Technical Manual*, Navy Environmental Health Center [NEHC-TM-OEM 6260.01a]).

VALGANCICLOVIR HCL is available as a 450 mg tablet; VALGANCICLOVIR HCL is a white to off-white crystalline powder.

VITRASERT®57 is an implant containing GANCICLOVIR.

GANCICLOVIR (CYTOVENE®56) capsules (250 mg and 500 mg) and is available as an injection/IV.

GANCICLOVIR (CYTOVENE®56) capsules (250 mg and 500 mg) and is available as an injection/IV (a white to off-white lyophilized powder).

CYTOVENE®56 is supplied as green capsules and as yellow and green capsules.

First Aid/Medical Information/Occupational Exposure Limits

First Aid Measures to include: Use general first aid measures except for the following:

Ingestion: GANCICLOVIR—if ingested, rinse out mouth and drink plenty of water (if conscious and alert). Seek medical attention.

GANCICLOVIR SODIUM—*Ingestion*: Give moderate amount (8–12 oz) of water and immediately seek medical assistance.

Physician's note: Physician should treat symptomatically and supportively. Preserve blood and urine samples for analysis.

Medical Information:

Caution and Warning Statements: GANCICLOVIR is toxic, may cause heritable genetic damage, may harm unborn child, may impair fertility, may cause blood changes. May cause cancer based on animal data. May cause birth defects based on animal data. May cause reproductive systems effects (lower parental fertility—male reproductive toxicity [aspermatogenesis]). There is a danger of serious damage to health by prolonged exposure. GANCICLOVIR may cause damage to the following organs: digestive system, head, and muscle tissue.

GANCICLOVIR SODIUM is a possible carcinogen and is a birth defect hazard. This drug may cause respiratory tract, skin, and eye irritation; and may be harmful if ingested.

CYTOVENE®56 (GANCICLOVIR SODIUM) should be considered a potential carcinogen and teratogenic in humans. Animal studies have shown that this product was mutagenic in several standard mutagenicity assays. Caution should be exercised in the handling and preparation of CYTOVENE®56 (GANCICLOVIR SODIUM), since the reconstituted solution is alkaline (pH ~11) and acute (one-time) exposure may cause severe eye irritation and skin irritation. Repeated administration or overexposure to CYTOVENE®56 has the potential to cause blood disorders, reproductive systems disorders, and cancer; avoid ingestion, inhalation, skin contact, and eye contact.

GANCICLOVIR SODIUM: Animal and in vitro studies have shown that GANCICLOVIR should be considered a potential teratogen and carcinogen in humans. It may cause birth defects and/or death to the exposed fetus. All work practices must be designed to reduce human exposure to the lowest level.

GANCICLOVIR SODIUM: The most common dose-dependent adverse effects associated with therapeutic treatments include decrease in the number of neutrophils in the blood, decrease in the number of platelets in the blood, and elevated serum creatinine levels. Less common side effects include enlarged abdomen, weakness, chest pain, swelling, headache, fatigue, pain, abnormal liver function test, canker sores in the mouth, constipation, indigestion, pancytopenia, increased coughing, difficulty breathing, abnormal dreams, anxiety, confusion, depression, dizziness, dry mouth, insomnia, seizures, sleepiness, tremor, hair loss, dry skin, abnormal pressure, kidney failure, abnormal taste, ringing in the ears, weight loss, increased SGOT, increased SGPT, high blood pressure, kidney failure, abnormal kidney function, increased urination, pancreatitis, and sepsis.

Caution: Females and males planning to have a child, pregnant women, and nursing mothers should exercise caution regarding potential occupational exposure to this cytotoxic drug. No information or not enough information exists or was provided concerning occupational exposure that may potentially occur while handling this drug and its affects on reproductive systems, the fetus, and/or if it is secreted along with breast milk, which may harm nursing infants. Staff members should consult with the occupational health physician monitoring workers' health in your facility to be apprised of potential hazards and should be advised to avoid becoming pregnant and/or breastfeeding or should be transferred in accordance with policy/procedures to other duties that do not involve preparation, handling, and administering this drug.

Therapeutic Levels: GANCICLOVIR/GANCICLOVIR SODIUM may be teratogenic or embryo-

toxic at dose levels recommended for human use. There are no adequate and well-controlled studies in pregnant women.

Target Organs/Systems: GANCICLOVIR—Skin, eyes, head, digestive system, muscle tissue, hematopoietic/blood system/bone marrow, CNS, male reproductive systems/ prostate, and female reproductive systems

GANCICLOVIR SODIUM—Blood, bone marrow, reproductive systems, skin, and eyes

Medical Conditions Generally Aggravated by Exposure:

- GANCICLOVIR/GANCICLOVIR SODIUM—Any preexisting conditions related to skin, eyes, blood system, and pregnancy. Repeated exposure to a highly toxic material may produce general deterioration of health by an accumulation in one or more human organs.
- Reproductive and pregnancy issues.

Specific Medical Surveillance Information: Reproductive and pregnancy counseling.

Occupational Exposure Level/Limit (OEL) & Sampling Methods:

Environmental Sentinel Contamination Action Level (ESCAL): Not otherwise specified

Occupational Exposure Level (OEL) F. Hoffmann and La-Roche:

IOELV: 5 µg/m3 sampling on glass fiber and chemical determination of the active compound (EG HPLC).

(Method not listed or specified)

Occupational Exposure Level (OEL) Syntex (Ganciclovir)

5 µg/m3 (8 hr Time-Weighted Average [TWA])

Occupational Exposure Level (OEL) Roche:

0.005 mg/m3

(Method not listed or specified)

Supplemental Response Information

Extinguishing Media: Use extinguishing agent which is the most appropriate to extinguish surrounding fire (carbon dioxide, foam, dry chemical or water fog as extinguishing media). (Do not use water jet.)

Solubility: GANCICLOVIR *SODIUM*: GANCICLOVIR solubility is as follows: Hot water; water (2.67 g/l), acidic water; alkaline water.

CYTOVENE®56 (GANCICLOVIR SODIUM) is water soluble in hot water, acids, or bases.

Chemical Degradation/Neutralization Method: Not otherwise specified

Note: If a specific degradation or neutralization method is not provided on this table and you do not have other specific information that will guide you on how to clean up the specific material spilled, then follow the general spill procedure found at the introduction section of this table.

Incompatibility: GANCICLOVIR is incompatible with strong oxidizers (peroxides, permanganates, nitric acid, etc.), strong acids, and bases.

GEMTUZUMAB OZOGAMYCIN (1)
MYLOTARG®60
ANTI-CD33

> Chemical Abstract Service (CAS) Registry
> Number: 220578-59-6 (mixture)
> (Two Degradation Methods)

Health & Safety Hazards/US Department of Transportation (DOT)/US Environmental Protection Agency (EPA)—Sources

Cytotoxic—Box Instruction, Pregnancy Category D—US Food and Drug Administration.

MYLOTARG®60 is available as an injection.

First Aid/Medical Information/ Occupational Exposure Limits

First Aid Measures to include: Use general first aid measures.

Medical Information:

Caution and Warning Statements:

Caution: The toxicological properties of most cytotoxic drugs have not been fully investigated, particularly as it pertains to occupational exposure. GEMTUZUMAB OZOGAMYCIN (MYLOTARG®60) is one of the drugs that has little occupational hazards information available. Therefore, therapeutic dose information was extrapolated below to assist in determining occupational toxicity, and signs and symptoms of overexposure. Therefore, it is prudent to minimize occupational exposure to GEMTUZUMAB OZOGAMYCIN (MYLOTARG®60).

GEMTUZUMAB OZOGAMYCIN (MYLOTARG®60) may cause decrease in bone marrow production, low red blood cell counts (anemia), low blood platelets, infection, bleeding, swelling of the membrane inside the mouth, liver problems, kidney problems, joint pain (gout), chills, fever, nausea, vomiting, headache, changes in blood pressure, low levels of oxygen in the body, and rash.

Caution: Females and males planning to have a child, pregnant women, and nursing mothers should exercise caution regarding potential occupational exposure to this cytotoxic drug. No information or not enough information exists or was provided concerning occupational exposure that may potentially occur while handling this drug and its affects on reproductive systems, the fetus, and/or if it is secreted along with breast milk, which may harm nursing infants. Staff members should consult with the occupational health physician monitoring workers' health in your facility to be apprised of potential hazards and should be advised to avoid becoming pregnant and/or breastfeeding or should be transferred in accordance with policy/procedures to other duties that do not involve preparation, handling, and administering this drug.

Therapeutic Levels: Breastfeeding: it is not known if MYLOTARG®60 (GEMTUZUMAB OZOGAMYCIN) is excreted in human milk; a decision should be made whether to discontinue nursing or to avoid potential exposure because many drugs are excreted in human milk, and the potential for serious adverse reactions in nursing infants exists.

Target Organs/Systems: Bone marrow, blood, spleen, liver, and kidneys

Medical Conditions Generally Aggravated by Exposure:

- Liver disease and hypersensitivity to GEMTUZUMAB OZOGAMICIN or any of its components. Prior therapy with anti-CD33 antibodies and in those known to have hypersensitivity to compounds of its type or any constituents of its formulation.
- Reproductive and pregnancy issues.
- GEMTUZUMAB OZOGAMICIN may lower your body's resistance and there is a chance you might get the infection the immunization is meant to prevent. In addition, other persons living in your household should not take oral polio vaccine since there is a chance they could pass the polio virus on to you. Also, avoid persons who have taken oral polio vaccine within the last several months. Do not get close to them, and do not stay in the same room with them for very long. If you cannot take these precautions, you should consider wearing a protective face mask that covers the nose and mouth.
- GEMTUZUMAB OZOGAMICIN can temporarily lower the number of white blood cells in your blood, increasing the chance of getting an infection. It can also lower the

number of platelets, which is necessary for proper blood clotting.

Specific Medical Surveillance Information: Reproductive and pregnancy counseling.

If an overdose occurs, blood pressure and blood counts should be carefully monitored.

Occupational Exposure Level/Limit (OEL) & Sampling Methods:

Environmental Sentinel Contamination Action Level (ESCAL): Not otherwise specified
Occupational Exposure Level: MYLOTARG®60 GEMTUZUMAB OZOGAMICIN (American Home Products)
0.1 μg/m3
(Method not listed or specified)

Supplemental Response Information

Extinguishing Media: Use extinguishing agent which is the most appropriate to extinguish surrounding fire (carbon dioxide, foam, dry chemical or water fog as extinguishing media).

Solubility: MYLOTARG®60 (GEMTUZUMAB OZOGAMYCIN) is water soluble. (MYLOTARG®60) (GEMTUZUMAB OZOGANYCIN) has a pH of 7.4 when reconstituted as a solution.

Chemical Degradation/Neutralization Method: There are two degradation or neutralization procedures:

A manufacturer's (American Home Products) Material Safety Data Sheet (MSDS) recommends two degradation or neutralization procedures.

First recommended procedure is presented here and the second procedure is located below:

States that steam autoclaving at 128 deg. C for at least 2 hours can be used as an alternative decontamination procedure.

Decontamination using the above mixture destroys the enediyne "warhead" structure of calicheamicin, that portion of the molecule responsible for the DNA-damaging effects. In vivo toxicology, testing of NAC-epsilon calicheamicin (which is representative of the calicheamicin molecule in which the enediyne structure has been chemically destroyed) was found to be non-toxic in rats and dogs.

Wherever feasible both procedures should be utilized to provided additional safe guards to ensure that degradation or neutralization or decontamination has occurred along with environmental surface monitoring as verification.

Incompatibility: MYLOTARG®60 (GEMTUZUMAB OZOGAMICIN) is incompatible with bases, acids, sunlight and direct fluorescent light.

GEMTUZUMAB OZOGAMYCIN (2)

(gem-TOO-zoo-mab oh-zog-a-MY-sin)
MYLOTARG®60 (2)
FORMULA: Unknown
ANTI-CD33

Chemical Abstract Service (CAS) Registry Number: 220578-59-6 (mixture)
(Two Degradation Methods)

Health & Safety Hazards/US Department of Transportation (DOT)/US Environmental Protection Agency (EPA)—Sources

Cytotoxic—Box Instruction, Pregnancy Category (D)—US Food and Drug Administrative.
MYLOTARG®60 is available as an injection.

First Aid/Medical Information/ Occupational Exposure Limits

First Aid Measures to include: Use general first aid measures.

Medical Information:

Caution and Warning Statements:

Caution: The toxicological properties of most cytotoxic drugs have not been fully investigated, particularly as it pertains to occupational exposure. GEMTUZUMAB OZOGAMYCIN (MYLOTARG®60) is one of the drugs that has little occupational hazards information available. Therefore, therapeutic dose information was extrapolated below to assist in determining occupational toxicity, and signs and symptoms of overexposure. Therefore, it is prudent to minimize occupational exposure to GEMTUZUMAB OZOGAMYCIN (MYLOTARG®60).

GEMTUZUMAB OZOGAMYCIN (MYLOTARG®60) may cause decrease in bone marrow production, low red blood cell counts (anemia), low blood platelets, infection, bleeding, swelling of the membrane inside the mouth, liver problems, tested, spleen, kidney problems, joint pain (gout), chills, fever, nausea, vomiting, headache, changes in blood pressure, low levels of oxygen in the body, and rash. This drug may cause birth defects (based on animal data).

Caution: Females and males planning to have a child, pregnant women, and nursing mothers should exercise caution regarding potential occupational exposure to this cytotoxic drug. No information or not enough information exists or was provided concerning occupational exposure that may potentially occur while handling this drug and its affects on reproductive systems, the fetus, and/or if it is secreted along with breast milk, which may harm nursing infants. Staff members should consult with the occupational health physician monitoring workers' health in your facility to be apprised of potential hazards and should be advised to avoid becoming pregnant and/or breastfeeding or should be transferred in accordance with policy/procedures to other duties that do not involve preparation, handling, and administering this drug.

Therapeutic Levels: Breastfeeding: it is not known if MYLOTARG®60 (GEMTUZUMAB OZOGAMYCIN) is excreted in human milk; a decision should be made whether to discontinue nursing or to avoid potential exposure because many drugs are excreted in human milk, and the potential for serious adverse reactions in nursing infants exists.

Target Organs/Systems: Bone marrow, blood, spleen, liver and kidneys

Medical Conditions Generally Aggravated by Exposure:

- Reproductive and pregnancy issues.
- Liver disease and hypersensitivity to GEMTUZUMAB OZOGAMICIN or any of its components. Prior therapy with anti-CD33 antibodies and in those known to have hypersensitivity to compounds of its type or any constituents of its formulation.
- GEMTUZUMAB OZOGAMICIN may lower your body's resistance and there is a chance you might get the infection the immunization is meant to prevent. In addition, other persons living in your household should not take oral polio vaccine since there is a chance they could pass the polio virus on to you. Also, avoid persons who have taken oral polio vaccine within the last several months. Do not get close to them, and do not stay in the same room with them for very long. If you cannot take these precautions, you should consider wearing a protective face mask that covers the nose and mouth.
- GEMTUZUMAB OZOGAMICIN can temporarily lower the number of white blood cells in your blood, increasing the chance of getting an infection. It can also lower the number of platelets, which is necessary for proper blood clotting.

Specific Medical Surveillance Information: Reproductive and pregnancy counseling.

If an overdose occurs, blood pressure and blood counts should be carefully monitored.

Occupational Exposure Level/Limit (OEL) & Sampling Methods:

Environmental Sentinel Contamination Action Level (ESCAL): Not otherwise specified
Occupational Exposure Level (OEL)
MYLOTARG®60 GEMTUZUMAB OZOGAMICIN (American Home Products): 0.1 µg/m3
(Method not listed or specified)

Supplemental Response Information

Extinguishing Media: Use extinguishing agent which is the most appropriate to extinguish surrounding fire (carbon dioxide, foam, dry chemical or water fog as extinguishing media).

Solubility: MYLOTARG®60 (GEMTUZUMAB OZOGAMYCIN) is very water soluble. MYLOTARG ®60 (GEMTUZUMAB OZOGANYCIN) has a pH of 7.4 when reconstituted as a solution.

Chemical Degradation/Neutralization Method: There are two degradation or neutralization procedures.

A manufacturer's (American Home Products) Material Safety Data Sheet (MSDS) recommends two degradation or neutralization procedures.

First recommended procedure is listed above and the second procedure is as follows:

Decontaminate equipment, spills, and spill sites by using a 3% sodium hypochlorite (1:1 ratio of household bleach and water). Wet surfaces first prior to applying mixture. Allow to stand for 15 minutes. Wipe down surfaces and rinse with clean water.

Decontamination using the above mixture destroys the enediyne "warhead" structure of calicheamicin, that portion of the molecule responsible for the DNA-damaging effects. In vivo toxicology, testing of NAC-epsilon calicheamicin (which is representative of the calicheamicin molecule in which the enediyne structure has been chemically destroyed) was found to be non-toxic in rats and dogs.

Note: Whenever feasible both procedures should be utilized to provided additional safe guards to ensure that degradation or neutralization or decontamination has occurred along with environmental surface monitoring as verification. The second procedure is located below.

Incompatibility: MYLOTARG®60 (GEMTUZUMAB OZOGAMICIN) is incompatible with bases, acids, sunlight, and direct fluorescent light.

GEMZAR®61

51-53% CONCEN
GEMCITABINE HCL (gem-SIGHT-a-been)
GEMCIN®62
GEMTRO®63

Chemical Abstract Service (CAS) Registry
Numbers: 95058-81-4, 12211-03-9
RTECS: HA3840000
C_9-H_{11}-F_2-N_3-O_4 . Cl-H

Health & Safety Hazards/US Department of Transportation (DOT)/US Environmental Protection Agency (EPA)—Sources

Mutagen—Material Safety Data Sheet, Reproductive Effector—Material Safety Data Sheet, Teratogen—Material Safety Data Sheet, Skin Permeable—Material Safety Data Sheet, Cytotoxic—British Columbia Cancer Agency Canada, Nonvesicant—British Columbia Cancer Agency Canada, Pregnancy Category (D)—US Food and Drug Administration, National Fire Protection Association Health (2) Flammability (1) Instability/Reactivity (0) (R) = Reproductive and Blood Effects Special Hazards—Material Safety Data Sheet, UN 2811, Class 6.1, Group III.

GEMICITABINE is a colorless fluid from a white powder.

GEMCITABINE HCL is an off-white crystalline powder.

First Aid/Medical Information/ Occupational Exposure Limits

First Aid Measures to include: Use general first aid measures except for the following:

Ingestion: Do not induce vomiting. If available and the victim is conscious and alert, administer activated charcoal (6–8 heaping teaspoons) with two to three glasses of water. Seek medical assistance.

Medical Information: GEMZAR®61 is skin permeable, an irritant, reproductive effector, and causes blood effects. Effects of exposure may include decreased fertility, fetal changes, and decrease blood cell counts. Elevated liver enzymes and flu-like syndrome; decrease sperm formation and decreased fertility in males and reproductive tissue changes. Dosed toxic to the mother depresses fetal viability, weight, and malformations. Absorption occurs through the skin in amounts capable of producing systemic toxicity and may be irritating to the eyes and skin (GEMZAR®61).

Effects of exposure due to therapeutic use may include, but not limited to, decreased blood cell counts, nausea, vomiting, edema, rash, elevated liver enzymes, and flu-like syndrome.

Caution: Females and males planning to have a child, pregnant women, and nursing mothers should exercise caution regarding potential occupational exposure to this cytotoxic drug. No information or not enough information exists or was provided concerning occupational exposure that may potentially occur while handling this drug and its affects on reproductive systems, the fetus, and/or if it is secreted along with breast milk, which may harm nursing infants. Staff members should consult with the occupational health physician monitoring workers' health in your facility to be apprised of potential hazards and should be advised to avoid becoming pregnant and/or breastfeeding or should be transferred in accordance with policy/procedures to other duties that do not involve preparation, handling, and administering this drug.

Target Organs/Systems: Skin, reproductive systems, blood effects (decreased red blood cell, white blood cell, and platelet counts), bone marrow, liver, and fetus

Medical Conditions Generally Aggravated by Exposure:

- Reproductive and pregnancy issues.

Specific Medical Surveillance Information: Reproductive and pregnancy counseling. GEMCITABINE may result in toxicities of other bodily systems including the hepatic (liver), renal (kidneys), and pulmonary (lungs) systems. For this reason the function of these systems should be monitored throughout treatment to prevent severe complications.

Occupational Exposure Level/Limit (OEL) & Sampling Methods:

Environmental Sentinel Contamination Action Level (ESCAL): Air, surface
Occupational Exposure Level (OEL) Lilly Exposure
Guidance/Method:
GEMCITABINE (95058-81-4)
Leg 0.3 µg/m3 TWA for 8 hours,
Leg 0.2 µg/m3 for 12 hours; Excursion Limit
2.4 µg/m3 for no more than a total of 30 minutes.
(Method not listed or specified)

Supplemental Response Information

Extinguishing Media: Use extinguishing agent which is the most appropriate to extinguish surrounding fire (carbon dioxide, foam, dry chemical or water fog as extinguishing media).

Solubility: GEMZAR®61 is water soluble with a pH of ~2.3; slightly soluble in methanol; and insoluble in polar organic solvents.

Chemical Degradation/Neutralization Method: Not otherwise specified

Note: If a specific degradation or neutralization method is not provided on this table and you do not have other specific information that will guide you on how to clean up the specific material spilled, then follow the general spill procedure found at the introduction section of this table.

Incompatibility: GEMCITABINE HYDROCHLORIDE may react with strong oxidizing agents (e.g., peroxides, permanganates, nitric acid, etc.).

GOSERELIN ACETATE
ZOLADEX®64

Chemical Abstract Service (CAS) Registry
Number: 145781-92-6

GOSERELIN (GOE-se-rel-in)

Chemical Abstract Service (CAS) Registry
Number: 65807-02-5
RTECS: OK6369900
$C_{59}-H_{84}-N_{18}-O_{14}$
$C_{59}H_{84}N_{18}O_{14} \cdot (C_2H_4O_2)$

Health & Safety Hazards/US Department of Transportation (DOT)/US Environmental Protection Agency (EPA)—Sources

Reproductive Effector—Material Safety Data Sheet, Pregnancy Category (X)—US Food and Drug Administration and US Navy), Developmental Male and Female—US California Proposition 65, Hazardous Materials Identification System (R) and/or US Department of Defense System Health (1) Flammability (0) Instability/Reactivity (0) Personal Protection Code (-) (None Stated)—Material Safety Data Sheet, National Fire Protection Association Health (1) Flammability (0) Instability/Reactivity (0)—Material Safety Data Sheet.

GOSERELIN are available as implants (10.8 mg).

GOSEREOIN ACETATE—Avoid pregnancy for 12 weeks after discontinuing use; breastfeeding is con-traindicated because of potential for reproductive and developmental harm (*A Guide for Occupational Health Professionals Technical Manual*, Navy Environmental Health Center [NEHC-TM-OEM 6260.01a]).

First Aid/Medical Information/ Occupational Exposure Limits

First Aid Measures to include: Use general first aid measures.

Medical Information:

Caution and Warning Statements: May cause reproductive effects in males and females and may impair fertility. Exposure to GOSERELIN ACETATE (ZOLADEX®64) may cause hot flashes, pain, gynecomastia, pelvic pain, bone pain, hypotension, headache, depression, gout, hyperglycemia, and asthenia.

Caution: Females and males planning to have a child, pregnant women, and nursing mothers should exercise caution regarding potential occupational exposure to this cytotoxic drug. No information or not enough information exists or was provided concerning occupational exposure that may potentially occur while handling this drug and its affects on reproductive systems, the fetus, and/or if it is secreted along with breast milk, which may harm nursing infants. Staff members should consult with the occupational health physician monitoring workers' health in your facility to be apprised of potential hazards and should be advised to avoid becoming pregnant and/or breastfeeding or should be transferred in accordance with policy/procedures to other duties that do not involve preparation, handling, and administering this drug.

Target Organs/Systems: Fetus and reproductive systems

Medical Conditions Generally Aggravated by Exposure:

- Reproductive and pregnancy issues.

Specific Medical Surveillance Information: Reproductive and pregnancy counseling.

Occupational Exposure Level/Limit (OEL) & Sampling Methods:

Environmental Sentinel Contamination Action Level (ESCAL): Not otherwise specified
Occupational Exposure Level (OEL)
ASTRAZENCA:
ZOLADEX®64 (GOSERELIN ACETATE)
0.0025 mg/m3 STEL/Ceiling
(Method not listed or specified)

Supplemental Response Information

Extinguishing Media: Use extinguishing agent which is the most appropriate to extinguish surrounding fire (carbon dioxide, foam, dry chemical or water fog as extinguishing media).

Solubility: GOSERELIN ACETATE (ZOLA-DEX®64) is water soluble. It is freely soluble in glacial acetic acid.

Chemical Degradation/Neutralization Method: Not otherwise specified

Note: If a specific degradation or neutralization method is not provided on this table and you do not have other specific information that will guide you on how to clean up the specific material spilled, then follow the general spill procedure found at the introduction section of this table.

Incompatibility: Incompatible with oxidizing agents.

H

HYDROXYUREA (*hi-DROX-e-u-ria*)

HU
HYDREA®65
HYDROYCARBAMIDE (hi-DROX-e-car-ba-mide)
DROXIA®66

Chemical Abstract Service (CAS) Registry
   Number: 127-07-1
$CH_4N_2O_2$

HYDROXYUREA

RTECS: YT4900000

Health & Safety Hazards/US Department of Transportation (DOT)/US Environmental Protection Agency (EPA)—Sources

Carcinogen G3—International Agency for Research on Cancer, Mutagen—University of Maryland at College Park, Teratogen—University of Maryland at College Park, Pregnancy Category (D)—US Food and Drug Administration, Developmental—US California Proposition 65, Toxic—Material Safety Data Sheet, Teratogen—Material Safety Data Sheet, Irritant—Material Safety Data Sheet, Reproductive Effector—Material Safety Data Sheet, National Fire Protection Association Health (0) Flammability (0) Instability/Reactivity (1)—Material Safety Data Sheet, National Fire Protection Association Health (1) Flammability (0) Instability/Reactivity (0)—Material Safety Data Sheet, National Fire Protection Association Health (2) Flammability (0) Instability/Reactivity (0)—Material Safety Data Sheet, National Fire Protection Association Health (2) Flammability (1) Instability/Reactivity (0)—Material Safety Data Sheet, Hazardous Materials Identification System (R) and/or US Department of Defense System Health (2) Fire Hazard (1) Reactivity (0) Personal Protection Code (E) (Safety Glasses, Chemical Gloves, Dust Respirator)—Material Safety Data Sheet, Hazardous Materials Identification System (R) and/or US Department of Defense System Health (0★) with additional chronic hazards present Fire Hazard (0) Reactivity (1) Personal Protection Code (-) (None stated)—Material Safety Data Sheet, UN 1851.

HYDROXYCARBAMIDE is manufactured as a pink/green 500 mg capsules.

HYDROXYCABAMIDE is a white or off-white hydroscopic crystalline powder, it exhibits polymorphism.

HYDROXYUREA—Male: testicular atrophy, impaired spermatogenesis; embryotoxic, fetal malformations; breastfeeding is contraindicated and is incompatible because the drug is excreted in human milk. This drug poses reproductive and developmental hazards if exposed to it (*A Guide for Occupational Health Professionals Technical Manual*, Navy Environmental Health Center [NEHC-TM-OEM 6260.01a]).

First Aid/Medical Information/ Occupational Exposure Limits

First Aid Measures to include: Use general first aid measures except for the following:

Ingestion: If victim is conscious and alert, give 2–4 cups of milk or water. Seek medical attention.

Physician's note: Induce vomiting if ingested within 3 hours. Treat symptomatically and supportively.

Dermal contact: Follow general first aid measures first. Cover the irritated skin with an emollient (antibacterial cream). Seek medical attention.

Medical Information:

Caution and Warning Statements: HYDROXYUREA is harmful: possible risk of irreversible effects through inhalation, in contact with skin, and if swallowed. There is a risk of impaired fertility. Exposure may cause heritable genetic and may cause harm to unborn child. HYDROXYUREA is harmful by inhalation, in contact with skin, and if swallowed. May cause eye and skin irritation. RTECS lists HYDROXYUREA as a suspected cardiovascular or blood toxicant.

Exposure to HYDROXYUREA can cause reduced resistance to infection, increased bleeding tendency, anemia, weakness, nausea, vomiting, diarrhea, sore mouth, and stomach pain. At higher levels, hair loss and skin rash may occur along with liver, kidney, and nervous system damage.

Caution: Females and males planning to have a child, pregnant women, and nursing mothers should exercise caution regarding potential occupational exposure to this cytotoxic drug. No information or not enough information exists or was provided concerning occupational exposure that may potentially occur while handling this drug and its affects on reproductive systems, the fetus, and/or if it is secreted along with breast milk, which may harm nursing infants. Staff members should consult with the occupational health physician monitoring workers' health in your facility to be apprised of potential hazards and should be advised to avoid becoming pregnant and/or breastfeeding or should be transferred in accordance with policy/procedures to other duties that do not involve preparation, handling, and administering this drug.

Target Organs/Systems: Bone marrow, blood, GI tract, skin, reproductive and upper respiratory systems, liver and kidneys, fetus, CNS, and eyes

Medical Conditions Generally Aggravated by Exposure:

- Anemia, leukopenia, and thrombocytopenia.
- Reproductive and pregnancy issues.

Specific Medical Surveillance Information: Reproductive and pregnancy counseling.

If symptoms develop and/or overexposure is suspected, order a complete blood count (repeat at least monthly if there is frequent exposure), liver and kidney functions tests, and an examination of the nervous system.

Occupational Exposure Level/Limit (OEL) & Sampling Methods:

Environmental Sentinel Contamination Action Level (ESCAL): Air

Occupational Exposure Level (OEL) Bristol-Myers Squibb:

OEL/exposure guidelines

0.1 mg/m3 8 hour TWA

Adherence to the exposure guideline will ensure that a worker is not exposed to more than 0.1% of the lowest recommended oral therapeutic dose of HYDROXYUREA and should protect employees who handle HYDROXYUREA from experiencing pharmacological affects of this drug. This substance is a weak mutagen. Adherence to the exposure guideline should minimize the potential for mutagenic changes to occur in cells of persons who handle this material. (Method not listed or specified)

Supplemental Response Information

Extinguishing Media: Use extinguishing agent which is the most appropriate to extinguish surrounding fire (carbon dioxide, foam, dry chemical or water fog as extinguishing media).

Solubility: HYDROXYUREA is freely water soluble: >10 g/100 ml at 21 c, pH is 6.1 (2% solution of HYDROXYUREA). HYDROXYUREA is practically insoluble to slightly soluble in alcohol; freely soluble in hot alcohol.

Chemical Degradation/Neutralization Method: Not otherwise specified

Note: If a specific degradation or neutralization method is not provided on this table and you do not have other specific information that will guide you on how to clean up the specific material spilled, then follow the general spill procedure found at the introduction section of this table.

Incompatibility: HYDROXYUREA is incompatible with strong oxidizing agents and moisture.

I

IBRITUMOMAB TIUXETAN
(ib-rih-TOO-mo-mab)
ZEVALIN®67

Chemical Abstract Service (CAS) Registry Numbers: 206181-63-7, 174722-31-7

$C_{6382}H_{9830}N_{1672}O_{1979}S_{54}$

Health & Safety Hazards/US Department of Transportation (DOT)/US Environmental Protection Agency (EPA)—Sources

Pregnancy Category (None)—US Food and Drug, National Fire Protection Association Health (0) Flammability (0) Instability/Reactivity (0)—Material Safety Data Sheet.

IBRITUMOMAB TIUXETAN is available as an injection.

First Aid/Medical Information/Occupational Exposure Limits

First Aid Measures to include: Use general first aid measures except for the following:

Ingestion/inhalation/skin: Antidote—Remove source of exposure, administer acetaminophen, diphenhydramine, and occasionally intravenous saline or bronchodilators.

Medical Information:

Caution and Warning Statements: Exposure may be irritating to eyes, respiratory system, and skin. This material is not readily absorbed through skin. Toxicological properties have not yet been thoroughly investigated.

Therapeutic doses may cause severe lung problems (hypoxia, pulmonary infiltrates, ARDS), heart problems (cardiogenic shock, Mi, ventricular fibrillation), and blood disorders (cytopenias). Other serious side effects are dizziness (lightheadedness), irregular heartbeat, or chest pain.

Target Organs/Systems: Eyes, respiratory system, heart, blood, and skin

Medical Conditions Generally Aggravated by Exposure:

- Patient information: medical history, especially of blood disorders (e.g., anemia, neutropenia, and thrombocytopenia), previous bone marrow therapy (myeloablative), current infections, and any allergies.
- Patient information: this medication is not recommended for use during pregnancy; it may cause fetal harm. Women of childbearing age, and men, are recommended to use effective birth control methods during and for up to 1 year after treatment with this drug.

Specific Medical Surveillance Information: Not otherwise specified

Occupational Exposure Level/Limit (OEL) & Sampling Methods: Not otherwise specific

Environmental Sentinel Contamination Action Level (ESCAL): Not otherwise specified

Supplemental Response Information

Extinguishing Media: Use extinguishing agent which is the most appropriate to extinguish surrounding fire (carbon dioxide, foam, dry chemical or water fog as extinguishing media).

Solubility: Not otherwise specified

Chemical Degradation/Neutralization Method: Not otherwise specified

Note: If a specific degradation or neutralization method is not provided on this table and you do not have other specific information that will guide you on how to clean up the specific material spilled, then follow the general spill procedure found at the introduction section of this table.

Incompatibility: Not otherwise specified

IDARUBICIN (*eye-da-ROO-bi-cin*)
IDAMYCIN®68

Chemical Abstract Service (CAS) Registry
Number: 58957-92-9

IDARUBICIN

$C_{26}H_{27}NO_9$.HCL
Chemical Abstract Service (CAS) Registry
Number: 57852-57-0

IDARUBICIN HCL

RTECS: HB7877000

Health & Safety Hazards/US Department of Transportation (DOT)/US Environmental Protection Agency (EPA)—Sources

Carcinogen—International Agency for Research on Cancer, Highly Toxic—Material Safety Data Sheet, Teratogen—Material Safety Data Sheet, Cytotoxic—Material Safety Data Sheet, Cytotoxic—British Columbia Cancer Agency Canada, Mutagen—Material Safety Data Sheet, Reproductive Effector—Material Safety Data Sheet, Vesicant—British Columbia Cancer Agency Canada, Pregnancy Category (D)—US Food and Drug Administration, Developmental Male—US California Proposition 65, National Fire Protection Association Health (3) Flammability (0) Instability/Reactivity (0)—Material Safety Data Sheet, National Fire Protection Association Health (3) Flammability (1) Instability/Reactivity (0)—Material Safety Data Sheet, Hazardous Materials Identification System (R) and/or US Department of Defense System (3★) with additional chronic hazards present Fire Hazard (0) Reactivity (0) Personal Protection Code (-) (None stated)—Material Safety Data Sheet, UN 2811, Class 6.1.

IDARUBICIN is a red fluid from powder or as a red capsules of 5 mg or red and white capsules of 10 mg and white capsules of 25 mg.

IDARUBICIN HYDROCHLORIDE: Embryotoxic and teratogenic in rats; breastfeeding is contraindicated and should be discontinued prior to taking drug or potential exposure, because of possible reproductive and developmental harm (*A Guide for Occupational Health Professionals Technical Manual*, Navy Environmental Health Center [NEHC-TM-OEM 6260.01a]).

First Aid/Medical Information/Occupational Exposure Limits

First Aid Measures to include: Use general first aid measures except for the following:

Physician's note: The treatment of IDARUBICIN HYDROCHLORIDE overdose is supportive and may include the following: platelet transfusions and antibiotics for severe and prolonged myelosuppression; symptomatic treatment of mucositis; and it is unlikely that dialysis would remove significant amounts of IDARUBICIN or its metabolites.

Medical Information:

Caution and Warning Statements: IDARUBACIN HYDROCHLORIDE is a cytotoxic agent. All work practices must be designed to reduce human exposure to the lowest level. IDARUBICIN will produce severe toxic effects on rapidly dividing tissues upon overexposure. It will cause severe tissue necrosis, myocardial toxicity, as manifested by potentially fatal congestive heart failure, acute life threatening arrhythmias or other cardiomyopathies, when given at therapeutical doses. Severe myelosuppression is the major toxicity associated with IDAMYCIN®68 therapies. IDARUBICIN exposure may cause skin, eye, mucous membranes, and upper respiratory tract irritation. If inhaled, may be harmful. If ingested, may be fatal. IDARUBICIN may be absorbed through the skin.

Caution: Females and males planning to have a child, pregnant women, and nursing mothers should exercise caution regarding potential occupational exposure to this cytotoxic drug. No information or not enough information exists or was provided concerning occupational exposure that may potentially occur while handling this drug and its affects on reproductive systems, the fetus, and/or if it is secreted along with breast milk, which may harm nursing infants. Staff members should consult with the occupational health physician monitoring workers' health in your facility to be apprised of potential hazards and should be advised to avoid becoming pregnant and/or breastfeeding or should be transferred in accordance with policy/procedures to other duties that do not involve preparation, handling, and administering this drug.

Therapeutic Levels: IDARUBICIN HYDROCHLORIDE is classified as a Food and Drug Administration Pregnancy Category (D). There are no adequate and well-controlled studies in pregnant women.

IDARUBICIN may cause congenital malformation in the fetus (teratogen), and laboratory experiments have shown mutagenic effects (mutagen). IDARUBICIN may cause reproductive disorders (reproductive hazard). This material readily absorbed by various body tissues, through the skin, intestinal tract, and transplacentally. BC Cancer Agency lists IDARUBICIN as a vesicant.

Target Organs/Systems: Bone marrow, heart, kidneys, liver, GI system, blood, skin, reproductive systems, fetus, nerves, and cancer.

Medical Conditions Generally Aggravated by Exposure:

- Skin, respiratory heart, liver, kidney, bone marrow, and reproductive disorders. Cardiac toxicity is more common in patients who have received prior anthracyclines or who have preexisting cardiac disease. Furthermore, hypersensivity to the material, chickenpox (including recent exposure) and herpes zoster.
- Reproductive and pregnancy issues.

Specific Medical Surveillance Information: Reproductive and pregnancy counseling.

Occupational Exposure Level/Limit (OEL) & Sampling Methods: Not otherwise specified

Environmental Sentinel Contamination Action Level (ESCAL): Not otherwise specified

Supplemental Response Information

Extinguishing Media: Use extinguishing agent which is the most appropriate to extinguish surrounding fire (carbon dioxide, foam, dry chemical or water fog as extinguishing media).

Solubility: IDARUBICIN is slightly to freely water soluble. IDARUBICIN is soluble in methyl alcohol and insoluble in acetone and in solvent ether (pH range of 3–7); slightly soluble in alcohol.

Chemical Degradation/Neutralization Method: A manufacturer's Material Safety Data Sheet (MSDS) and the IARC recommends treating spill surfaces with a 5.25% sodium hypochlorite (bleach) solution after absorbing liquids with inert absorbent pads or removing any powder present: allow solution to stand for up to one hour, and then thoroughly wash spilled surfaces with soap and water; sample to determine if surface contamination is still present (if sampling method is available).

If drug is still present, repeat above steps; dispose of wastes in accordance with your local procedures, state, and federal regulations.

Incompatibility: IDARUBICIN is incompatible with strong oxidizing agents.

IFOSFAMIDE (*eye-FOSS-fa-mide*)
IFOSPHAMIDE®69
IFEX®70

Chemical Abstract Service (CAS) Registry
    Numbers: 3778-73-2, 66849-33-0, 66849-34-1, 84711-20-6, 19767-45-4 (mixture)
RTECS: RP5788693
RTECS: RP6050000
C_7-H_{15}-CL_2-N_2-O_2-P

Health & Safety Hazards/US Department of Transportation (DOT)/US Environmental Protection Agency (EPA)—Sources

Carcinogen—Berkeley University Hazardous Chemical List, Carcinogen G3—International Agency for Research on Cancer, Teratogen—University of Maryland at College Park, Reproductive Effector—Material Safety Data Sheet, Acutely Toxic—US National Institute of Health (NIH) and Material Safety Data Sheet, Teratogen—US National Institute of Health (NIH) and Material Safety Data Sheet, Embryotoxic—US National Institute of Health (NIH) and Material Safety Data Sheet, Mutagen—US National Institute of Health (NIH) and Material Safety Data Sheet, Possible Carcinogen—US National Institute of Health (NIH) and Material Safety Data Sheet, Nonvesicant—British Columbia Cancer Agency Canada, Cytotoxic—Material Safety Data Sheet, Cytotoxic—British Columbia Cancer Agency Canada, Pregnancy Category (D)—US Food and Drug Administration and US Navy, Developmental—US California Proposition 65, US California Environmental Protection Agency Listed, Hazardous Materials Identification System (R) and/or US Department of Defense System Health (2) Fire Hazard (0) Reactivity (0) Personal Protective Code (X) (ask supervisor)—Material Safety Data Sheet, National Fire Protection Association Health (1) Flammability (0) Instability/Reactivity (0)—Material Safety Data Sheet, UN 3249, Class 6.1; UN 1851, Class 6.1; Toxic Solid, Organic, Not otherwise Specified (IFOSFAMIDE), UN 2811, Class 6.1, Group III.

(IFOSFAMIDE & MESNA)

IFOSFAMIDE—Breastfeeding is contraindicated and incompatible because of potential for reproductive and developmental harm (*A Guide for Occupational Health Professionals Technical Manual*, Navy Environmental Health Center [NEHC-TM-OEM 6260.01a]).

IFOSFAMIDE is a clear fluid from a white or almost white crystalline powder with sterile water.

First Aid/Medical Information/ Occupational Exposure Limits

First Aid Measures to include: Use general first aid measures except for the following:

Ingestion: If swallowed, drink plenty of water or milk. Vomiting may be induced if person is conscious, alert, and not experiencing convulsions. Seek medical assistance.

Physician's note (A): Refer for gastric lavage. IFOSFAMIDE is a mutagen and a cytotoxic drug. When administered parenterally, it is a toxic drug with a low therapeutic index.

Physician's note (B): Overdose treatment: since there is no antidote for IFOSFAMIDE overdose, treatment should be supportive, including appropriate treatment for any concurrent infection, myelosuppression, or cardiac toxicity, should it occur. Liberal fluid intake and frequent urination are advised to reduce the risk of cystitis, but care must be taken to avoid water retention and intoxication.

Physician's note (C): After absorbing larger amounts of substance: early endoscopy in order to assess mucosa lesions in the esophagus and stomach which may appear. Suck away leftover substance. Start dialysis of the blood and monitoring of hemogram. Monitor kidney function and electrolyte metabolism. This product contains an active substance, cytostatic, and oxazaphosphorine.

Dermal contact: Avoid rubbing of skin or increasing its temperature. Skin should not be washed with organic solvents.

Medical Information:

Caution and Warning Statements: IFOSFAMIDE is a potential carcinogen. Exposure by ingestion is acutely toxic. Important dose-dependent effects include bone marrow suppression, genital-urinary, lung and cardiac toxicity. Dermal exposure may result in possible allergic rash. Exposure to eyes may cause conjunctivitis. This material has been shown to have the following characteristics: carcinogenicity, mutagenicity, teratogenicity, and reproductive effects. RTECS lists IFOSFAMIDE as a suspected cardiovascular or blood toxicant; as a gastrointestinal or liver toxicant; and as a skin or sense organ toxicant.

Caution: Females and males planning to have a child, pregnant women, and nursing mothers should exercise caution regarding potential occupational exposure to this cytotoxic drug. No information or not enough information exists or was provided concerning occupational exposure that may potentially occur while handling this drug and its affects on reproductive systems, the fetus, and/or if it is secreted along with breast milk, which may harm nursing infants. Staff members should consult with the occupational health physician monitoring workers' health in your facility to be apprised of potential hazards and should be advised to avoid becoming pregnant and/or breastfeeding or should be transferred in accordance with policy/procedures to other duties that do not involve preparation, handling, and administering this drug.

Target Organs/Systems: Skin, heart, eyes, blood, kidneys, urinary bladder, bone marrow, genital-urinary tract, CNS, male reproductive systems, and delay temporary sterility

Medical Conditions Generally Aggravated by Exposure:

- Therapeutic doses of this material may aggravate blood disorders. Personnel with impaired renal function may be at increased risk following therapeutic exposure. Individuals with severely depressed bone marrow function or hypersensitivity to IFOSFAMIDE. Disorders involving the target organs of this product can be aggravated by exposures to this product (especially in doses approaching therapeutic levels for this product). Hypersensitivity to the material, impaired liver or kidney function, bone marrow depression, chickenpox (including recent exposure), herpes zoster, previous cytotoxic drug or radiation therapy, and infection. May aggravate blood disorders. IFOSFAMIDE is a toxicological synergistic product: IFOSFAMIDE may potentiate the toxicity of other antineoplastic agents and vice versa. Mesnex (2-mercaptoethane sulfonic acid monosodium salt) antagonizes the hemorrhagic cystitis effects of IFOSFAMIDE.
- Reproductive and pregnancy issues.

Specific Medical Surveillance Information: Reproductive and pregnancy counseling.

A complete blood count, including differential; these tests may be taken to provide a baseline. Pe-riodic follow-up examinations should be given in accordance with institutional policy, overseen by a physician thoroughly knowledgeable about both the toxicity of the substances and the extent of workplace exposure.

Occupational Exposure Level/Limit (OEL) & Sampling Methods:

> *Environmental Sentinel Contamination Action Level (ESCAL)*: Not otherwise specified
> Occupational Exposure Level (OEL) Bristol-Myers Squibb:
> IFOSFAMIDE 0.1 μ/m3* TWA
> *Bristol-Myers Squibb dust control target
> Exposure guideline summary: IFOSFAMIDE is a cytotoxic drug used alone or in combination with other chemotherapeutic drugs to treat various types of cancer. A dust control target of 0.1 μ/m3 in air (8-hour time-weighted average concentration) has been established for workplace exposure to IFOSFAMIDE. Adherence to this target level should protect most employees who handle this drug from experiencing adverse effects from this material; however, exposure to this substance should be maintained as low as reasonably possible.

(Method not listed or specified)

Supplemental Response Information

Extinguishing Media: Use extinguishing agent which is the most appropriate to extinguish surrounding fire (carbon dioxide, foam, dry chemical or water fog as extinguishing media).

Solubility: INFOSFAMIDE is completely (freely) water soluble (100 g/l); very soluble in alcohol, in methyl alcohol, in isopropyl alcohol; freely soluble in dichloromethane (5% solution has a pH of 5.5), pH range from 5.0–8.0 very soluble in alcohol, in ethyl acetate, in methanol, and in methylene chloride, very slightly soluble in hexanes.

Chemical Degradation/Neutralization Method: The IARC recommends treating spill surfaces with a 5.25% sodium hypochlorite (bleach) solution after absorbing liquids with inert absorbent pads or removing any powder present: allow solution to stand for up to one hour, and then thoroughly wash spilled surfaces with soap and water; sample to determine if surface contamination is still present (if sampling method is available). If drug is still present, repeat above steps; dispose of wastes in accordance with your local procedures, state, and federal regulations.

Incompatibility: IFOSFAMIDE is incompatible with strong oxidizers and bleach. Avoid exposure to heat.

IMATINIB MESYLATE
(*eye-MAT-eh-nib mez-i-late*)
IMATINIB
GLEEVEC®71

Chemical Abstract Service (CAS) Registry
Number: 152459-95-5
CH_3-SO_3-H
$C_{29}-H_{31}-N_7-O$
C29H31N7O. H4SO3

STI-571
IMATINIB

Chemical Abstract Service (CAS) Registry
Number: 220127-57-1

IMATINIB MESYLATE

Health & Safety Hazards/US Department of Transportation (DOT)/US Environmental Protection Agency (EPA)—Sources

Pregnancy Category (D)—US Food and Drug Administration

GLEEVEC®71 is available as tablets and capsules.

IMATINIB MESYLATE is a white to off-white to brownish or yellowish tinged crystalline powder.

First Aid/Medical Information/ Occupational Exposure Limits

First Aid Measures to include: Use general first aid measures.

Medical Information:

Caution and Warning Statements:

Caution: The toxicological properties of most cytotoxic drugs have not been fully investigated, particularly as it pertains to occupational exposure. IMATINIB MESYLATE (GLEEVEC®71) is one of the drugs that has little occupational hazards information available. Therefore, therapeutic dose information was extrapolated below to assist in determining occupational toxicity, and signs and symptoms of overexposure. Therefore, it is prudent to minimize occupational exposure to IMATINIB MESYLATE (GLEEVEC®71).

Commonly reported side effects include nausea, vomiting, fluid retention (sometimes severe), muscle cramps, skin rash, diarrhea, heartburn, muscle or bone pain, and headache. Although some of the serious side effects occur less frequently, severe side effects include severe fluid retention (edema), liver problems, and the potential for bleeding (hemorrhage), especially in the elderly.

Caution: Females and males planning to have a child, pregnant women, and nursing mothers should exercise caution regarding potential occupational exposure to this cytotoxic drug. No information or not enough information exists or was provided concerning occupational exposure that may potentially occur while handling this drug and its affects on reproductive systems, the fetus, and/or if it is secreted along with breast milk, which may harm nursing infants. Staff members should consult with the occupational health physician monitoring workers' health in your facility to be apprised of potential hazards and should be advised to avoid becoming pregnant and/or breastfeeding or should be transferred in accordance with policy/procedures to other duties that do not involve preparation, handling, and administering this drug.

Food and Drug Administration Pregnancy Category (D).

Target Organs/Systems: Blood, liver, and possibly fetus
Medical Conditions Generally Aggravated by Exposure:

- If hypersensitivity with IMATNIB MESYLATE exists, or any other component of GLEEVEC®71, anemia or platelet problems or white blood cell problems—may worsen and affect the decision to continue therapy; chickenpox (including recent exposure) or herpes zoster (shingles)—risk of severe disease affecting other parts of the body, liver disease—effects may be increased because of slower removal of IMATINIB from the body; and infection—IMATINIB may decrease your body's ability to fight infection.
- This drug is listed as having possible reactions and side effects if alcohol is consumed.
- Reproductive and pregnancy issues.

Specific Medical Surveillance Information: Reproductive and pregnancy counseling.

Metabolism of IMATINIB occurs in the liver and the main metabolite, N-demethylated piperazine derivative is active. The major route of elimination is in the bile; only a small portion is excreted in the urine. Most of IMATINIB eliminated as metabolites; only

25% is eliminated unchanged. The half-life including the main metabolite is 18–40 hrs respectively (www .answers.com) during treatment with GLEEVEC®71; frequent blood tests are required. These tests are for measuring blood counts and checking liver function.

Occupational Exposure Level/Limit (OEL) & Sampling Methods: Not otherwise specified

Environmental Sentinel Contamination Action Level (ESCAL): Not otherwise specified

Supplemental Response Information

Extinguishing Media: Use extinguishing agent which is the most appropriate to extinguish surrounding fire (carbon dioxide, foam, dry chemical or water fog as extinguishing media).

Solubility: GLEEVEC®71 (IMATINIB MESYLATE) is very water soluble.

Chemical Degradation/Neutralization Method: Not otherwise specified

Note: If a specific degradation or neutralization method is not provided on this table and you do not have other specific information that will guide you on how to clean up the specific material spilled, then follow the general spill procedure found at the introduction section of this table.

Incompatibility: Not otherwise specified

M

METHYL-GAG®82
MITOGUAZONE

MGBG

Chemical Abstracts Service (CAS) Registry Numbers: 459-86-9 7059-23-6

Registry of Toxic Effects of Chemical Substance (RTECS): MF3860000

National Cancer Institute: NSC 32946

$C_5H_{14}Cl_2N_8$

Health & Safety Hazards/US Department of Transportation (DOT)/US Environmental Protection Agency (EPA)—Sources

Mutagen—Registry of Toxic Effects of Chemical Substance, Mutagen—ToxReport, Reproductive Effector—ToxReport, Pregnancy Category (None)—Food and Drug Administration.

First Aid/Medical Information/ Occupational Exposure Limits

First Aid Measures to include: Use general first aid measures.

Medical Information:

Caution and Warning Statements:

Caution: The toxicological properties of most cytotoxic drugs have not been fully investigated, METHYL-GAG®82 (MITOGUAZONE), particularly as it pertains to occupational exposure. MITOGUAZONE is one of the drugs that has little occupational hazards information available. Therefore, therapeutic dose information was extrapolated below to assist in determining occupational toxicity, and signs and symptoms of overexposure. Therefore, it is prudent to minimize occupational exposure to METHYL-GAG®82 (MITOGUAZONE).

Sign and symptoms of overexposure may include signs of infection (fever, chills, sore throat); pain, numbness, and tingling in fingers or toes; severe muscle weakness; nausea and vomiting, and yellowing of the skin or eyes; unresolved mouth sores; mental status changes (euphoria, drowsiness, anxiety, emotional instability); unusual bleeding or bruising; and skin rash or itching.

The dose-limiting toxicity of MGBG is muscle weakness. The most common side effect of MGBG is flushing primarily on the face during infusion. Other toxicities associated with MGBG are usually mild, consisting of somnolence, tingling in the face or extremities, ringing in the ears, euphoria, mouth ulcers, nausea, vomiting, and fatigue.

Target Organs/Systems: Blood, liver, and bone marrow

Medical Conditions Generally Aggravated by Exposure:

- Any immunizations, liver disease, chicken pox, shingles, peripheral neuropathy (tingling and weakness in hands or feet), suppressed immune system, stomach ulcers, mouth sores, or a history of allergic reactions to various drugs.

Specific Medical Surveillance Information: At therapeutic levels, typical laboratory testing consists of white blood cell count, liver, and bone marrow function.

Occupational Exposure Level/Limit (OEL) & Sampling Methods: Not otherwise specified

Environmental Sentinel Contamination Action Level (ESCAL): Not otherwise specified

Supplemental Response Information

Extinguishing Media: Use extinguishing agent which is the most appropriate to extinguish surrounding fire (carbon dioxide, foam, dry chemical or water fog as extinguishing media).

Solubility: METHYL-GAG®82 (MGBG is >100 mg/ml in water). Completely water soluble.

Chemical Degradation/Neutralization Method: Not otherwise specified

Note: If a specific degradation or neutralization method is not provided on this table and you do not have other specific information that will guide you on how to clean up the specific material spilled, then follow the general spill procedure found in the introduction section of this handbook.

Incompatibility: Not otherwise specified

MITOMYCIN C (1) *(mye-toe-MYE-sin C)*
MUTAMYCIN®84
MITOMYCIN
STREPTOZOTOCIN
AMETYCIN

Chemical Abstracts Service (CAS) Registry
Number: 50-07-7
Registry of Toxic Effects of Chemical Substance
(RTECS): CN0700000
National Cancer Institute: NSC 26980
$C_{15}H_{18}N_4O_5$
(Three Degradation Methods)

Health & Safety Hazards/US Department of Transportation (DOT)/US Environmental Protection Agency (EPA)—Sources

Carcinogen G2B—International Agency Research on Cancer, Carcinogen—University of Maryland at College Park, Carcinogen—Berkeley University Hazardous Chemical List, Reproductive Effector— Reproductive Effector—US National Institute of Environmental Health Sciences (NIEHS), Teratogen— University of Maryland at College Park, Mutagen— US New Jersey Department of Health and Senior Services Hazardous Substances Fact Sheet, Highly Toxic—Material Safety Data Sheet, Lactation—Avoid Breastfeeding—US Navy, Carcinogen—US California Proposition 65, National Fire Protection Association Health (4) Flammability (1) Instability (0)—Material Safety Data Sheet, Materials Identification System (R)

and/or US Department of Defense System Health (4★) with additional chronic hazards present Fire Hazard (1) Reactivity (0) Personal Protection Code (A)(Safety Glasses)—Material Safety Data Sheet, ORAL RAT: LD50: 30 mg/kg; ORAL MOUSE: LD50: 23 mg/kg; Title III, U010, UN 2811, Class 6.1, MIDI: HW01— (http://usaphcapps.amedd.army.mil/midi/), US California Environmental Protection Agency Listed.

MITOMYCIN is a purple fluid from powder.

MITOMYCIN is a blue-violet crystalline powder.

MITOYCIN: Safety has not been established (teratological changes in animals) (facts and comparisons); breastfeeding is contraindicated because of potential reproductive and developmental harm (*A Guide for Occupational Health Professionals Technical Manual*, Navy Environmental Health Center [NEHC-TM-OEM 6260.01a]).

MITOMYCIN is an antineoplastic antibiotic produced by the growth of streptomyces caespitosus.

First Aid/Medical Information/ Occupational Exposure Limits

First Aid Measures to include: Use general first aid measures.

Medical Information:

Caution and Warning Statements: Routes of exposure are ingestion, inhalation, skin contact, and eye contact.

Ingestion may cause blood and kidney changes, microrangiopathic hemolytic anemic and lung changes. Ingestion is similar to inhalation effects, while skin contact may result in sensitization, rash, tissue necrosis and irritation. Contact with eyes may cause conjunctivitis. RTECS lists MITOMYCIN C as a suspected gastrointestinal or liver toxicant, and as a neurotoxicant. MITOMYCIN C may damage the testes (male reproductive glands) causing abnormal sperm shape.

MITOMYCIN C exposure can cause irritation of the skin and eyes. Higher exposure may cause poor appetite, fever, nausea, headache, fatigue, and drowsiness. Repeated contact at high exposure may damage the eye, liver, kidneys, and blood cells.

Caution: Females and males planning to have a child, pregnant women, and nursing mothers should exercise caution regarding potential occupational exposure to this cytotoxic drug. No information or not enough information exists or was provided concerning occupational exposure that may potentially occur while handling this drug and its affects on reproductive systems, the fetus, and/or if it is secreted along with breast milk, which may harm nursing infants. Staff members should consult with the occupational health physician monitoring workers' health in your facility to be apprised of potential hazards and should be advised to avoid becoming pregnant and/or breastfeeding or should be transferred in accordance with policy/procedures to other duties that do not involve preparation, handling, and administering this drug.

Target Organs/Systems: Blood, bone marrow, liver, kidneys, skin, eyes, possible reproductive system, and fetus

Medical Conditions Generally Aggravated by Exposure:

- Individuals who have demonstrated a hypersensitivity or idiosyncratic reaction to MITOMYCIN in the past. Individuals with thrombocytopenia, coagulation disorder,
- Or an increase in bleeding tendency due to other causes.
- Reproductive and pregnancy issues.

Specific Medical Surveillance Information: Reproductive and pregnancy counseling.

A pre-placement physical examination and history (noting any risk factors) for all employees with potential exposure to MUTAMYCIN®84 is recommended. A complete blood count, including differential, may be taken to provide a baseline.

If symptoms develop and/or overexposure is suspected, a complete blood count should be performed along with liver and kidney functions tests.

Occupational Exposure Level/Limit (OEL) & Sampling Methods: Not otherwise specified

Environmental Sentinel Contamination Action Level (ESCAL): Not otherwise specified

Supplemental Response Information

Extinguishing Media: Use extinguishing agent which is the most appropriate to extinguish surrounding fire (carbon dioxide, foam, dry chemical or water fog as extinguishing media).

Solubility: MITOMYCIN C (MUTAMYCIN®84) is slightly to moderately water soluble. MITOMYCIN C is sparingly soluble in methyl alcohol, freely soluble in organic solvents; pH range of 6.0–8.0.

Chemical Degradation/Neutralization Method: See below for additional degradation methods—A manufacturer's Material Safety Data Sheet (MSDS) recommends using a 2 fold molar excess of 1% potassium permanganate (KMNO4) to clean spill surfaces after absorbing liquids with inert absorbent pads or removing any powder present: repeat using soap and water; sample to determine if surface contamination is still present (if

sampling method is available). If the drug is still present, repeat above steps; dispose of wastes in accordance with your local procedures, state, and federal regulations.

Incompatibility: MITOMYCIN C is incompatible with strong acids, strong bases, and strong oxidizing agents.

MITOMYCIN C (2) (*my-toe-MY-sin C*)
MUTAMYCIN®84

Chemical Abstracts Service (CAS) Registry
Number: 50-07-7
Registry of Toxic Effects of Chemical Substance
(RTECS): CN0700000
National Cancer Institute: NSC 26980
$C_{15}H_{18}N_4O_5$
(Three Degradation Methods)

Health & Safety Hazards/US Department of Transportation (DOT)/US Environmental Protection Agency (EPA)—Sources

Carcinogen G2B International Agency for Research on Cancer, Carcinogen—University of Maryland at College Park, Carcinogen—Berkeley University Hazardous Chemical List, Reproductive Effector—US National Institute of Environmental Health Sciences (NIEHS), Teratogen—University of Maryland at College Park, Mutagen—US New Jersey Department of Health and Senior Services Hazardous Substances Fact Sheet, Highly Toxic—Material Safety Data Sheet, Carcinogen—US California Proposition 65, National Fire Protection Association Health (4) Flammability (1) Instability (0)—Material Safety Data Sheet, Materials Identification System (R) and/or US Department of Defense System Health (4★) with additional chronic hazards present Fire Hazard (1) Reactivity (0) Personal Protection Code (A) (Safety Glasses)—Material Safety Data Sheet, DOT: Title III, U010, UN 2811, Class 6.1, EPA: US California Environmental Protection Agency Listed, ORAL RAT: LD50: 30 mg/kg; ORAL MOUSE: LD50: 23 mg/kg; MIDI: HW01—(http://usaphcapps.amedd.army.mil/midi/).

MITOMYCIN is a purple fluid from powder.

MITOMYCIN is a blue-violet crystalline powder.

MITOYCIN: Safety has not been established (teratological changes in animals) (facts and comparisons); breastfeeding is contraindicated because of potential for reproductive and developmental harm (*A Guide for Occupational Health Professionals Technical Manual*, Navy Environmental Health Center [NEHC-TM-OEM 6260.01a]).

MITOMYCIN is an antineoplastic antibiotic produced by the growth of streptomyces caespitosus.

First Aid/Medical Information/ Occupational Exposure Limits

First Aid Measures to include: Use general first aid measures.

Medical Information:

Caution and Warning Statements: Routes of exposure are ingestion, inhalation, skin contact, and eye contact.

Ingestion may cause blood and kidney changes, microrangiopathic hemolytic anemic and lung changes. Ingestion is similar to inhalation effects, while skin contact may result in sensitization, rash, tissue necrosis and irritation. Contact with eyes may cause conjunctivitis. RTECS lists MITOMYCIN C as a suspected gastrointestinal or a liver toxicant, and as a neurotoxicant. MITOMYCIN C may damage the testes (male reproductive glands) causing abnormal sperm shape.

MITOMYCIN C exposure can cause irritation of the skin and eyes. Higher exposure may cause poor appetite, fever, nausea, headache, fatigue, and drowsiness. Repeated contact at high exposure may damage the eye, liver, kidneys, and blood cells.

Caution: Females and males planning to have a child, pregnant women, and nursing mothers should exercise caution regarding potential occupational exposure to this cytotoxic drug. No information or not enough information exists or was provided concerning occupational exposure that may potentially occur while handling this drug and its affects on reproductive systems, the fetus, and/or if it is secreted along with breast milk, which may harm nursing infants. Staff members should consult with the occupational health physician monitoring workers' health in your facility to be apprised of potential hazards and should be advised to avoid becoming pregnant and/or breastfeeding or should be transferred in accordance with policy/procedures to other duties that do not involve preparation, handling, and administering this drug.

Target Organs/Systems: Blood, bone marrow, liver, kidneys, skin, eyes, possible reproductive system, and fetus

Medical Conditions Generally Aggravated by Exposure:

- Individuals who have demonstrated a hypersensitivity or idiosyncratic reaction to MITOMYCIN in the past. Individuals with thrombocytopenia, coagulation disorder,
- Or an increase in bleeding tendency due to other causes.
- Reproductive and pregnancy issues.

Specific Medical Surveillance Information: Reproductive and pregnancy counseling.

A pre-placement physical examination and history (noting any risk factors) for all employees with potential exposure to MUTAMYCIN®84 is recommended. A complete blood count, including differential, may be taken to provide a baseline.

If symptoms develop and/or overexposure is suspected, a complete blood count should be performed along with liver and kidney functions tests.

Occupational Exposure Level/Limit (OEL) & Sampling Methods: Not otherwise specified

Environmental Sentinel Contamination Action Level (ESCAL): Not otherwise specified

Supplemental Response Information

Extinguishing Media: Use extinguishing agent which is the most appropriate to extinguish surrounding fire (carbon dioxide, foam, dry chemical or water fog as extinguishing media).

Solubility: MITOMYCIN C (MUTAMYCIN®84) is slightly to moderately water soluble. MITOMYCIN C is sparingly soluble in methyl alcohol freely soluble in organic solvents; pH range of 6.0–8.0.

Chemical Degradation/Neutralization Method: There are three recommended procedures: alkaline soap/detergent, bleach [sodium hypochlorite], and potassium permanganate (KMNO4) for MITOMYCIN C (MUTAMYCIN®84). See below and above for additional degradation methods.

A manufacturer's Material Safety Data Sheet (MSDS) recommends using a 30 fold molar excess of bleach (5.25% NAOCL) to clean spill surfaces after absorbing liquids with inert absorbent pads or removing any powder present: repeat using soap and water; sample to determine if surface contamination is still present (if sampling method is available). If the drug is present, repeat above steps; dispose of wastes in accordance with your local procedures, state, and federal regulations.

Incompatibility: MITOMYCIN C is incompatible with strong acids, strong bases, and strong oxidizing agents.

MITOMYCIN C (3) *(mye-toe-MYE-sin C)*
MUTAMYCIN®84

Chemical Abstracts Service (CAS) Registry
   Number: 50-07-7
Registry of Toxic Effects of Chemical Substance
   (RTECS): CN0700000
National Cancer Institute: NSC 26980

$C_{15}H_{18}N_4O_5$
(Three Degradation Methods)

Health & Safety Hazards/US Department of Transportation (DOT)/US Environmental Protection Agency (EPA)—Sources

Carcinogen G2B—International Agency for Research on Cancer, Carcinogen—University of Maryland at College Park, Carcinogen—Berkeley University Hazardous Chemical List, Reproductive Effector—Reproductive Effector—US National Institute of Environmental Health Sciences (NIEHS), Teratogen—University of Maryland at College Park, Mutagen—US New Jersey Department of Health and Senior Services Hazardous Substances Fact Sheet, Highly Toxic—Material Safety Data Sheet, Lactation—Avoid Breastfeeding—US Navy, Carcinogen—US California Proposition 65, National Fire Protection Association Health (4) Flammability (1) Instability (0)—Material Safety Data Sheet, Materials Identification System (R) and/or US Department of Defense System Health (4★) with additional chronic hazards present Fire Hazard (1) Reactivity (0) Personal Protection Code (A) (Safety Glasses)—Material Safety Data Sheet, ORAL RAT: LD50: 30 mg/kg; ORAL MOUSE: LD50: 23 mg/kg; MIDI:HW01—(http://usaphcapps.amedd.army.mil/midi/), DOT: Title III; U010, UN 2811, Class 6.1, EPA: US California Environmental Protection Agency Listed.

MITOMYCIN is a purple fluid from powder.

MITOMYCIN is a blue-violet crystalline powder.

MITOYCIN: Safety has not been established (teratological changes in animals) (facts and comparisons); breastfeeding is contraindicated because of potential for reproductive and developmental harm (*A Guide for Occupational Health Professionals Technical Manual*, Navy Environmental Health Center [NEHC-TM-OEM 6260.01a]).

MITOMYCIN is an antineoplastic antibiotic produced by the growth of streptomyces caespitosus.

First Aid/Medical Information/ Occupational Exposure Limits

First Aid Measures to include: Use general first aid measures.

Medical Information:

Caution and Warning Statements: Routes of exposure are ingestion, inhalation, skin contact, and eye contact.

Ingestion may cause blood and kidney changes, microrangiopathic hemolytic anemic and lung changes. Ingestion is similar to inhalation effects, while skin contact may result in sensitization, rash, tissue necrosis and irritation. Contact with eyes may cause conjunctivitis. RTECS lists MITOMYCIN C as a suspected gastro-intestinal or a liver toxicant, and as a neurotoxicant. MITOMYCIN C may damage the testes (male reproductive glands) causing abnormal sperm shape.

MITOMYCIN C exposure can cause irritation of the skin and eyes. Higher exposure may cause poor appetite, fever, nausea, headache, fatigue, and drowsiness. Repeated contact at high exposure may damage the eye, liver, kidneys, and blood cells.

Caution—Females and males planning to have a child, pregnant women, and nursing mothers should exercise caution regarding potential occupational exposure to this cytotoxic drug. No information or not enough information exists or was provided concerning occupational exposure that may potentially occur while handling this drug and its affects on reproductive systems, the fetus, and/or if it is secreted along with breast milk, which may harm nursing infants. Staff members should consult with the occupational health physician monitoring workers' health in your facility to be apprised of potential hazards and should be advised to avoid becoming pregnant and/or breastfeeding or should be transferred in accordance with policy/procedures to other duties that do not involve preparation, handling, and administering this drug.

Target Organs/Systems: Blood, bone marrow, liver, kidneys, skin, eyes, possible reproductive system, and fetus

Medical Conditions Generally Aggravated by Exposure:

- Individuals who have demonstrated a hypersensitivity or idiosyncratic reaction to MITOMYCIN in the past. Individuals with thrombocytopenia, coagulation disorder,
- Or an increase in bleeding tendency due to other causes.
- Reproductive and pregnancy issues.

Specific Medical Surveillance Information: Reproductive and pregnancy counseling.

A pre-placement physical examination and history (noting any risk factors) for all employees with potential exposure to MUTAMYCIN®84 is recommended. A complete blood count, including differential, may be taken to provide a baseline.

If symptoms develop and/or overexposure is suspected, a complete blood count should be performed along with liver and kidney functions tests.

Occupational Exposure Level/Limit (OEL) & Sampling Methods: Not otherwise specified

Environmental Sentinel Contamination Action Level (ESCAL): Not otherwise specified

Supplemental Response Information

Extinguishing Media: Use extinguishing agent which is the most appropriate to extinguish surrounding fire (carbon dioxide, foam, dry chemical or water fog as extinguishing media).

Solubility: MITOMYCIN C (MUTAMYCIN®84) is slightly to moderately water soluble. MITOMYCIN C is sparingly soluble in methyl alcohol, freely soluble in organic solvents; pH range of 6.0–8.0.

Chemical Degradation/Neutralization Method: See above for additional degradation methods—There are three recommended procedures: alkaline soap/detergent, bleach (sodium hypochlorite), and potassium permanganate (KMNO4) for MITOMYCIN C (MUTAMYCIN®84).

A manufacturer's Material Safety Data Sheet (MSDS) recommends using alkaline soap/detergent and water to clean spill surfaces after absorbing liquids with inert absorbent pads or removing any powder present: repeat using soap and water; sample to determine if surface contamination is still present (if sampling method is available). If the drug is present, repeat above steps; dispose of wastes in accordance with your local procedures, state, and federal regulations.

Incompatibility: MITOMYCIN C is incompatible with strong acids, strong bases, and strong oxidizing agents.

MITOTANE (*MYE-toe-tane*)
LYSODREN®85
MJ7236
0,P-DDD

> Chemical Abstracts Service (CAS) Registry Number: 53-19-0 (Mixture)
> Registry of Toxic Effects of Chemical Substance (RTECS): KH7880000
> National Cancer Institute: NSC 38721
> $C_{14}H_{10}Cl_4$

Health & Safety Hazards/US Department of Transportation (DOT)/US Environmental Protection (EPA)—Sources

Pregnancy Category (C)—US Food and Drug Administration, Tumorigenic—ToxReport, Mutagen—ToxReport Reproductive Effector—ToxReport, Carcinogen—US California Proposition 65—MC, Weak Carcinogen—Material Safety Data Sheet.

MITOTANE is available in tablet form.

MITOTANE is a white crystalline powder with a slight aromatic odor.

First Aid/Medical Information/Occupational Exposure Limits

First Aid Measures to include: Use general first aid measures except for the following:

Ingestion: Vomiting may be induced if person is conscious and not experiencing convulsions.

Physician's note: This product contains a drug that suppresses adrenal function and is used to treat neoplasm of the adrenal cortex.

Medical Information:

Caution and Warning Statements: MITOTANE studies conducted by NCI in animals found to have weak, slightly positive carcinogenic potential. Mutagenicity potential has not been characterized. It is not known whether MITOTANE can cause fetal harm when administered to pregnant women. Reproductive effects have not been performed with MITOTANE. It is not known whether MITOTANE is distributed into milk. Approximately 35–40% of an oral dose of MITOTANE is absorbed from the gastrointestinal tract. Eye contact may cause conjunctivitis. Toxicological synergistic effects may occur when administered with other drugs. Ingestion of a therapeutic dose may result in symptoms such as anorexia, nausea, vomiting, diarrhea, lethargy, somnolence, dizziness, or vertigo. No information is available on inhalation symptoms.

RTECS lists MITOTANE as a suspected cardiovascular or blood toxicant; as a gastrointestinal or liver toxicant; as a neurotoxicant; and as a skin or sense organ toxicant.

Caution: Females and males planning to have a child, pregnant women, and nursing mothers should exercise caution regarding potential occupational exposure to this cytotoxic drug. No information or not enough information exists or was provided concerning occupational exposures that may potentially occur while handling this drug and its affects on reproductive systems, the fetus, and/or if it is secreted along with breast milk, which may harm nursing infants. Staff members should consult with the occupational health physician monitoring workers' health in your facility to be apprised of potential hazards and should be advised to avoid becoming pregnant and/or breastfeeding or should be transferred in accordance with policy/procedures to other duties that do not involve preparation, handling, and administering this drug.

Target Organs/Systems: Adrenal cortex, CNS, and fetus

Medical Conditions Generally Aggravated by Exposure:

- May aggravate shock or severe trauma by adrenal suppression.
- Pregnancy.

Specific Medical Surveillance Information: Reproductive and pregnancy counseling.

A complete blood count, including differential and serum electrolytes, may be taken to provide a baseline. Periodic follow-up examination is recommended.

Occupational Exposure Level/Limit (OEL) & Sampling Methods: Not otherwise specified

Environmental Sentinel Contamination Action Level (ESCAL): Not otherwise specified

Supplemental Response Information

Extinguishing Media: Use extinguishing agent which is the most appropriate to extinguish surrounding fire (carbon dioxide, foam, dry chemical or water fog as extinguishing media).

Solubility: MITOTANE is practically water insoluble but soluble in alcohol, ethanol, iso-octane, and carbon tetrachloride.

Chemical Degradation/Neutralization Method: A manufacturer's Material Safety Data Sheet (MSDS) recommends using alkaline soap/detergent and water to clean spill surfaces after absorbing liquids with inert absorbent pads or removing any powder present: repeat using soap and water; sample to determine if surface contamination is still present (if sampling method is available). If the drug is present, repeat above steps; dispose of wastes in accordance with your local procedures, state, and federal regulations.

Incompatibility: Not otherwise specified

MITOXANTRONE (1)

(*mye-toe-ZAN-trone*)
MITOXANTRONE HYDROCHLORIDE
NOVANTRONE®86
DHAD

Chemical Abstracts Service (CAS) Registry
Number: 70476-82-3
$C_{22}H_{30}Cl_2N_4O_6$
$C_{22}H_{30}Cl_2N_4O_6 \cdot 2CL\text{-}H$

MITOXANTRONE HYDROCHLORIDE

Chemical Abstracts Service (CAS) Registry
Number: 70476-82-3
National Cancer Institute: NSC 301739

MITOXANTRONE HYDROCHLORIDE

Chemical Abstracts Service (CAS) Registry
Number: 65271-80-9

MITOXANTRONE

Registry of Toxic Effects of Chemical Substance
(RTECS): CB0386900
(Two Degradation Methods)

Health & Safety Hazards/US Department of Transpiration (DOT)/US Environmental Protection Agency (EPA)—Sources

Carcinogen G2B—International Agency For Research on Cancer, Teratogen—Material Safety Data Sheet, Cytotoxic—Material Safety Data Sheet, Toxic—Material Safety Data Sheet, Mutagen—Toxic, and Irritant—British Columbia Cancer Agency Canada, Cytotoxic—British Columbia Cancer Agency Canada, Pregnancy Category (D)—US Food and Drug Administration, Developmental—US California Proposition 65, National Fire Protection Association Health (2) Flammability (0) Instability (0) Special Toxic, Materials Identification System (R) and/or US Department of Defense System Health (2) Fire Hazard (0) Reactivity (0) Personal Protection Code (–) (None stated)—Material Safety Data Sheet, Cardiotoxicity—Drugs.com and Material Safety Data Sheet.

MITOXANTRONE is a dark blue odorless fluid.

MITROXANTRONE HYDROCHLORIDE is a dark-blue, electrostatic, hygroscopic powder.

MITOXANTRONE is available as an injection.

MITOXANTRONE HCL may cause fetal harm; breastfeeding should be discontinued because of potential for reproductive and developmental harm (*A Guide for Occupational Health Professionals Technical Manual*, Navy Environmental Health Center [NEHC-TM-OEM 6260.01a]).

(UV Detection: 254 nm; Color Unknown, 241 nm)

First Aid/Medical Information/Occupational Exposure Limits

First Aid Measures to include: Use general first aid measures except for the following:

Ingestion: If conscious, induce vomiting, as directed by medical personnel.

Physician's note: Acute overdose treatment—There is no specific antidote for MITOXANTRONE overdose. Treatment is symptomatic and supportive with close patient monitoring. This material is unlikely to be significantly removed by dialysis.

Medical Information:

Caution and Warning Statements: This material (drug) is toxic and may cause heritable genetic damage. Exposure may cause harm to the unborn child. Inhalation may be mildly irritating. Ingestion may cause GI irritation. Skin and eyes exposure may cause irritation. Chronic exposure may cause cardiovascular and birth defects. This material (drug) is cytotoxic.

Caution: Females and males planning to have a child, pregnant women, and nursing mothers should exercise caution regarding potential occupational exposure to this cytotoxic drug. No information or not enough information exists or was provided concerning occupational exposures that may potentially occur while handling this drug and its affects on reproductive systems, the fetus, and/or if it is secreted along with breast milk, which may harm nursing infants. Staff members should consult with the occupational health physician monitoring workers' health in your facility to be apprised of potential hazards and should be advised to avoid becoming pregnant and/or breastfeeding or should be transferred in accordance with policy/procedures to other duties that do not involve preparation, handling, and administering this drug.

Therapeutic Levels: The Food and Drug Administration lists this drug as a Pregnancy Category (D). Avoid possible exposure if you are pregnant or if you planning to become pregnant or if you are breastfeeding. Exposure to this drug may harm the fetus (unborn child) or child.

Target Organs/Systems: Heart, bone marrow, CNS, kidney, liver, spleen, thymus, fetus, lymph nodes, and GI system

Medical Conditions Generally Aggravated by Exposure:

- Prior hypersensitivity to NOVANTRONE®86.
- Hypersensitivity to MITOXANTRONE HYDROCHLORIDE severely impaired liver function, bone marrow depression, chickenpox, (including recent exposure), herpes zoster, gout or kidney stones, infection, heart disease, and previous cytotoxic drug or radiation therapy.
- Reproductive and pregnancy issues.

Specific Medical Surveillance Information: Reproductive and pregnancy counseling.

Occupational Exposure Level/Limit (OEL) & Sampling Methods:

Environmental Sentinel Contamination Action Level (ESCAL): Not otherwise specified

Occupational Exposure Level (OEL) AHPC-OEG: (NOVANTRONE®86) MITOXANTRONE HCL:

0.2 μg/m3
(No specific method listed)

Occupational Exposure Level (OE) Lederle Laboratories:
(NOVANTRONE®86) MITOXANTRONE HCL
ACCO PEL:
0.016 mg/m3 once/month
0.003 mg/m3 5 consecutive exposures per month
(No specific method listed)

Supplemental Response Information

Extinguishing Media: Use extinguishing agent which is the most appropriate to extinguish surrounding fire (carbon dioxide, foam, dry chemical or water fog as extinguishing media).

Solubility: MITOXANTRONE is sparingly water soluble. Slightly to sparingly soluble in methanol, insoluble in acetonitrile, chloroform and acetone (pH = 3–4.5); MITOXANTRONE HYDROCHLORIDE is water soluble at (5–10 mg/ml).

Chemical Degradation/Neutralization Method:

Warning: Do not use bleach for neutralizing; toxic gas is generated when mixed with bleach unless measures are taken to ventilate the area.

There are two recommended procedures for MITOXANTRONE. See below for methods.

A manufacturer's Material Safety Data Sheet (MSDS) recommends decontaminate with 5.5 parts calcium hypochlorite in 13 parts by weight of water for each 1 part of MITOXANTRONE HCL.

Repeat using soap and water to rinse the spill area; sample to determine if surface contamination is still present (if sampling method is available at your facility). If the drug is present, repeat above steps; dispose of wastes in accordance with your local procedures, state, and federal regulations.

Caution: Chlorine gas may be produced during decontamination.

Incompatibility: MITOXANTRONE: HYDROCHLORIDE or permananganate is incompatible with strong oxidizing agents (bleach) and moisture.

Chlorine gas is liberated when degraded with calcium hypochlorite.

MITOXANTRONE (2)

(mye-toe-ZAN-trone)
MITOXANTRONE HYDROCHLORIDE
NOVANTRONE®86
DHAD

Chemical Abstracts Service (CAS) Registry
Number: 70476-82-3
$C_{22}H_{30}Cl_2N_4O_6$
$C_{22}H_{30}Cl_2N_4O_6 \cdot 2CL-H$

MITOXANTRONE HYDROCHLORIDE

Chemical Abstracts Service (CAS) Registry
Number: 70476-82-3
National Cancer Institute: NSC 301739

MITOXANTRONE HYDROCHLORIDE

Chemical Abstracts Service (CAS) Registry
Number: 65271-80-9

MITOXANTRONE

Registry of Toxic Effects of Chemical Substance
(RTECS): CB0386900
(Two Degradation Methods)

Health & Safety Hazards/US Department of Transportation (DOT)/US Environmental Protection Agency (EPA)—Sources

Carcinogen G2B—International Agency for Research on Cancer, Teratogen—Material Safety Data Sheet, Cytotoxic—Material Safety Data Sheet, Toxic—Material Safety Data Sheet, Mutagen—Toxic and Irritant—British Columbia Cancer Agency Canada, Cytotoxic—British Columbia Cancer Agency Canada, Pregnancy Category (D), US Food and Drug Administration, Developmental—US California Proposition 65, National Fire Protection Association Health (2) Flammability (0) Instability (0)—Material Safety Data Sheet, Materials Identification System (R) and/or US Department of Defense System Health (2) Fire Hazard (0) Reactivity (0)—Material Safety Data Sheet, Material Safety Data Sheet, Cardiotoxicity—Drugs.com and Material Safety Data Sheet.

MITOXANTRONE is a dark blue fluid.

MITROXANTRONE HYDROCHLORIDE is a dark-blue, electrostatic, hygroscopic powder.

MITOXANTRONE is available as an injection.

MITOXANTRONE HCL may cause fetal harm; breastfeeding should be discontinued because of potential for reproductive and developmental hazards (*A Guide for Occupational Health Professionals Technical Manual*, Navy Environmental Health Center [NEHC-TM-OEM 6260.01a]).

(UV Detection: 254 nm; Color Unknown, 241 nm)

First Aid/Medical Information/ Occupational Exposure Limits

First Aid Measures to include: Use general first aid measures except for the following:

Ingestion: If conscious, induce vomiting, as directed by medical personnel.

Physician's note: Acute overdose treatment: there is no specific antidote for MITOXANTRONE overdose. Treatment is symptomatic and supportive with close patient monitoring. This material is unlikely to be significantly removed by dialysis.

Medical Information:

Caution and Warning Statements: This material (drug) is toxic and may cause heritable genetic damage. Exposure may cause harm to the unborn child. Inhalation may be mildly irritating. Ingestion may cause GI irritation. Skin and eyes exposure may cause irritation. Chronic exposure may cause cardiovascular and birth defects. This material (drug) is cytotoxic. BC Cancer Agency lists MITOXANTRONE as an irritant.

Caution: Females and males planning to have a child, pregnant women, and nursing mothers should exercise caution regarding potential occupational exposure to this cytotoxic drug. No information or not enough information exists or was provided concerning occupational exposures that may potentially occur while handling this drug and its affects on reproductive systems, the fetus, and/or if it is secreted along with breast milk, which may harm nursing infants. Staff members should consult with the occupational health physician monitoring workers' health in your facility to be apprised of potential hazards and should be advised to avoid becoming pregnant and/or breastfeeding or should be transferred in accordance with policy/procedures to other duties that do not involve preparation, handling, and administering this drug.

Therapeutic Levels: The Food and Drug Administration lists this drug as a Pregnancy Category (D). Avoid possible exposure if you are pregnant or if you planning to become pregnant or if you are breastfeeding. Exposure to this drug may harm the fetus (unborn child) or child.

Target Organs/Systems: Heart, bone marrow, CNS, kidney, liver, spleen, thymus, lymph nodes, fetus, and GI system

Medical Conditions Generally Aggravated by Exposure:

- Prior hypersensitivity to NOVANTRONE®86. Hypersensitivity to MITOXANTRONE HYDROCHLORIDE severely impaired liver function, bone marrow depression, chickenpox (including recent exposure), herpes zoster, gout or kidney stones, infection, heart disease, and previous cytotoxic drug or radiation therapy.

- Reproductive and pregnancy issues.

Specific Medical Surveillance Information: Reproductive and pregnancy counseling.

Occupational Exposure Level/Limit (OEL) & Sampling Methods:

Environmental Sentinel Contamination Action Level (ESCAL): Not otherwise specified
Occupational Exposure Level (OEL) AHPC-OEG (NOVANTRONE®86) MITOXANTRONE HCL:
0.1 μg/m3
(No specific method listed)

Occupational Exposure Level (OEL) Lederle Laboratories (NOVANTRONE®86) MITOXANTRONE HCL:
Acco Pel:
0.016 mg/m3 once/month
0.1 mg/m3 5 consecutive exposures per month
(No specific method listed)

Supplemental Response Information

Extinguishing Media: Use extinguishing agent which is the most appropriate to extinguish surrounding fire (carbon dioxide, foam, dry chemical or water fog as extinguishing media).

Solubility: MITOXANTRONE is sparingly water soluble. Slightly to sparingly soluble in methanol; in-soluble in acetonitrile, chloroform, and acetone (pH = 3–4.5); MITOXANTRONE HYDROCHLORIDE is water soluble at (5–10 mg/ml).

Chemical Degradation/Neutralization Method:

Warning: Do not use bleach for neutralizing because toxic gas is generated when mixed with bleach unless measures are taken to ventilate the area.

There are two recommended procedures for MITOXANTRONE. See below and above for methods.

A manufacturer's Material Safety Data Sheet (MSDS) recommends wetting the spill with a mixture of water and household dish detergent, adding bleach until the blue color disappears (slight foaming may be observed). The amounts of water, detergent, and bleach used to validate this method were arbitrarily set at approximately 25:1:50, but variation on these proportions should still accomplish the decontamination provided the blue color is eliminated.

Repeat using soap and water; sample to determine if surface contamination is still present (if sampling method is available at your facility). If the drug is present, repeat above steps; dispose of wastes in accordance with your local procedures, state, and federal regulations.

Caution: Chlorine gas may be produced during decontamination.

Incompatibility: MITOXANTRONE: HYDROCHLORIDE or permananganate is incompatible with strong oxidizing agents (bleach) and moisture.

Chlorine gas is liberated when degraded with calcium hypochlorite.

N

NILUTAMIDE (*ni-LOO-ta-mide*)
NILANDRON®87

Chemical Abstracts Service (CAS) Registry Number: 63612-50-0
Registry of Toxic Effects of Chemical Substance (RTECS): NI9453300
RU 23908
$C_{12}H_{10}F_3N_3O_4$

Health & Safety Hazards/US Department of Transportation (DOT)/US Environmental Protection Agency (EPA)—Sources

Potential Teratogen—Drugs.com, Toxic—Material Safety Data Sheet, Reproductive Effector—Material Safety Data Sheet, Pregnancy Category (C)—US Food and Drug Administration, Materials Identification System (R) and/or US Department of Defense System Health (2★) with additional chronic hazards present Fire Hazard (0) Reactivity (0) Personal Protection Code (-) (None stated)—Material Safety Data Sheet, National Fire Protection Association Health (2) Flammability (0) Instability (0)—Material Safety Data Sheet, DOT: UN 2811, CLASS 6.1, GROUP III.

NILUTAMIDE is available as a white tablet.

First Aid/Medical Information/ Occupational Exposure Limits

First Aid Measures to include: Use general first aid measures except for the following:

Ingestion: If vomiting does not occur spontaneously, it should be induced if the patient is conscious and alert. General supportive care, including frequent monitoring of the vital signs and close observation of the patient, is indicated.

Medical Information:

Caution and Warning Statements: Signs and symptoms of exposure by ingestion may include nausea and vomiting, malaise, headache, and dizziness.

Caution: Females and males planning to have a child, pregnant women, and nursing mothers should exercise caution regarding potential occupational exposure to this cytotoxic drug. No information or not enough information exists or was provided concerning occupational exposures that may potentially occur while handling this drug and its affects on reproductive systems, the fetus, and/or if it is secreted along with breast milk, which may harm nursing infants. Staff members should consult with the occupational health physician monitoring workers' health in your facility to be apprised of potential hazards and should be advised to avoid becoming pregnant and/or breastfeeding or should be transferred in accordance with policy/procedures to other duties that do not involve preparation, handling, and administering this drug.

Therapeutic Levels: The Food and Drug Administration lists NILUTAMIDE as a Pregnancy Category (C). This means that it is not known whether NILUTAMIDE will harm an unborn baby. NILUTAMIDE is not indicated for use by women.

Target Organs/Systems: Vision (eye), liver, gastrointestinal, and possibly fetus

Medical Conditions Generally Aggravated by Exposure:

- Known hypersensitivity to NILUTAMIDE, severe low RBC (anemia) or severe liver failure.
- Consumption of alcohol may have a possible disculfram-like reaction (5–20%) (increases toxicity of drug).
- Reproductive and pregnancy issues.

Specific Medical Surveillance Information: Reproductive and pregnancy counseling.

Occupational Exposure Level/Limit (OEL) & Sampling Methods: Not otherwise specified

Environmental Sentinel Contamination Action Level (ESCAL): Not otherwise specified

Supplemental Response Information

Extinguishing Media: Use extinguishing agent which is the most appropriate to extinguish surrounding fire (carbon dioxide, foam, dry chemical or water fog as extinguishing media).

Solubility: NILUTAMIDE is freely soluble in ethyl acetate, acetone, chloroform, ethyl alcohol, dichloromethane, and methanol.

Chemical Degradation/Neutralization Method: Not otherwise specified

Note: If a specific degradation or neutralization method is not provided on this table and you do not have other specific information that will guide you on how to clean up the specific material spilled, then follow the general spill procedure found in the introduction section of this handbook.

Incompatibility: NILUTAMIDE is incompatible with strong oxidizing agents.

O

OXALIPLATIN (*ox-AL-i-PLA-tin*)
ELOXATIN®88
TRANS-I-DIAMINOCYCLOHEXANE OXALATOPLATINUM

Chemical Abstracts Service (CAS) Registry
    Number: 61825-94-3
Registry of Toxic Effects of Chemical Substance
    (RTECS): TP2275850
$C_8H_{12}N_2O_4Pt$

Health & Safety Hazards/US Department of Transportation (DOT)/US Environmental Protection Agency (EPA)—Sources

Reproductive Effector—Material Safety Data Sheet, Fetotoxic—Material Safety Data Sheet, Cytotoxic—Box Instruction, Carcinogen Limited Effect—Material Safety Data Sheet, Cytotoxic—British Columbia Cancer Agency Canada, Nonvesicant—British Columbia Cancer Agency Canada, Pregnancy Category (D)—US Food and Drug Administration,

National Fire Protection Association Health (3) Flammability (0) Instability (0)—Material Safety Data Sheet, National Fire Protection Association Health (3) Flammability (0) Instability (0)—Material Safety Data Sheet, Materials Identification System (R) and/or US Department of Defense System Health (3★) Fire Hazard (0) Reactivity (0) Personal Protection Code (-) (None stated)—Material Safety Data Sheet.

OXALIPLATIN is a clear fluid from powdered form.

OXALIPLATIN is a white or almost white crystalline powder.

First Aid/Medical Information/ Occupational Exposure Limits

First Aid Measures to include: Use general first aid measures except for the following:

Medical Information:

Caution and Warning Statements: ELOXATIN®88 may cause cancer; may cause heritable genetic damage; may impair fertility; may cause harm to the unborn child; may be an ocular irritant; toxic drug; danger of serious damage to health by prolonged exposure through inhalation and if swallowed. Exposure may be irritating to eyes, respiratory system, and skin. Exposure may cause sensitization by inhalation and skin contact. Limited evidence of a carcinogenic effect has been documented.

Caution: Females and males planning to have a child, pregnant women, and nursing mothers should exercise caution regarding potential occupational exposure to this cytotoxic drug. No information or not enough information exists or was provided concerning occupational exposures that may potentially occur while handling this drug and its affects on reproductive systems, the fetus, and/or if it is secreted along with breast milk, which may harm nursing infants. Staff members should consult with the occupational health physician monitoring workers' health in your facility to be apprised of potential hazards and should be advised to avoid becoming pregnant and/or breastfeeding or should be transferred in accordance with policy/procedures to other duties that do not involve preparation, handling, and administering this drug.

Target Organs/Systems: Liver and kidneys, peripheral nervous system, bone marrow, testes, female reproductive toxicity, and cancer

Medical Conditions Generally Aggravated by Exposure:

▪ Pregnancy issues.

Specific Medical Surveillance Information: Reproductive and pregnancy counseling.

Occupational Exposure Level/Limit (OEL) & Sampling Methods:

Environmental Sentinel Contamination Action Level (ESCAL): Not otherwise specified

Occupational Exposure Level (OEL) & Sampling Methods: Sanofi Winthrop Inc:

ELOXATIN®88 lyophilized

Exposure band: 0.1–5 μg/m3

Exposure limit: 10 mg/m3

(No specific method listed)

Supplemental Response Information

Extinguishing Media: Use extinguishing agent which is the most appropriate to extinguish surrounding fire (carbon dioxide, foam, dry chemical or water fog as extinguishing media).

Solubility: OXALIPLATIN (ELOXATIN®88) is slightly soluble in water at 6 mg/ml; practically insoluble in dehydrated alcohol; very slightly soluble in methanol and practically insoluble in ethanol and acetone. OXALIPLATIN pH range is 4.8–5.7 (in 2 mg/ml aqueous solution).

Chemical Degradation/Neutralization Method: A manufacturer's Material Safety Data Sheet (MSDS) recommends treating spill surfaces with a 5–10% sodium hypochlorite (bleach) solution after absorbing liquids with inert absorbent pads or removing any powder present: allow solution to stand for up to one hour, and then thoroughly wash spilled surfaces with soap and water; sample to determine if surface contamination is still present (if sampling method is available). If the drug is present, repeat above steps; dispose of wastes in accordance with your local procedures, state, and federal regulations.

Incompatibility: OXALIPLATIN is incompatible with oxidizing and reducing agents. Materials to avoid:

Incompatibility of this material has not been thoroughly investigated. Keep from contact with oxidizing materials, highly oxygenated or halogenated solvents and organic compounds containing reducible functional groups.

P

PCNU
1-(2-CHLOROETHYL)-3-(2,6-DIOXO-3-PIPERIDYL)-1-NITROSOUREA
UREA

Chemical Abstracts Service (CAS) Registry
Number: 13909-02-9
Registry of Toxic Effects of Chemical Substance
(RTECS): YS4915000
National Cancer Institute: NSC-95466
$C_8H_{11}ClN_4O_4$

Health & Safety Hazards/US Department of Transportation (DOT)/US Environmental Protection Agency (EPA)—Sources

Toxic—US National Institute of Health (NIH) and Material Safety Data Sheet, Mutagen—US National Institute of Health (NIH) and Material Safety Data Sheet, Mutagen—Sax's "Dangerous Properties of Industrial Materials," Mutagen—University of Maryland at College Park, Pregnancy Category (None)—US Food and Drug Administration.

(UV Detection: 254 nm; Color Unknown, 230 nm)

First Aid/Medical Information/ Occupational Exposure Limits

First Aid Measures to include: Use general first aid measures except for the following:

Dermal Contact: Various body tissues readily absorb this material. Avoid rubbing of skin or increasing its temperature. If skin contact occurs, the skin should not be washed with organic solvents.

Medical Information:

Caution and Warning Statements: Not otherwise specified

Target Organs/Systems: Not otherwise specified

Medical Conditions Generally Aggravated by Exposure: Not otherwise specified

Specific Medical Surveillance Information: Not otherwise specified

Occupational Exposure Level/Limit (OEL) & Sampling Methods: Not otherwise specified

Environmental Sentinel Contamination Action Level (ESCAL): Not otherwise specified

Supplemental Response Information

Extinguishing Media: Use extinguishing agent which is the most appropriate to extinguish surrounding fire (carbon dioxide, foam, dry chemical or water fog as extinguishing media).

Solubility: PCNU is somewhat water soluble (<1 mg/ml).

Chemical Degradation/Neutralization Method: Not otherwise specified

Note: If a specific degradation or neutralization method is not provided on this table and you do not have other specific information that will guide you on how to clean up the specific material spilled, then follow the general spill procedure found in the introduction section of this handbook.

Incompatibility: PCNU is incompatible with alkali and elevated temperature.

PEGASPARGASE (*peg-AS-par-jase*)
ONCASPAR®89
AFRINOL
PEG-ASPARGASE

Chemical Abstracts Service (CAS) Registry
Number: 130167-69-0
$C_{1377}-H_{2208}-N_{382}-O_{442}-S_{17}$

Health & Safety Hazards/US Department of Transportation (DOT)/US Environmental Protection Agency (EPA)—Sources

Pregnancy Category (C)—US Food and Drug Administration

PEGASPARGASE is a clear injection.

First Aid/Medical Information/ Occupational Exposure Limits

First Aid Measures to include: Use general first aid measures except for the following:

Physician's note: Toxicology studies have shown material to be of very low acute toxicity. There is no specific antidote. Treatment of overexposure should be directed at the control of symptoms and clinical condition. Anaphylactic reactions require immediate use of epinephrine, oxygen, intravenous steroids, and antihistamines. Consult the physicians' desk reference for additional details.

Medical Information:

Caution and Warning Statements: PEG-ASPARGASE (ONCASPAR®89) is an irritant to mucous membranes. This material may cause eye and skin irritation.

Caution: Females and males planning to have a child, pregnant women, and nursing mothers should exercise caution regarding potential occupational exposure to this cytotoxic drug. No information or not enough information exists or was provided concerning occupational exposures that may potentially occur while handling this drug and its affects on reproductive systems, the fetus, and/or if it is secreted along with breast milk, which may harm nursing infants. Staff members should consult with the occupational health physician monitoring workers' health in your facility to be apprised of potential hazards and should be advised to avoid becoming pregnant and/or breastfeeding or should be transferred in accordance with policy/procedures to other duties that do not involve preparation, handling, and administering this drug.

Therapeutic Levels: The Food and Drug Administration lists this drug as a Pregnancy Category (C). Animal reproduction studies have not been conducted with ONCASPAR®89. It is also not known whether ONCASPAR®89 can cause fetal harm when administered to a pregnant woman or can affect reproduction capacity.

Target Organs/Systems: Hypersensitivity, allergic reactions, and fetus

Medical Conditions Generally Aggravated by Exposure:

- As with all proteins, hypersensitivity and allergic reactions are possible.
- Reproductive and pregnancy issues.

Specific Medical Surveillance Information: Reproductive and pregnancy counseling.

Occupational Exposure Level/Limit (OEL) & Sampling Methods: Not otherwise specified

Environmental Sentinel Contamination Action Level (ESCAL): Not otherwise specified

Supplemental Response Information

Extinguishing Media: Use extinguishing agent which is the most appropriate to extinguish surrounding fire (carbon dioxide, foam, dry chemical or water fog as extinguishing media).

Solubility: ONCASPAR®89 (PEG-ASPARGASE) is completely water soluble.

pH = 7.3

Chemical Degradation/Neutralization Method: Not otherwise specified

Note: If a specific degradation or neutralization method is not provided on this table and you do not have other specific information that will guide you on how to clean up the specific material spilled, then follow the general spill procedure found in the introduction section of this handbook.

Incompatibility: Not otherwise specified

PENTAMIDINE (*pen-TAM-i-deen*)
PENTAMINDINE ISETHIONATE
MJ7236
PENTAM 300

Chemical Abstracts Service (CAS) Registry Number: 140-64-7
Registry of Toxic Effects of Chemical Substance (RTECS): CV6500000
$C_{21}H_{30}N_4O_6S$

Health & Safety Hazards/US Department of Transportation (DOT)/US Environmental Agency (EPA)—Sources

Pregnancy Category (C)—US Food and Drug Administration, Mutagen—University of Maryland at College Park, Corrosive—Material Safety Data Sheet, Harmful and Irritant—Material Safety Data Sheet, Materials Identification System (R) and/or US Department of Defense System Health (3★) with additional chronic hazards present Fire Hazard (0) Reactivity (1) Personal Protection Code (-) (None stated)—Material Safety Data Sheet, National Fire Protection Association Health (3) Flammability (0) Instability (1)—Material Safety Data Sheet.

PENTAMIDINE ISETHIONATE is prepared as a solution and lyophilized in its final container prior to injection (300 mg).

First Aid/Medical Information/ Occupational Exposure Limits

First Aid Measures to include: Use general first aid measures except for the following:

Medical Information:

Caution and Warning Statements: PENTAMIDINE ISETHIONATE is an irritant/corrosive to the eyes. Inhalation is the major route of entry. Signs and symptoms of overexposure are chest pain, coughing, skin rash, wheezing, shortness of breath, drowsiness, nausea, headache, metallic fume fever, and metallic taste. This drug may cause allergic skin reaction. Occupational exposure has not been fully investigated. RTECS lists PENTAMIDINE as a suspected endocrine toxicant and as a skin or sense organ toxicant.

Caution: Females and males planning to have a child, pregnant women, and nursing mothers should exercise caution regarding potential occupational exposure to this cytotoxic drug. No information or not enough information exists or was provided concerning occupational exposures that may potentially occur while handling this drug and its affects on reproductive systems, the fetus, and/or if it is secreted along with breast milk, which may harm nursing infants. Staff members should consult with the occupational health physician monitoring workers' health in your facility to be apprised of potential hazards and should be advised to avoid becoming pregnant and/or breastfeeding or should be transferred in accordance with policy/procedures to other duties that do not involve preparation, handling, and administering this drug.

Therapeutic Levels: The Food and Drug Administration lists PENTAMIDINE as a Pregnancy Category (C). This means that it is not known whether PENTAMIDINE will harm an unborn baby. It is not known whether PENTAMIDINE passes into breast milk.

Target Organs/Systems: Kidneys, pancreas, heart, cardiovascular system, glucose metabolism, hematopoietic system, liver, gastrointestinal tract, respiratory system, and possibly fetus

Medical Conditions Generally Aggravated by Exposure:

- Hypersensitivity to PENTAMIDINE ISETHIONATE, renal injury, cardiac or cardiovascular disease, diabetic conditions, hematologic abnormalities, liver aliments, gastrointestinal ailments, respiratory lesions and pancreatic disease, eye lesions, and Stevens-Johnson syndrome; preexisting skin and respiratory conditions.
- Reproductive and pregnancy issues.

Specific Medical Surveillance Information: Reproductive and pregnancy counseling.

Occupational Exposure Level/Limit (OEL) & Sampling Methods:

Environmental Sentinel Contamination Action Level (ESCAL): Not otherwise specified
Occupational Exposure Level (OEL) Abbott Lab: 0.1 mg/m3
(Method not listed or specified)

Supplemental Response Information

Extinguishing Media: Use extinguishing agent which is the most appropriate to extinguish surrounding fire (carbon dioxide, foam, dry chemical or water fog as extinguishing media).

Solubility: PENTAMIDINE (PENTAMIDINE ISETHIONATE) is water soluble with a pH range from 4.5 to 7.5 (reconstituted). Furthermore it is soluble in glycerol; slightly soluble in alcohol; insoluble in ether, in acetone, in chloroform, and in liquid petroleum.

Chemical Degradation/Neutralization Method: A manufacturer's Material Safety Data Sheet (MSDS) recommends using alkaline soap/detergent and water to clean spill surfaces after absorbing liquids with inert absorbent pads or removing any powder present: repeat using soap and water; sample to determine if surface contamination is still present (if sampling method is available). If the drug is present, repeat above steps; dispose of wastes in accordance with your local procedures, state, and federal regulations.

Incompatibility: PENTAMIDINE is incompatible with strong oxidizing agents, strong acids, and strong bases. Protect from light and moisture.

PENTOSTATIN (*PEN-toe-stat-in*)
PD-ADI
NIPENT®90

Chemical Abstracts Service (CAS) Registry Number: 53910-25-1 (mixture)
Registry of Toxic Effects of Chemical Substance (RTECS): NI2931000
$C_{11}H_{16}N_4O_4$

Health & Safety Hazards/US Department of Transportation (DOT)/US Environmental Protection Agency (EPA)—Sources

Mutagen—University of Maryland at College Park, Teratogen—University of Maryland at College Park, Teratogen—Sax's "Dangerous Properties of Industrial Materials," Hematoxic—Material Safety Data Sheet, Pregnancy Category (D)—US Food and Drug Administration, Carcinogen, Developmental and other Reproductive Harm—US California Proposition 65, National Fire Protection Association Health (2) Flammability (0) Instability (0)—Material Safety Data Sheet, National Fire Protection Association Health (2) Flammability (1) Instability (0)—Material Safety Data Sheet, UN3249 or UN 2811 (Air), Class 6.1 (Air), Packing Group III.

PENTOSTATIN is a clear colorless fluid from powder.

PENTOSTATIN can cause fetal harm; breastfeeding should be discontinued because of potential for reproductive and developmental harm (*A Guide for*

Occupational Health Professionals Technical Manual, Navy Environmental Health Center [NEHC-TM-OEM 6260.01a]).

First Aid/Medical Information/ Occupational Exposure Limits

First Aid Measures to include: Use general first aid measures except for the following:

Eye Contact: Remove any contact lenses. Immediately flush eyes with water for at least 15 minutes while keeping eye lids open. Do not use an eye ointment. Seek medical help.

Medical Information:

Caution and Warning Statements:

Caution: The toxicological properties of most cytotoxic drugs have not been fully investigated, particularly as it pertains to occupational exposure. PENTOSTATIN is one of the drugs that has little occupational hazards information available. Therefore, therapeutic dose information was extrapolated below to assist in determining occupational toxicity, and signs and symptoms of overexposure. Therefore, it is prudent to minimize occupational exposure to PENTOSTATIN.

Commonly reported side effects include an allergic reaction (shortness of breath; closing of throat; difficulty breathing; swelling of lips, face, or tongue; or hives); nervous system problems, such as a burning, pricking, or tingling feeling, or twitching; severe skin rash; confusion, dizziness, extreme sleepiness; signs of infection such as fever, chills, or sore throat; sudden shortness of breath, difficulty breathing, or increased coughing; or unusual bleeding or bruising; nausea, vomiting, diarrhea, or decreased appetite; mouth sores; itching; muscle or joint aches and pains; or headache.

Several references listed PENTOSTATIN as having mutagenic and teratogenic properties. PENTOSTATIN exposure caused hepatotoxicity and lymphopenia, thrombocytopenia, reticulocytopenia, leukocytosis, and elevated serum live enzymes in animals. Toxicological properties are not fully understood. Individuals must use prudent practices when handling and storing drug.

Caution: Females and males planning to have a child, pregnant women, and nursing mothers should exercise caution regarding potential occupational exposure to this cytotoxic drug. No information or not enough information exists or was provided concerning occupational exposures that may potentially occur while handling this drug and its affects on reproductive systems, the fetus, and/or if it is secreted along with breast milk, which may harm nursing infants. Staff members should consult with the occupational health physician monitoring workers' health in your facility to be apprised of potential hazards and should be advised to avoid becoming pregnant and/or breastfeeding or should be transferred in accordance with policy/procedures to other duties that do not involve preparation, handling, and administering this drug.

Target Organs/Systems: Blood, immune system, and possibly fetus

Medical Conditions Generally Aggravated by Exposure:

- Immune system and vaccines (live strains).
- Reproductive and pregnancy issues.

Specific Medical Surveillance Information: Reproductive and pregnancy counseling.

Treatment in humans has been associated with immunosuppression and the resulting infectious complications—reduced white blood cells (lymphopenia). Important ill effects found in clinical treatment of patients are low white blood counts, low platelet count, anemia, kidney damage, eye irritation, nausea, and vomiting.

Occupational Exposure Level/Limit (OEL) & Sampling Methods:

Environmental Sentinel Contamination Action Level (ESCAL): Not otherwise specified
Occupational Exposure Level (OEL) Warner-Lambert: 0.014 mg/m3 Time-Weighted Average (TWA) (Method not listed or specified)

Supplemental Response Information

Extinguishing Media: Use extinguishing agent which is the most appropriate to extinguish surrounding fire (carbon dioxide, foam, dry chemical or water fog as extinguishing media).

Solubility: NIPENT®90 (PENTOSTATIN) is freely water soluble with a pH range from 7.0 to 8.5.

Chemical Degradation/Neutralization Method: A manufacturer's Material Safety Data Sheet (MSDS) recommends treating spill surfaces with a 10% sodium hypochlorite (bleach) solution after absorbing liquids with inert absorbent pads or removing any powder present: allow solution to stand for up to one hour (at least 30 minutes), and then thoroughly wash spilled surfaces with soap and water; sample to determine if surface contamination is still present (if sampling method is available). If the drug is present, repeat above steps; dispose of wastes in accordance with your local procedures, state, and federal regulations.

Incompatibility: PENTOSTATIN is incompatible with strong oxidizing materials.

PLICAMYCIN (*ply-kuh-MY-sin*)
MITHRAMYCIN
MITHRACIN®91
A-2371

Chemical Abstracts Service (CAS) Registry
Number: 18378-89-7 (mixture)
Registry of Toxic Effects of Chemical Substance
(RTECS): PZ2800000
$C_{52}H_{76}O_{24}$

Health & Safety Hazards/US Department of Transportation (DOT)/US Environmental Protection Agency (EPA)—Sources

Carcinogen—Material Safety Data Sheet, Teratogen—Material Safety Data Sheet, Reproductive Effector—Material Safety Data Sheet, Highly Toxic—Material Safety Data Sheet, Mutagen—Material Safety Data Sheet, Vesicant—British Columbia Cancer Agency Canada, Pregnancy Category (X)—US Food and Drug Administration, Developmental—US California Proposition 65, Materials Identification System (R) and/or US Department of Defense System Health (2★) with additional chronic hazards present Fire Hazard (0) Reactivity (0) Personal Protection Code (-) (None stated)—Material Safety Data Sheet, National Fire Protection Association Health (2) Flammability (0) Instability (0), Material Safety Data Sheet, National Fire Protection Association Health (2) Flammability (0) Instability (1)—Material Safety Data Sheet, National Fire Protection Association Health (2★) with additional chronic hazards present Flammability (1) Instability (0).

PLICAMYCIN is a yellow odorless hygroscopic crystalline powder.

PLICAMYCIN is available as an injection.

PLICAMYCIN (MITHRACIN®91) may cause fetal harm; breastfeeding should be discontinued because of potential for reproductive and developmental hazards (*A Guide for Occupational Health Professionals Technical Manual*, Navy Environmental Health Center [NEHC-TM-OEM 6260.01a]).

PLICAMYCIN is an antineoplastic antibiotic produced by the growth of Streptomyces Argillaceus, s. Plicatus and s. Tanashiensis.

(UV fluorescence at 280 nm—strong yellow color)

First Aid/Medical Information/ Occupational Exposure Limits

First Aid Measures to include: Use general first aid measures except for the following:

Physician's note: Acute overdose treatment: there is no specific antidote for PLICAMYCIN. Overdose treatment is generally supportive and may include the use of antiemetics to treat nausea and vomiting.

Emergency and First Aid Procedures: Discontinue use. Blood transfusions if needed. Treat bone marrow depression. If infiltrated, inject saline and lidocaine locally. Use ice bag. Follow platelets, hemoglobin, liver and renal function.

Medical Information:

Caution and Warning Statements: PLICAMYCIN (MITHRAMYCIN) is poisonous by intravenous, subcutaneous, and other routes. An experimental teratogen, experimental reproductive effects (human mutagenic data). Decreased white and red blood cell counts, liver and kidney damage and decrease serum calcium, phosphorus, and/or potassium. RTECS lists PLICAMYCIN as a suspected cardiovascular or blood toxicant. This drug is a possible mutagen and limited evidence of carcinogenic effect; and a possible risk of irreversible effects. Avoid prolonged or repeated exposure. BC Cancer Agency lists PLICAMYCIN as a vesicant.

Caution: Females and males planning to have a child, pregnant women, and nursing mothers should exercise caution regarding potential occupational exposure to this cytotoxic drug. No information or not enough information exists or was provided concerning occupational exposures that may potentially occur while handling this drug and its affects on reproductive systems, the fetus, and/or if it is secreted along with breast milk, which may harm nursing infants. Staff members should consult with the occupational health physician monitoring workers' health in your facility to be apprised of potential hazards and should be advised to avoid becoming pregnant and/or breastfeeding or should be transferred in accordance with policy/procedures to other duties that do not involve preparation, handling, and administering this drug.

Target Organs/Systems: Blood, bone marrow, nerves, reproductive, GI system, liver, kidneys, and possible fetus

Medical Conditions Generally Aggravated by Exposure:

- Hypersensitivity to PLICAMYCIN, blood dyscrasias, depressed bone marrow function, existing or recent chickenpox exposure, herpes zoster, severe liver or kidney function impairment, previous cytotoxic drug or radiation therapy, scheduled dental work, recent immunization with live virus vaccines, and coagulation disorders or increased susceptibility to bleeding due to other causes, such as ingestion of aspirin within the past week.

- Reproductive and pregnancy issues.

Specific Medical Surveillance Information: Reproductive and pregnancy counseling.

In case of exposure, treat bone marrow depression and follow, platelet, hemoglobin, liver, and renal function tests.

Occupational Exposure Level/Limit (OEL) & Sampling Methods: Not otherwise specified

Environmental Sentinel Contamination Action Level (ESCAL): Not otherwise specified

Supplemental Response Information

Extinguishing Media: Use extinguishing agent which is the most appropriate to extinguish surrounding fire (carbon dioxide, foam, dry chemical or water fog as extinguishing media).

Solubility: PLICAMYCIN (MITHRAMYCIN) is slightly too moderately water soluble, very slightly soluble in alcohol (a 0.05% solution in water has a pH of 4.5 to 5.5).

Chemical Degradation/Neutralization Method: Not otherwise specified

Note: If a specific degradation or neutralization method is not provided on this table and you do not have other specific information that will guide you on how to clean up the specific material spilled, then follow the general spill procedure found in the introduction section of this handbook.

Incompatibility: PLICAMYCIN is incompatible with strong oxidizers, avoid contact with divalent cations, especially iron; avoid exposure to light, heat, and moisture.

PREDNISONE (*pred-NIS-one*)

Chemical Abstracts Service (CAS) Registry Number: 53-03-2

DELTASONE®92

Registry of Toxic Effects of Chemical Substance (RTECS): TU4154100
$C_{21}H_{26}O_5$

Health & Safety Hazards/US Department of Transportation (DOT)/US Environmental Protection Agency (EPA)—Sources

Ca G3—International Agency for Research on Cancer, Carcinogen—Berkeley University Hazardous Chemical List, Carcinogen—University of Maryland at College Park, Teratogen—University of Maryland at College Park, Sensitizer—Material Safety Data Sheet, Cardiotoxic—Material Safety Data Sheet, Lactation Small Amount in Breast Milk—Material Safety Data Sheet, Pregnancy Category (C)—US Food and Drug Administration and Drugs.com, National Fire Protection Association Health (1) Flammability (1) Instability (0)—Material Safety Data Sheet, Materials Identification System (R) and/or US Department of Defense System Health (1) Fire Hazard (1) Reactivity (0) Personal Protection Code (E) (Safety Glasses, Chemical Gloves, Dust Respirator)—Material Safety Data Sheet.

PREDNISONE is available as an oral solution or syrup; tablets of 2.5, 5, 10, 20, and 50 mg. Oral solutions or syrup of 5mg/5ml.

PREDNISIONE appearance is a white crystalline powder.

First Aid/Medical Information/Occupational Exposure Limits

First Aid Measures to include: Use general first aid measures.

Medical Information:

Caution and Warning Statements:

Therapeutic Levels: PREDNISONE decreases inflammation by preventing white blood cells from completing an inflammatory reaction. This drug can cause lymphocytes, a type of white blood cell, to break apart and die.

PREDNISONE may cause adverse reproductive effects and cancer based on animal test data. This drug may affect genetic material (mutagenic). Human: small amount excreted in maternal milk.

Acute potential health effects—skin: may cause skin irritation. PREDNISONE may cause skin sensitization and/or an allergic reaction. Eyes: may cause eye irritation. Inhalation: may cause respiratory tract irritation. *Ingestion*: may cause gastritis with nausea, vomiting, abdominal distention, ulcerative esophagitis, increased sweating. May affect metabolism and cause disturbance of electrolyte balance, which is manifest in the retention of sodium and water, with edema and hypertension, and in the increased excretion of potassium with the possibility of hypokalemic alkalosis. Cardiac failure may be induced in sensitive individuals.

Chronic potential health effects—skin: prolonged or repeated skin contact may cause sensitization, an allergic reaction. Eyes: prolonged contact with eyes may affect vision (cataracts); inhalation/ingestion: may cause anaphylaxis, an allergic reaction. Prolonged or repeated inhalation or ingestion of corticosteroids may also cause thinning of the skin, impaired wound healing, and other dermatologic reactions (erythema, petechiae, and ecchymoses). Ingestion: prolonged or repeated ingestion of corticosteroids may cause nausea, vomiting, abdominal distention, peptic ulcer with possible perforation and hemorrhage, possible hypersensitization, swelling of the feet and lower legs due to electrolyte imbalance and sodium retention, irregular heartbeat, acute adrenal insufficiency, osteoporosis, muscle weakness, loss of muscle mass, vertebral compression fractures, pathologic fracture of long bones, aseptic necrosis of femoral and humeral heads, effect glucose tolerance (causing decreased carbohydrate tolerance resulting in manifestations of latent diabetes mellitus, increased requirements for insulin or oral hypoglycemic agents in diabetes), the liver, pancreas (pancreatitis), eyes/vision (cataracts, glaucoma, increased intraocular pressure), behavior/central nervous system/nervous system (mental disturbances such as psychosis, euphoria, depression, vertigo, headache, convulsions, increased intracranial pressure with papilledema). It may also affect the immune system (immunosuppressant). Repeated large doses of corticosteroids may produce cushingoid symptoms typical of hyperactivity of the adrenal cortex, with moon-face, sometimes hirsutism, buffalo hump, flushing, increased bruising, ecchymoses, striae, and acne.

Caution: Females and males planning to have a child, pregnant women, and nursing mothers should exercise caution regarding potential occupational exposure to this cytotoxic drug. Prednisone has been assigned a Pregnancy Category (C) by the Food and Drug Administration. No information or not enough information exists or was provided concerning occupational exposures that may potentially occur while handling this drug and its affects on reproductive systems, the fetus, and/or if it is secreted along with breast milk, which may harm nursing infants. Staff members should consult with the occupational health physician monitoring workers' health in your facility to be apprised of potential hazards and should be advised to avoid becoming pregnant and/or breastfeeding or should be transferred in accordance with policy/procedures to other duties that do not involve preparation, handling, and administering this drug.

Therapeutic Levels: Corticosteroids cross the placenta into the fetus. Compared to other corticosteroids, however, prednisone is less likely to cross the placenta. (Small amounts excreted in maternal milk.) Chronic use of corticosteroids during the first trimester of pregnancy may cause cleft palate.

Corticosteroids are secreted in breast milk and can cause side effects in the nursing infant. Prednisone is less likely than other corticosteroids to be secreted in breast milk, but it may still pose a risk to the infant.

Target Organs/Systems: May cause adrenal insufficiency, skin, fetus, and immune system

Medical Conditions Generally Aggravated by Exposure:

- PREDNISONE: if diabetic, this medicine will increase blood sugar levels. Hypersensivity to material, ocular herpes simplex, active alcoholism, aids or HIV infection, heart disease or hypertension, diabetes mellitus, myasthenia gravis, impaired kidney or liver.
- Reproductive and pregnancy issues.

Specific Medical Surveillance Information: Reproductive and pregnancy counseling.

Occupational Exposure Level/Limit (OEL) & Sampling Methods: Not otherwise specified

Environmental Sentinel Contamination Action Level (ESCAL): Not otherwise specified

Supplemental Response Information

Extinguishing Media: Use extinguishing agent which is the most appropriate to extinguish surrounding fire (carbon dioxide, foam, dry chemical or water fog as extinguishing media). (Do not use water jet.)

Solubility: PREDNISONE is very slightly water soluble. Furthermore, PREDNISONE is slightly soluble in alcohol, in chloroform, in dioxane, and in methanol.

Chemical Degradation/Neutralization Method: Not otherwise specified

Note: If a specific degradation or neutralization method is not provided on this table and you do not have other specific information that will guide you on how to clean up the specific material spilled, then follow the general spill procedure found in the introduction section of this handbook.

Incompatibility: PREDNISONE is incompatible with oxidizing agents.

PROCARBAZINE HYDROCHLORIDE (*pro-CAR-ba-zeen*)
MATULANE®93

Chemical Abstracts Service (CAS) Registry Number: 366-70-1

$C_{12}H_{20}ClN_3O$
$C_{12}H_{19}N_3O$

PROCARBAZINE HYDROCHLORIDE

RETC XS4725000

Health & Safety Hazards/US Department of Transportation (DOT)/US Environmental Protection Agency (EPA)—Sources

Carcinogen G2A—International Agency for Research on Cancer, Carcinogen G1—International Agency for Research on Cancer, Carcinogen C2—US National Toxicology Program—US New Jersey Department of Health and Senior Services Hazardous Substances Fact Sheet and Material Safety Data Sheet, Carcinogen—Material Safety Data Sheet, Carcinogen—Berkeley University Hazardous Chemical List, Carcinogen—University Maryland at College Park, Teratogen—University of Maryland at College Park, Teratogen—Material Safety Data Sheet, Teratogen—Rx.com, Irritation—Material Safety Data Sheet, Reproductive Effector—Material Safety Data Sheet, Mutagen—University of Maryland at College Park, Lactation—Avoid Breastfeeding (World Health Organization), Pregnancy Category (D)—US Food and Drug Administration, Carcinogen and Developmental (PROCARBAZINE HCL)—US California Proposition 65, National Fire Protection Association Health (2) Flammability (0) Instability (0)—Material Safety Data Sheet.

PROCARBAZINE is manufactured in 50 mg cream-colored capsules.

PROCARBAZINE HCL—Male: azoospermia, can cause fetal harm; breastfeeding: do not nurse because of potential for reproductive and developmental harm (*A Guide for Occupational Health Professionals Technical Manual*, Navy Environmental Health Center [NEHC-TM-OEM 6260.01a]).

PROCARBAZINE HYDROCHLORIDE is a white to pale yellow crystalline powder.

First Aid/Medical Information/ Occupational Exposure Limits

First Aid Measures to include: Use general first aid measures except for the following:

Physician's note: Treatment of PROCARBAZINE HYDROCHLORIDE overdose may include the following:

1. Induce vomiting or perform gastric lavage (with protected airway) followed by instillation of charcoal slurry for recent ingestion;

2. Treat signs and symptoms of CNS stimulation with diazepam, administered intravenously and slowly;

3. Treat hypotension and vascular collapse with intravenous fluids and a dilute pressor agent;

4. Closely monitor and correct body temperature; maintain fluid and electrolyte balance and respiration;

5. Reduce symptoms of hypermetabolic state with intravenous Dantrolene Sodium at 2.5 mg per kg of body weight per day in divided doses. Carefully monitor for signs of liver toxicity and pleural or pericardial effusions;

6. Effects of massive overdose may persist for several days; recovery from mild overdose may take three to four days.

Medical Information:

Caution and Warning Statements: PROCARBAZINE HYDROCHLORIDE may cause cancer and is a teratogen based on animal data. Handle with extreme caution. May cause birth defects based on animal data and may cause male reproductive systems effects based on animal data. Exposure may cause skin and respiratory tract irritation. RTECS lists PROCARBAZINE as a suspected, cardiovascular or blood toxicant, as an endocrine toxicant, and as a respiratory toxicant.

Exposure to PROCARBAZINE HYDROCHLORIDE can cause nausea, vomiting, diarrhea, and stomach pain, loss of appetite, and loss of weight. Other symptoms are headache and nightmares, a feeling of being sleepy, confusion, and depression.

Caution: Females and males planning to have a child, pregnant women, and nursing mothers should exercise caution regarding potential occupational exposure to this cytotoxic drug. No information or not enough information exists or was provided concerning occupational exposures that may potentially occur while handling this drug and its affects on reproductive systems, the fetus, and/or if it is secreted along with breast milk, which may harm nursing infants. Staff members should consult with the occupational health physician monitoring workers' health in your facility to be apprised of potential hazards and should be advised to avoid becoming pregnant and/or breastfeeding or should be transferred in accordance with policy/procedures to other duties that do not involve preparation, handling, and administering this drug.

Therapeutic Levels: Females and males planning to have a child and pregnant women should exercise caution regarding potential exposure. It is advisable for nursing mothers to exercise caution regarding potential exposure. This material may cause impairment of mental and/or physical abilities, which are required to perform hazardous tasks, such as operating machinery or driving a motor vehicle.

Target Organs/Systems: Gastrointestinal system, CNS, peripheral nervous system, hematopoietic/blood system, male reproductive systems/prostate, immune, dermal, respiratory systems, and possibly fetus

Medical Conditions Generally Aggravated by Exposure:

- If you are taking antihistamines, sedatives, or any prescribed medications, notify your occupational health staff that you are potentially exposed to PROCARBAZINE HYDROCHLORIDE. Furthermore, alcohol consumption may cause severe nausea, vomiting, flushing, palpitations, and weakness. Animal studies have shown that the risks of secondary lung cancer from treatment appear to be multiplied by tobacco use.
- Hypersensitivity to material, active alcoholism or alcohol ingestion, heart problems, severely impaired liver or kidney function, pheochromocytoma, bone marrow depression, existing or recent chickenpox or herpes zoster, severe or frequent headaches, infection, hyperexcitable personality states, and previous cytotoxic drug or radiation therapy.
- Reproductive and pregnant issues.

Specific Medical Surveillance Information: Reproductive and pregnancy counseling.

If symptoms develop and/or overexposure is suspected, a complete blood count should be performed.

Occupational Exposure Level/Limit (OEL) & Sampling Methods: Not otherwise specified

Environmental Sentinel Contamination Action Level (ESCAL): Air
(OSHA Salt Lake Lab method)

Supplemental Response Information

Extinguishing Media: Use extinguishing agent which is the most appropriate to extinguish surrounding fire (carbon dioxide, foam, dry chemical or water fog as extinguishing media).

Solubility: PROCARBAZINE HCL is completely water soluble and 95% soluble in methanol and ethanol.

Chemical Degradation/Neutralization Method: The IARC recommends treating PROCARBAZINE HYDROCHLORIDE spill surfaces with a solution of 0.3 mol/liter potassium permanganate/3 mol/liter of sulfuric acid solution over the contaminated area and allow to react overnight or longer after absorbing liquids with inert absorbent pads or removing any powder present: after allowing the solution to stand for the required time and then thoroughly washing spilled surfaces with soap and water; sample to determine if surface contamination is still present (if sampling method is available). If the drug is present, repeat above steps; dispose of wastes in accordance with your local procedures, state, and federal regulations.

Incompatibility: PROCARBAZINE HYDROCHLORIDE is incompatible with alcohols and manganese or cupric ions in the presence of oxidizing agents. Void exposure to light, heat, and moisture.

R

RAZOXANEB
ZINECARD®94
ICRF-187
DEXRAZOXANE (deks-ray-ZOKS-ane)
$C_{11}H_{16}N_4O_4$

Chemical Abstracts Service (CAS) Registry Number: 21416-67-1, 83713-23-9 (mixture with hydrochloric acid)
Registry of Toxic Effects of Chemical Substance (RTECS): TL6389900

Health & Safety Hazards/US Department of Transportation (DOT)/US Environmental Protection Agency (EPA)—Sources

Mutagen—University of Maryland at College Park, Mutagen—Sax's "Dangerous Properties of Industrial Materials," Carcinogen—Berkeley University Hazardous Chemical List, Reproductive Effector—Material Safety Data Sheet, Cytotoxic—British Columbia Cancer Agency Canada, Nonvesicant—British Columbia Cancer Agency Canada, Pregnancy Category (C)—US Food and Drug Administration,

DEXRAZOXANE (RAZOXANE) is available as an injection.

First Aid/Medical Information/ Occupational Exposure Limits

First Aid Measures to include: Use general first aid measures.

Medical Information:

Caution and Warning Statements: Primary routes of exposure are skin contact, eye contact, ingestion, and inhalation. DEXRAZOXANE (ZINECARD®94) has caused adverse reproductive effects in animals.

Caution: Females and males planning to have a child, pregnant women, and nursing mothers should exercise caution regarding potential occupational exposure to this cytotoxic drug. No information or not enough information exists or was provided concerning occupational exposures that may potentially occur while handling this drug and its affects on reproductive systems, the fetus, and/or if it is secreted along with breast milk, which may harm nursing infants. Staff members should consult with the occupational health physician monitoring workers' health in your facility to be apprised of potential hazards and should be advised to avoid becoming pregnant and/or breastfeeding or should be transferred in accordance with policy/procedures to other duties that do not involve preparation, handling, and administering this drug.

Therapeutic Levels: The Food and Drug Administration lists this drug as a Pregnancy Category (C). There are no adequate and well-controlled studies in pregnant women. ZINECARD®94 should be used during pregnancy only if the potential benefit justifies the potential risk to the fetus. Nursing mothers—it is not known whether DEXRAZOXANE is excreted in human milk.

Target Organs/Systems: Reproductive systems
Medical Conditions Generally Aggravated by Exposure:

- Reproductive and pregnancy issues.

Specific Medical Surveillance Information: Reproductive and pregnancy counseling.
Occupational Exposure Level/Limit (OEL) & Sampling Methods: Not otherwise specified

Environmental Sentinel Contamination Action Level (ESCAL): Not otherwise specified

Supplemental Response Information

Extinguishing Media: Use extinguishing agent which is the most appropriate to extinguish surrounding fire (carbon dioxide, foam, dry chemical or water fog as extinguishing media).

Solubility: ZINECARD®94 is slightly water soluble (10–12 mg/ml).

Chemical Degradation/Neutralization Method: Not otherwise specified

Note: If a specific degradation or neutralization method is not provided on this table and you do not have other specific information that will guide you on how to clean up the specific material spilled, then follow the general spill procedure found in the introduction section of this handbook.

Incompatibility: Not otherwise specified

REMICADE®95
CHIMERIC ANT-TNF MONOCLONAL ANTI-BODY
INFLIXIMAB (in-FLIX-i-mab)

Chemical Abstracts Service (CAS) Registry Numbers: 170277-31-3, 331731-18-1
$C_{6428}H_{9912}N_{1694}O_{1987}S_{46}$

Health & Safety Hazards/US Department of Transportation (DOT)/US Environmental Protection Agency (EPA)—Sources

Pregnancy Category (B)—US Food and Drug Administration.

REMICADE®95 (INFLIXIMAB) is available as an injection (injection lyophilized powder).

First Aid/Medical Information/ Occupational Exposure Limits

First Aid Measures to include: Use general first aid measures.

Medical Information:

Cautions and Warnings: Material Safety Data Sheet (MSDS) claims that REMICADE®95 contains no hazardous components as defined in OSHA 29 CFR 1910.1200. Avoid direct contact and significant aerosol/lyophilized powder exposure, which has the remote possibility of eliciting an allergic response. If a person with an allergy to mouse proteins might have a remote possibility for an allergic reaction upon contact with drug (pH = 7.2).

Food and Drug Administration Pregnancy Category (B); Since INFLIXIMAB does not cross-react with TNF (alpha) in species other than humans and chimpanzees; animal reproduction studies have not been conducted with (REMICADE®95). No evidence of maternal toxicity, embryotoxicity, or teratogenicity was observed in a developmental toxicity study conducted in mice using an analogous antibody that selectively inhibits the functional activity of mouse TNF (alpha).

Target Organs/Systems: REMICADE®95 has possible allergic reaction upon repeated exposure. Liver failure has occurred at therapeutic doses

Medical Conditions Generally Aggravated by Exposure:

- Allergic reaction to drug or/and mouse proteins.

Specific Medical Surveillance Information: Not otherwise specified

Occupational Exposure Level/Limit (OEL) & Sampling Methods: Not otherwise specified

Environmental Sentinel Contamination Action Level (ESCAL): Not otherwise specified

Supplemental Response Information

Extinguishing Media: Use extinguishing agent which is the most appropriate to extinguish surrounding fire (carbon dioxide, foam, dry chemical or water fog as extinguishing media).

Solubility: REMICADE®95 is water soluble (~pH 7.2).

Chemical Degradation/Neutralization Method: A manufacturer's material safety data sheet Material Safety Data Sheet (MSDS) recommends treating spill surfaces with a ~2 mol/liter (~8 g/100 ml), aqueous caustic soda (sodium hydroxide) solution after absorbing liquids with inert absorbent pads or removing any powder present: allow solution to stand for up to one hour, and then thoroughly wash spilled surfaces with soap and water; sample to determine if surface contamination is still present (if sampling method is available). If the drug is present, repeat above steps; dispose of wastes in accordance with your local procedures, state, and federal regulations.

Incompatibility: Not otherwise specified

RITUXAN®96

RITUXIMAB (*ri-TUK-si-mab*)
IDEC 102
IBRITUMOMAB

Chemical Abstracts Service (CAS) Registry Number: 174722-31-7
$C_{6416}-H_{9874}N_{1688}-O_{1987}-S_{44}$
$C_{6382}-H_{9830}-N_{1672}-O_{1979}-S_{54}$
IDEC-C2B8

Health & Safety Hazards/US Department of Transportation (DOT)/US Environmental Protection Agency (EPA)—Sources

Cytotoxic—British Columbia Cancer Agency Canada, Nonvesicant—British Columbia Cancer Agency Canada, Pregnancy Category (C)—US Food and Drug Administration, National Fire Protection Association Health (0) Flammability (0) Instability (0)—Material Safety Data Sheet.

RITUXIMAB (RITUXAN) is available as an injection (a clear fluid after being diluted).

First Aid/Medical Information/ Occupational Exposure Limits

First Aid Measures to include: Use general first aid measures.

Medical Information:

Caution and Warning Statement:

Caution: The toxicological properties of most cytotoxic drugs have not been fully investigated, particularly as it pertains to occupational exposure. RITUXAN (RITUXIMAB) is one of the drugs that has little occupational hazards information available. Therefore, therapeutic dose information was extrapolated below to assist in determining occupational toxicity, and signs and symptoms of overexposure. Therefore, it is prudent to minimize occupational exposure to RITUXAN (RITUXIMAB) (Healthline).

RITUXAN may be irritating to eyes, respiratory system, and skin. This material is not readily absorbed through skin. RITUXAN is clear (colorless) liquid. Single-agent RITUXAN therapy has not been associated with clinically significant hepatic or renal toxicity, through mild, transient increases in liver function tests have occurred. No long term toxicological studies have been performed. RITUXAN target CD20-positive B lymphocytes (box instructions).

Caution: Females and males planning to have a child, pregnant women, and nursing mothers should exercise caution regarding potential occupational exposure to this cytotoxic drug. No information or not enough information exists or was provided concerning occupational exposures that may potentially occur while handling this drug and its affects on reproductive systems, the fetus, and/or if it is secreted along with breast milk, which may harm nursing infants. Staff members should consult with the occupational health physician monitoring workers' health in your facility to be apprised of potential hazards and should be advised to avoid becoming pregnant and/or breastfeeding or should be transferred in accordance with policy/procedures to other duties that do not involve preparation, handling, and administering this drug.

Therapeutic Levels: The Food and Drug Administration list this drug as a Pregnancy Category (C); animal reproduction studies have not been conducted with RITUXAN. It is not known whether RITUXAN can cause fetal harm when administered to a pregnant woman or whether it can affect reproductive capacity. Human IGG is known to pass the placental barrier, and thus may potentially cause fetal B-cell depletion.

Target Organs/System: Lung, heart, kidney, skin, immune system hypersensitive response, and possibly fetus

Medical Conditions Generally Aggravated by Exposure:

- Hepatitis B virus (HBV)—Reported reactivation of the hepatitis B virus (HBV) during therapeutic treatments, and pregnancy.

Specific Medical Surveillance Information: Reproductive and pregnancy counseling. Complete blood count (CBC) and platelet counts.

Occupational Exposure Level/Limit (OEL) & Sampling Methods:

Environmental Sentinel Contamination Action Level (ESCAL): Not otherwise specified
Occupational Exposure Level (OEL) Hoffmann-La Roche:
Threshold value (Roche) Air—Category 1 (Roche group directive K1, annex 3): IOELV >500 µg/m3
(Method not listed or specified)

Supplemental Response Information

Extinguishing Media: Use extinguishing agent which is the most appropriate to extinguish surrounding fire (carbon dioxide, foam, dry chemical or water fog as extinguishing media).

Solubility: RITUXAN is water soluble (pH = 6.5 for 1 % RITUXIMAB solution with excipients).

Chemical Degradation/Neutralization Method: Not otherwise specified

Note: If a specific degradation or neutralization method is not provided on this table and you do not have other specific information that will guide you on how to clean up the specific material spilled, then follow the general spill procedure found in the introduction section of this handbook.

Incompatibility: Not otherwise specified

S

SEMUSTINE
METHYL-CCNU
ME-CCNU

Chemical Abstracts Service (CAS) Registry Numbers: 13909-09-6 33073-59-5 33185-87-4 56748-54-0
National Cancer Institute: NSC95441
C_{10}-H_{18}-CL-N_3-O_2
$C_{10}H_{18}ClN_3O_2$

METHYL-CCNU

Registry of Toxic Effects of Chemical Substance (RTECS): Ys5000000

Health & Safety Hazards/US Department of Transportation (DOT)/US Environmental Protection Agency (EPA)—Sources

Toxic—US National Institute of Health (NIH) and Material Safety Data Sheet, Carcinogen G1—International Agency for Research on Cancer, Carcinogen—US National Institute of Health (NIH) and Material

Safety Data Sheet, Carcinogen C1—US National Toxicology Program, Carcinogen—University of Maryland at College Park, Teratogen—US National Institute of Health (NIH) and Material Safety Data Sheet, Mutagen—US National Institute of Health (NIH) and Material Safety Data Sheet, Mutagen—University of Maryland at College Park, Mutagen—ToxReport, Tumorigenic—ToxReport, Carcinogen—US California Proposition 65, Carcinogen—Material Safety Data Sheet, UN 2811, Class 6.1, Group II, US California Environmental Protection Agency Listed.

SEMUSTINE is a light yellow powder.

First Aid/Medical Information/Occupational Exposure Limits

First Aid Measures to include: Use general first aid measures except for the following:

Dermal Contact: Avoid rubbing of skin or increasing its temperature.

Medical Information:

Caution and Warning Statements: The toxicological properties have not been thoroughly investigated. May cause cancer and may cause heritable genetic damage.

Absorbed by various body tissues, skin (primary irritant), respiratory and intestinal, and transplacentally. Irritates the skin and eyes. RTECS lists SEMUSTINE as a suspected cardiovascular or blood toxicant; as a gastrointestinal or liver toxicant; and as a kidney toxicant.

Signs and symptoms of possible overexposure at therapeutic exposure levels are myelosuppression, the damage to white blood cells and platelets. Such damage may result in infection and bleeding, respectively. The myelosuppression from SEMUSTINE is prolonged, meaning that it takes longer for blood cells to recover than is seen with many other anticancer drugs. Therefore, the interval between courses of SEMUSTINE is longer than with other agents. SEMUSTINE also causes nausea and vomiting. Sometimes anorexia, or loss of appetite, persists after nausea and vomiting. As noted above, SEMUSTINE has also been associated with the development of secondary leukemia.

Target Organs/Systems: Kidneys, blood, bone marrow, and cancer

Medical Conditions Generally Aggravated by Exposure:

- The toxicological properties have not been thoroughly investigated—investigational drug, not widely used in the United States. Chicken pox, gout, heart disease, congestive heart failure, shingles, kidney stones, liver disease, or other forms of cancer.

Specific Medical Surveillance Information: The toxicological properties have not been thoroughly investigated—investigational drug, not widely used in the United States.

Exposure to METHYL-CCNU can lower the blood counts (white blood cells, red blood cells, and platelets).

Occupational Exposure Level OEL)/Limit & Sampling Methods: Not otherwise specified.

Environmental Sentinel Contamination Action Level (ESCAL): Not otherwise specified

Supplemental Response Information

Extinguishing Media: Use extinguishing agent which is the most appropriate to extinguish surrounding fire (carbon dioxide, foam, dry chemical or water fog as extinguishing media).

Solubility: SEMUSTINE (ME-CCNU) is very slightly water soluble (<0.1 g/100 ml at 18 c), soluble in absolute ethanol, lipids, and nonpolar organic solvents.

Chemical Degradation/Neutralization Method: Not otherwise specified

Note: If a specific degradation or neutralization method is not provided on this table and you do not have other specific information that will guide you on how to clean up the specific material spilled, then follow the general spill procedure found in the introduction section of this handbook.

Incompatibility: SEMUSTINE is incompatible with strong oxidizing agents, alkali, and elevated temperature. Avoid/protect from moisture.

SPIROMUSTINE
SPIROHYDANTOIN MUSTARD

Chemical Abstracts Service (CAS) Registry
Number: 56605-16-4
Registry of Toxic Effects of Chemical Substance
(RTECS): HM2508000
National Cancer Institute: NSC172112
C_{14}-H_{23}-C_{12}-N_3-O_2

Health & Safety Hazards/US Department of Transportation (DOT)/US Environmental Protection Agency (EPA)—Sources

Pregnancy Category (None)—US Food and Drug Administration, Mutagen ToxReport.

First Aid/Medical Information/ Occupational Exposure Limits

First Aid Measures to include: Use general first aid measures.

Medical Information:

Caution and Warning Statements:

Caution: The toxicological properties of most cytotoxic drugs have not been fully investigated, particularly as it pertains to occupational exposure. SPIROMUSTINE (SPIROHYDANTOIN MUSTARD) is one of the drugs that has little occupational hazards information available. Therefore, it is prudent to minimize occupational exposure to SPIROMUSTINE (SPIROHYDANTOIN MUSTARD).

Target Organs/Systems: Not otherwise specified

Medical Conditions Generally Aggravated by Exposure: Not otherwise specified

Specific Medical Surveillance Information: Not otherwise specified

Occupational Exposure Level/Limit (OEL) & Sampling Methods: Not otherwise specified

Environmental Sentinel Contamination Action Level (ESCAL): Not otherwise specified

Supplemental Response Information

Extinguishing Media: Use extinguishing agent which is the most appropriate to extinguish surrounding fire (carbon dioxide, foam, dry chemical or water fog as extinguishing media).

Solubility: MUSTARD has a very poor solubility in water.

Chemical Degradation/Neutralization Method: Not otherwise specified

Note: If a specific degradation or neutralization method is not provided on this table and you do not have other specific information that will guide you on how to clean up the specific material spilled, then follow the general spill procedure found in the introduction section of this handbook.

Incompatibility: Not otherwise specified

T

TAMOXIFEN CITRATE
(*ta-MOKS-i-fen*)
NOLVADEX®98

Chemical Abstracts Service (CAS) Registry Number: 54965-24-1

TAMOXIFEN (FREE BASE)

Chemical Abstracts Service (CAS) Registry Number: 10540-29-1 (free base)
$C_{26}H_{29}NO$

TAMOXIFEN CITRATE SALT

Chemical Abstracts Service (CAS) Registry Number: 54965-24-1
$C_{32}H_{37}NO_8$

NOLVADEX®98

Registry of Toxic Effects of Chemical Substance (RTECS): KH2387000
$C_{26}H_{29}NO.C_6H_8O_7$

Health & Safety Hazards/US Department of Transportation (DOT)/US Environmental Protection Agency (EPA)—Sources

Carcinogen G1—International Agency for Research on Cancer, Carcinogen C1—US National Toxicology Program, Tumorigenic—Material Safety Data Sheet, Reproductive Effector—Material Safety Data Sheet, Fetotoxic—Material Safety Data Sheet, Toxic—Material Safety Data Sheet, Pregnancy Category (D)—US Food and Drug Administration, Carcinogen (Tamoxifen)—US California Proposition 65, Developmental—US California Proposition 65, Irritant—Material Safety Data Sheet, National Fire Protection Association Health (1) Flammability (0) Instability (0)—Material Safety Data Sheet, National Fire Protection Association Health (1) Flammability (0) Instability (1)—Material Safety Data Sheet, National Fire Protection Association Health (1) Flammability (1) Instability (0)—Material Safety Data Sheet, National Fire Protection Association Health (2) Flammability (1) Instability (0)—Material Safety Data Sheet, National Fire Protection Association Health (1) Flammability (1) Instability (0)—Material Safety Data Sheet, Materials Identification System (R) and/or US Department of Defense System Health (2) Fire Hazard (1) Reactivity (0) Personal Protection Code (E) (Safety Glasses, Chemical Gloves, Dust Respirator)—Material Safety Data Sheet, Materials Identification System (R) and/or US Department of Defense System Health (1★) with additional chronic hazards present Fire Hazard (0) Reactivity (1) Personal Protection Code (-) (None stated)—Material Safety Data Sheet.

TAMOXIFEN CITRATE is a white or almost white, polymorphic, crystalline powder.

TAMOXIFEN (NOLVADEX®98) is available as 10 mg and 20 mg tablets and oral solution.

TAMOXIFEN may cause fetal harm; breastfeeding should be discontinued because of potential for reproductive and developmental harm (*A Guide for Occupational Health Professionals Technical Manual*, Navy Environmental Health Center [NEHC-TM-OEM 6260.01a]).

First Aid/Medical Information/ Occupational Exposure Limits

First Aid Measures to include: Use general first aid measures except for the following:

Ingestion: Do not induce vomiting. If conscious and alert, rinse mouth and drink 2–4 cups of milk or water.

Physician's note: Treat symptomatically and supportively; TAMOXIFEN CITRATE use has shown to increase the risk of endometrial cancer. Animal studies have shown genotoxic and carcinogenic effects.

Administer activated charcoal. Induce vomiting if person is conscious.

Dermal Contact: Perform general first aid measure, then cover the irritated skin with an emollient (antibacterial cream). Seek medical attention.

Medical Information:

Caution and Warning Statements:

Warning: TAMOXIFEN CITRATE is a human carcinogen and a reproductive hazard.

Caution: Not to be handled by female personnel.

Toxic: TAMOXIFEN CITRATE is harmful if swallowed, potential cancer hazard. Exposure to this drug may be irritating to eyes and skin. This drug may cause skin irritation in sensitive individuals. Exposure may have a possible risk of irreversible effects. Exposure to TAMOXIFEN CITRATE has a possible risk of impaired fertility and risk of harm to the unborn child. May cause harm to breastfeeding babies. TAMOXIFEN CITRATE may cause cancer (tumorigenic). TAMOXIFEN CITRATE may affect genetic material. Exposure may cause adverse reproductive effects (paternal and maternal effects; female fertility). RTECS lists TAMOXIFEN as a suspected skin or sense organ toxicant. The toxicological properties of this material have not been fully investigated. Because of the physical presentation of the product, the risk to health in the normal handling of the product is expected to be low.

Caution: Females and males planning to have a child, pregnant women, and nursing mothers should exercise caution regarding potential occupational exposure to this cytotoxic drug. No information or not enough information exists or was provided concerning occupational exposures that may potentially occur while handling this drug and its affects on reproductive systems, the fetus, and/or if it is secreted along with breast milk, which may harm nursing infants. Staff members should consult with the occupational health physician monitoring workers' health in your facility to be apprised of potential hazards and should be advised to avoid becoming pregnant and/or breastfeeding or should be transferred in accordance with policy/procedure to other duties that do not involve preparation, handling, and administering this drug.

Therapeutic Levels: TAMOXIFEN CITRATE may affect genetic material and may cause adverse reproductive effects (paternal and maternal effects; female fertility). Avoid possible exposure if you are pregnant or if you planning to become pregnant or if you are breastfeeding. Exposure to this drug may harm the fetus (unborn child) or child.

Target Organs/Systems: Liver, kidneys, cataracts, reproductive systems (male and female), and fetus (unborn child)

Medical Conditions Generally Aggravated by Exposure:

- TAMOXIFEN CITRATE is contraindicated in patients with known hypersensitivity to the drug.
- Reproductive and pregnancy issues.

Specific Medical Surveillance Information: Reproductive and pregnancy counseling.

Occupational Exposure Level/Limit (OEL) & Sampling Methods:

Environmental Sentinel Contamination Action Level (ESCAL): Air, surface
Occupational Exposure Level (OEL) Zeneca: TAMOXIFEN (NOLVADEX®98) 0.01 mg/m3 Time-Weighted Average (TWA) (Method not listed or specified)

Supplemental Response Information

Extinguishing Media: Use extinguishing agent which is the most appropriate to extinguish surrounding fire (carbon dioxide, foam, dry chemical or water fog as extinguishing media).

Solubility: TAMOXIFEN CITRATE (NOLVADEX®98) is reported to be insoluble to partially soluble in cold water; soluble in methyl alcohol. TAMOXIFEN CITRATE is soluble in methanol, acetone, and ethanol. TAMOXIFEN CITRATE has a water solubility of 0.0005 g/l @ 37 deg c. Very slightly soluble in alcohol and chloroform.

Chemical Degradation/Neutralization Method: Not otherwise specified

Note: If a specific degradation or neutralization method is not provided on this table and you do not have other specific information that will guide you on how to clean up the specific material spilled, then follow the general spill procedure found in the introduction section of this handbook.

Incompatibility: TAMOXIFEN CITRATE is incompatible with oxidizing agents. Avoid exposure to light, air, or moisture over prolonged periods.

TAXOL®99 *(0.6 WT %)*
PACLITAXEL (1) (*PAK-li-taks-el*)
TAX

Chemical Abstracts Service (CAS) Registry Number: 33069-62-4 (mixture)

Registry of Toxic Effects of Chemical Substance (RTECS): WX1272100, DA8340700, DA8340750

National Cancer Institute: NSC 125973

$C_{47}H_{51}NO_{14}$

(Two Degradation Methods)

Health & Safety Hazards/US Department of Transportation (DOT)/US Environmental Protection Agency (EPA)—Sources

Potential Carcinogen—Material Safety Data Sheet, Possible Mutagen (Animal Data)—Material Safety Data Sheet, Possible Teratogen—Material Safety Data Sheet, Possible Reproductive Effector—Material Safety Data Sheet, Reproductive Effector—Material Safety Data Sheet, Development and Toxic—US California Environmental Protection Agency, Highly Toxic—Material Safety Data Sheet, Cytotoxic—Material Safety Data Sheet, Cytotoxic—British Columbia Cancer Agency Canada, Flammable—Material Safety Data Sheet, Vesicant—British Columbia Cancer Agency Canada, Irritant—British Columbia Cancer Agency Canada, Pregnancy Category (D)—US Food and Drug Administration, Developmental Male and Female—US California Proposition 65, National Fire Protection Association Health (3) Flammability (0) Instability (0)—Material Safety Data Sheet, Materials Identification System (R) and/or US Department of Defense System Health (2★) with additional chronic hazards present Fire Hazard (1) Reactivity (0) Personal Protective Code (E) (Safety Glasses, Chemical Gloves, Dust Respirator)—Material Safety Data Sheet, National Fire Protection Association Health (2) Flammability (1) Instability (0)—Material Safety Data Sheet, Materials Identification System (R) and/or US Department of Defense System Health (3★) with additional chronic hazards present Fire Hazard (0) Reactivity (0) Personal Protection Code (–) (None stated)—Material Safety Data Sheet, Material Identification System (R) and/or US Department of Defense System Health (1) with additional chronic hazards present Fire Hazard (1) Reactivity (0) Personal Protection Code (E) (Safety Glasses, Chemical Gloves, Dust Respirator)—Material Safety Data Sheet, National Fire Protection Association Health (1) Flammability (1) Instability (0)—Material Safety data Sheet, National Fire Protection Association Health (1) Flammability (1) Instability/Reactivity (0), Materials Identification System (R) and/or US Department of Defense System Health (1) Fire Hazard (1) Reactivity (0) Personal Protection Code (E) (Safety Glasses, Chemical Gloves, Dust Respirator)—Material Safety Data Sheet, Lactation Breastfeeding not recommended due to the potential secretion into breast milk—British Columbia Cancer Agency Canada, SARA 313—US Environmental Protection Agency.

PACLITAXEL is a white to off-white powder.

TAXOL®99 is a colorless fluid.

TAXOL®99 (PACLITAXEL) is available as an injection.

PACLITAXEL can cause fetal harm; breastfeeding should be discontinued because of potential for reproductive and developmental harm (*A Guide for Occupational Health Professionals Technical Manual*, Navy Environmental Health Center [NEHC-TM-OEM 6260.01a]).

First Aid/Medical Information/ Occupational Exposure Limits

First Aid Measures to include: Use general first aid measures except for the following:

Physician's note: This product is used in the treatment of certain types of cancer and is highly toxic after systemic injection. It inhibits the function of microtubules in cells therefore interfering with cell division. Information concerning the therapeutic uses of this drug substance should be obtained from formulated product package inserts and other appropriate references. When used therapeutically, adverse effects on the bone marrow, heart (arrhythmias), and peripheral nervous system have been reported. At high doses, it may have potential to affect fertility as well as the fetus. There is no known antidote for PACLITAXEL overdosage. Treat symptomatically and supportively.

Medical Information:

Caution and Warning Statements:

Caution: Chronic toxicity of TAXOL®99 has not been fully characterized. Available information states that TAXOL®99 may be harmful to fetus. Repeated exposure may affect reproductive systems. Exposure to (TAXOL®99) may be irritating to respiratory system and skin. There is a risk of serious damage to eyes. There is a possible risk of impaired fertility. There is a possible risk of irreversible effects from exposure to TAXOL®99. This material may be a mutagen and possibility a reproductive effector. Furthermore, this drug may cause sensitization by inhalation and skin contact.

Contact dermatitis may cause allergic skin reaction (sensitization). Severe cardiotoxicity and bone marrow suppression has been noted. Research has indicated that male and female reproductive toxicity is a possible concern (CAL EPA). Exposure may cause the following: respiratory difficulty, loss of muscle coordination, weight loss, nausea, vomiting, alopecia, hypersensitivity reactions, hypotension, bronchospasm, erythematous rashes, ulceration of the esophagus, decrease number of leukocytes; and thrombocytes in the blood and peripheral neuropathy. BC Cancer Agency lists PACLITAXEL as an irritant but states to treat as a vesicant.

Caution: Females and males planning to have a child, pregnant women, and nursing mothers should exercise caution regarding potential occupational exposure to this cytotoxic drug. No information or not enough information exists or was provided concerning occupational exposures that may potentially occur while handling this drug and its affects on reproductive systems, the fetus, and/or if it is secreted along with breast milk, which may harm nursing infants. Staff members should consult with the occupational health physician monitoring workers' health in your facility to be apprised of potential hazards and should be advised to avoid becoming pregnant and/or breastfeeding or should be transferred in accordance with policy/procedures to other duties that do not involve preparation, handling, and administering this drug.

Target Organs/Systems: Bone marrow, peripheral nervous system (nerves), kidneys, liver, GI tract, fetus, cardiovascular, reproductive systems, eyes, and skin

Medical Conditions Generally Aggravated by Exposure:

- Reproductive and pregnancy issues.
- Workers with preexisting asthma, anemia, lung conditions, other forms of bone marrow suppression, and cardiac arrhythmia should not work with TAXOL®99 without medical evaluation.

Specific Medical Surveillance Information: Reproductive and pregnancy counseling.

Workers with preexisting asthma, anemia, lung conditions, other forms of bone marrow suppression, and cardiac arrhythmia should not work with TAXOL®99 without medical evaluation.

Occupational Exposure Level/Limit (OEL) & Sampling Methods:

Environmental Sentinel Contamination Action Level (ESCAL): Air, surface
OEL Bristol-Myers Squibb
PACLITAXEL 0,0000 mg/m3 Time-Weighted Average (8 hour TWA)
BMS dust control★ target
★PACLITAXEL is a potent stabilizer of microtubules in vitro and in vivo. It is quite

toxic when administered systemically and has potential to cause chromosome damage in human cells. It is being evaluated in clinical trials as a therapy for various types of cancer, especially ovarian and breast cancer. A dust control target of 0.0008 mg/m3 in air (8-hour time-weighted average concentration in air) has been established for workplace exposure to PACLITAXEL. Adherence to this target level should protect most employees who handle this drug from experiencing adverse effects from this substance. However, exposure to this substance should be maintained as low as reasonably possible.
(Method not listed or specified)

Supplemental Response Information

Extinguishing Media: Use extinguishing agent which is the most appropriate to extinguish surrounding fire (carbon dioxide, foam, dry chemical or water fog as extinguishing media).

Solubility: TAXOL®99 range from insoluble in water to slightly water soluble; soluble in alcohol
(pH range from 3 to 8). (Highly lipophilic.)
Solubility in water (25°C) (for bulk PACLITAXEL [TAXOL®99]):
0.252 mg/l at pH: 5
0.172 mg/l at pH: 7
0.249 mg/l at pH: 9.

Chemical Degradation/Neutralization Method: See below for additional degradation methods—A TAXOL®99 Material Safety Data Sheet (MSDS) recommends that spilled area to be washed twice with detergent and water. Neutralizing agent can be made from sodium carbonate solution/methanolic potassium hydroxide.

Incompatibility: TAXOL®99 is incompatible with strong oxidizing agents. Protect from light, excess heat, sparks, and open flame.

TAXOL®99 *(0.6 WT %)*
PACLITAXEL (2) *(PAK-li-taks-el)*
(TAX)

Chemical Abstracts Service (CAS) Registry Number: 33069-62-4 (mixture)
Registry of Toxic Effects of Chemical Substance (RTECS): WX1272100, DA8340700, DA8340750
National Cancer Institute: NSC 125973
$C_{47}H_{51}NO_{14}$
(Two Degradation Methods)

Health & Safety Hazards/US Department of Transportation (DOT)/US Environmental Protection Agency (EPA)—Sources

Potential Carcinogen—Material Safety Data Sheet, Possible Mutagen (Animal Data)—Material Safety Data Sheet, Possible Teratogen—Material Safety Data Sheet, Possible Reproductive Effector—Material Safety Data Sheet, Reproductive Effector—Material Safety Data Sheet, Developmental and Toxic—US California Environmental Protection Agency, Highly Toxic—Material Safety Data Sheet, Cytotoxic—Material Safety Data Sheet, Cytotoxic—British Columbia Cancer Agency Canada, Flammable—Material Safety Data Sheet, Vesicant—British Columbia Cancer Agency Canada, Irritant—British Columbia Cancer Agency Canada, Pregnancy Category (D)—US Food and Drug Administration, Developmental Male and Female—US California Proposition 65, National Fire Protection Association Health (3) Flammability (0) Instability (0)—Material Safety Data Sheet, Materials Identification System (R) and/or US Department of Defense System Health (2) with additional chronic hazards present Fire Hazard (1) Reactivity (0) Personal Protection Code (E) (Safety Glasses, Chemical Gloves, Dust Respirator)—Material Safety Data Sheet, National Fire Protection Association Health (2) Flammability (1) Instability (0)—Material Safety Data Sheet, Materials Identification System (R) and/or US Department of Defense System Health (3) with additional chronic hazards present Fire Hazard (0) Reactivity (0) Personal Protection Code (-) (None stated)—Material Safety Data Sheet. Material Identification System (R) and/or US Department of Defense System Health (1) with additional chronic hazards present Fire Hazard (1) Reactivity (0) Personal Protection Code (E) (Safety Glasses, Chemical Gloves, Dust Respirator)—Material Safety Data Sheet, National Fire Protection Association Health (1) Flammability (1) Instability (0)—Material Safety Data Sheet, National Fire Protection Association Health (1) Flammability (1) Instability/Reactivity (0), Materials Identification System (R) and/or US Department of Defense System Health (1) Fire hazard (1) Reactivity (0) Personal Protection Code (E) (Safety Glasses, Chemical Gloves, Dust Respirator)—Material Safety Data Sheet, Lactation Breastfeeding not recommended due to the potential secretion into breast milk—British Columbia Cancer Agency Canada, SARA 313—US Environmental Protection Agency.

PACLITAXEL is a white to off-white powder.

TAXOL®99 is a colorless fluid.

TAXOL®99 (PACLITAXEL) is available as an injection.

PACLITAXEL can cause fetal harm; breastfeeding is discontinued because of potential for reproductive and developmental harm (*A Guide for Occupational Health Professionals Technical Manual*, Navy Environmental Health Center [NEHC-TM-OEM 6260.01a]).

First Aid/Medical Information/Occupational Exposure Limits

First Aid Measures to include: Use general first aid measures except for the following:

Physician's note: This product is used in the treatment of certain types of cancer and is highly toxic after systemic injection. It inhibits the function of microtubules in cells therefore interfering with cell division. Information concerning the therapeutic uses of this drug substance should be obtained from formulated product package inserts and other appropriate references. When used therapeutically, adverse effects on the bone marrow, heart (arrhythmias), and peripheral nervous system have been reported. At high doses, it may have potential to affect fertility as well as the fetus. Treat symptomatically and supportively.

Medical Information:

Caution and Warning Statements: Contact dermatitis may cause allergic skin reaction (sensitization). Severe cardiotoxicity and bone marrow suppression has been noted. Research has indicated that male and female reproductive toxicity may be a concern (CAL EPA). Exposure may cause the following: respiratory difficulty, loss of muscle coordination, weight loss, nausea, vomiting, alopecia, hypersensitivity reactions, hypotension, bronchospasm, erythematous rashes, ulceration of the esophagus, decrease number of leukocytes and thrombocytes in the blood, and peripheral neuropathy. BC Cancer Agency Canada lists PACLITAXEL as an irritant but states to treat as a vesicant.

Caution: Chronic toxicity of TAXOL®99 has not been fully characterized. Available information states that TAXOL®99 may be harmful to fetus. Repeated exposure may affect reproductive systems. Exposure to TAXOL®99 may be irritating to respiratory system and skin. There is a risk of serious damage to eyes. There is a possible risk of impaired fertility. There is a possible risk of irreversible effects from exposure to TAXOL®99. This material may be a mutagen and possibility a reproductive effector. TAXOL®99 may cause sensitization by inhalation and skin contact.

Caution: Females and males planning to have a child, pregnant women, and nursing mothers should exercise caution regarding potential occupational exposure to this cytotoxic drug. No information or not enough information exists or was provided concerning occupational exposures that may potentially occur while handling this drug and its affects on reproductive systems, the fetus, and/or if it is secreted along with breast milk, which may harm nursing infants. Staff members should consult with the occupational health physician monitoring workers' health in your facility to be apprised of potential hazards and should be advised to avoid becoming pregnant and/or breastfeeding or should be transferred in accordance with policy/procedures to other duties that do not involve preparation, handling, and administering this drug.

Target Organs/Systems: Bone marrow, peripheral nervous system (nerves), kidneys, liver, GI tract, fetus, cardiovascular system, reproductive systems, eyes, and skin

Medical Conditions Generally Aggravated by Exposure:

- Reproductive and pregnancy issues.
- Workers with preexisting asthma, anemia, lung conditions, other forms of bone marrow suppression, and cardiac arrhythmia should not work with TAXOL®99 without medical evaluation

Specific Medical Surveillance Information: Reproductive and pregnancy counseling.

Workers with preexisting asthma, anemia, lung conditions, other forms of bone marrow suppression, and cardiac arrhythmia should not work with TAXOL®99 without medical evaluation.

Occupational Exposure Level/Limit (OEL) & Sampling Methods:

Environmental Sentinel Contamination Action Level (ESCAL): Air, surface

Occupational Exposure Level (OEL) Bristol-Myers Squibb:

PACLITAXEL 0.0000 mg/m3 Time-Weighted Average (8 hours TWA)

BMS dust control★ target

★PACLITAXEL is a potent stabilizer of microtubules in vitro and in vivo. It is quite toxic when administered systemically and has potential to cause chromosome damage in human cells. It is being evaluated in clinical trials as a therapy for various types of cancer, especially ovarian and breast cancer. A dust control target of 0.0008 mg/m3 in air (8-hour time-weighted average concentration in air) has been established for workplace exposure to PACLITAXEL. Adherence to this target level should protect most employees who handle this drug from experiencing adverse effects from this material; however, exposure to this substance should be maintained as low as reasonably possible.

(Method not listed or specified)

Supplemental Response Information

Extinguishing Media: Use extinguishing agent which is the most appropriate to extinguish surrounding fire (carbon dioxide, foam, dry chemical or water fog as extinguishing media).

Solubility: TAXOL®99 range from insoluble in water to slightly water soluble; soluble in alcohol (pH range from 3 to 8). (Highly lipophilic.)

TAXOL®99 is solubility in water (25°C); for bulk PACLITAXEL (TAXOL®99):

0.252 mg/l at pH: 5

0.172 mg/l at pH: 7

0.249 mg/l at pH: 9.

Chemical Degradation/Neutralization Method: A manufacturer's Material Safety Data Sheet (MSDS) recommends treating spill surfaces with 10% sodium carbonate (soda ash) solution, after absorbing liquids with inert absorbent pads or removing any powder present. Allow solution to stand for up to one hour. Then thoroughly wash spilled surfaces with soap and water. Take a sample to determine if surface contamination is still present (if sampling method is available at your facility). If the drug is present, repeat above steps; dispose of wastes in accordance with your local procedures, state, and federal regulations.

Incompatibility: TAXOL®99 is incompatible with strong oxidizing agents. Protect from light, excess heat, sparks, and open flame.

TAXOTERE®100 (*tax-oh-tare*)
$C_{43}H_{55}NO_{13}$

DOCETAXEL (*doe-se-TAKS-sel*)

Chemical Abstracts Service (CAS) Registry Number: 114977-28-5 (mixture)

$C_{43}-H_{53}-NO_{14}$

ANHYDROUS DOCETAXEL

Registry of Toxic Effects of Chemical Substance
(RTECS): DA4172750

Health & Safety Hazards/US Department of Transportation (DOT)/US Environmental Protection Agency (EPA)—Sources

Cytotoxic—Material Safety Data Sheet, Moderate Toxic—Material Safety Data Sheet, Cytotoxic—British Columbia Cancer Agency Canada, Embryotoxic—Material Safety Data Sheet, Fetotoxic—Material Safety Data Sheet, Irritant—British Columbia Cancer Agency Canada, Pregnancy Category (D)—US Food and Drug Administration, National Fire Protection Association Health (1) Flammability (0) Instability (0)—Material Safety Data Sheet, Hazardous Materials Identification System (R) and/or US Department of Defense System Health (1) Fire Hazard (0) Reactivity (0) Personal Protection Code (-) (None stated), UN 1170.

DOCETAXEL (TAXOTERE®100) is a yellow/brown liquid when diluted from a clear solution; odorless white crystalline powder.

First Aid/Medical Information/ Occupational Exposure Limits

First Aid Measures to include: Use general first aid measures except for the following:

Medical Information:

Caution and Warning Statements: TAXOTERE®100 (DOCETAXEL) is moderately toxic. Exposure may cause skin, eyes, and mucous membranes and upper respiratory tract irritation. Taxotere®100 is a nervous system depressant and a hepatotoxin. BC Cancer Agency lists DOCETAXEL has an irritant.

Caution: Females and males planning to have a child, pregnant women, and nursing mothers should exercise caution regarding potential occupational exposure to this cytotoxic drug. No information or not enough information exists or was provided concerning occupational exposures that may potentially occur while handling this drug and its affects on reproductive systems, the fetus, and/or if it is secreted along with breast milk, which may harm nursing infants. Staff members should consult with the occupational health physician monitoring workers' health in your facility to be apprised of potential hazards and should be advised to avoid becoming pregnant and/or breastfeeding or should be transferred in accordance with policy/procedures to other duties that do not involve preparation, handling, and administering this drug.

Therapeutic Levels: TAXOTERE®100 can cause fetal harm when administered to pregnant women. Studies in both rats and rabbits at doses >/= 0.3 and 0.03 mg/kg/day, respectively (about 1/50 and 1/300 the daily maximum recommended human dose on a mg/m² basis), administered during the period of organogenesis, have shown that TAXOTERE®100 is embryotoxic and fetotoxic (characterized by intrauterine mortality, increased resorption, reduced fetal weight, and fetal ossification delay). The doses indicated above also caused maternal toxicity. There are no adequate and well-controlled studies in pregnant women using TAXOTERE®100. If TAXOTERE®100 is used during pregnancy, or if the patient becomes pregnant while receiving this drug, it is not known whether TAXOTERE®100 is excreted in human milk.

Target Organs/Systems: Potential for neurotoxicity, myelosuppression, and leucopenia, necrosis of the intestinal epithelium, testicular atrophy, and lymphoid organ depletion

Medical Conditions Generally Aggravated by Exposure:

- Workers with preexisting nervous system disorders and liver disease.
- Reproductive issues.

Specific Medical Surveillance Information: Reproductive and pregnancy counseling.

Occupational Exposure Level/Limit (OEL) & Sampling Methods: Not otherwise specified

Environmental Sentinel Contamination Action Level (ESCAL): Not otherwise specified

Supplemental Response Information

Extinguishing Media: Use extinguishing agent which is the most appropriate to extinguish surrounding fire (carbon dioxide, foam, dry chemical or water fog as extinguishing media).

Solubility: TAXOTERE®100 is miscible in water. (Approximately 0.1 mg/ml in water.) TAXOTERE®100 is soluble in methanol. The pH is approximately neutral.

Chemical Degradation/Neutralization Method: A TAXOTERE®100 Material Safety Data Sheet (MSDS) recommends that spilled liquid can be destroyed by mixing with a caustic ethanol solution (30% ethanol/70% water/1n sodium hydroxide) with sufficient caustic added to raise the solution pH above 11, stirring at room temperature for 5 hours. Solution volume must be sufficient to prevent precipitation of

DOCETAXEL. The residual destruction products of DOCETAXEL do not possess cytotoxic activity.

Incompatibility: TAXOTERE®100 is incompatible with acids and bases.

TEGAFUR

Chemical Abstracts Service (CAS) Registry Number: 17902-23-7

FTORAFUR

Chemical Abstracts Service (CAS) Registry Number: 37076-68-9

Registry of Toxic Effects of Chemical Substance (RTECS): YR0450000

National Cancer Institute: NSC 148958

$C_8H_9F-N_2O_3$

Health & Safety Hazards/US Department of Transportation (DOT)/US Environmental Protection Agency (EPA)—Sources

Teratogen—University of Maryland at College Park, Highly Toxic—Material Safety Data Sheet, Tumorigenic—ToxReport, Mutagen—ToxReport, Experimental reproductive effects—Material Safety Data Sheet, Pregnancy Category (None)—Food and Drug Administration, National Fire Protection Association Health (3) Flammability (1) Instability (0)—Material Safety Data Sheet, National Fire Protection Association Health (1) Flammability (0) Instability (0)—Material Safety Data Sheet, Materials Identification System (R) and/or US Department of Defense System Health (3) Fire Hazard (1) Reactivity (0) Personal Protection Code (E) (Safety Glasses, Chemical Gloves, Dust Respirator)—Material Safety Data Sheet, UN 2811, Class 6.1.

TEGAFUR is a white odorless crystalline powder.

First Aid/Medical Information/ Occupational Exposure Limits

First Aid Measures to include: Use general first aid measures except for the following:

Ingestion: If victim is conscious and alert, rinse mouth and drink 2-4 cups of milk or water. Do not induce vomiting. Seek medical assistance.

Inhalation: If victim is not breathing, give artificial respiration, but do not use mouth-to-mouth respiration.

Medical Information:

Caution and Warning Statements:

Warning: TEGAFUR exposure is harmful if inhaled, absorbed through the skin, or swallowed. Very hazardous in case of skin contact (permeator); severe overexposure can result in death. May be fatal is ingested or inhaled. Exposure to TEGAFUR may cause digestive tract irritation with nausea, vomiting, and diarrhea. Ingestion may cause encephalitis, muscular contractions, bone marrow depression, and neurological effects.

Target Organs/Systems: Bone marrow

Medical Conditions Generally Aggravated by Exposure:

- Repeated exposure to a highly toxic material may produce general deterioration of health by an accumulation in one or more human organs.

Specific Medical Surveillance Information: Not otherwise specified

Occupational Exposure Level OEL/Limit & Sampling Methods: Not otherwise specified

Environmental Sentinel Contamination Action Level (ESCAL): Not otherwise specified

Supplemental Response Information

Extinguishing Media: Use extinguishing agent which is the most appropriate to extinguish surrounding fire (carbon dioxide, foam, dry chemical or water fog as extinguishing media).

Solubility: TEGAFUR is soluble in hot water.

Chemical Degradation/Neutralization Method: Not otherwise specified

Note: If a specific degradation or neutralization method is not provided on this table and you do not have other specific information that will guide you on how to clean up the specific material spilled, then follow the general spill procedure found in the introduction section of this handbook.

Incompatibility: TEGAFUR is incompatible with oxidizing agents.

TEMOZOLOMIDE (*TEE-mo-ZOL-o-mide*)
TEMODAR®101
METHAZOLASTONE®102

Chemical Abstracts Service (CAS) Registry Number: 85622-93-1

Registry of Toxic Effects of Chemical Substance (RTECS): NJ5927050

$C_6H_6N_6O_2$

Health & Safety Hazards/US Department of Transportation (DOT)/US Environmental Protection Agency (EPA)—Sources

Cytotoxic—Box Instruction, Cytotoxic—Material Safety Data Sheet, Mutagen—Material Safety Data

Sheet, Carcinogen—Material Safety Data Sheet, Reproductive Effector Male—Material Safety Data Sheet, Pregnancy Category (D)—US Food and Drug Administration, National Fire Protection Association Health (3) Flammability (0) Instability (1)—Material Safety Data Sheet.

TEMOZOLOMIDE (TEMODAL) (TEMODAR®101) is available in 5 mg, 20 mg, 100 mg, and 250 mg.

First Aid/Medical Information/ Occupational Exposure Limits

First Aid Measures to include: Use general first aid measures except for the following:

Ingestion: If conscious, rinse mouth out, give copious amounts of water, and induce vomiting. Seek medical assistance.

Medical Information:

Caution and Warning Statements: TEMOZOLMIDE is a cytotoxic drug and causes DNA damage. TEMOZOLMIDE is mutagenic. This material may cause cancer. TEMOZOLMIDE may impair fertility.

Caution: Females and males planning to have a child, pregnant women, and nursing mothers should exercise caution regarding potential occupational exposure to this cytotoxic drug. No information or not enough information exists or was provided concerning occupational exposures that may potentially occur while handling this drug and its affects on reproductive systems, the fetus, and/or if it is secreted along with breast milk, which may harm nursing infants. Staff members should consult with the occupational health physician monitoring workers' health in your facility to be apprised of potential hazards and should be advised to avoid becoming pregnant and/or breastfeeding or should be transferred in accordance with policy/procedures to other duties that do not involve preparation, handling, and administering this drug.

TEMODAR®101 is in the Food and Drug Administration Pregnancy Category (D).

Target Organs/Systems: Blood forming system and male reproductive systems

Medical Conditions Generally Aggravated by Exposure:

- Patients who have a history of hypersensitivity reaction to TEMOZOLOMIDE or DACARBAZINE.
- Male reproductive disorder.

Specific Medical Surveillance Information: Reproductive and pregnancy counseling.

Occupational Exposure Level/Limit (OEL) & Sampling Methods:

Environmental Sentinel Contamination Action Level (ESCAL): Not otherwise specified
Occupational Exposure level (OEL) Schering: TEMODAR®101 Schering OEG: 2 μg/m3 (Method not listed or specified)

Supplemental Response Information

Extinguishing Media: Use extinguishing agent which is the most appropriate to extinguish surrounding fire (carbon dioxide, foam, dry chemical or water fog as extinguishing media).

Solubility: TEMOZOLOMIDE: Not otherwise specified

Chemical Degradation/Neutralization Method: Not otherwise specified

Note: If a specific degradation or neutralization method is not provided on this table and you do not have other specific information that will guide you on how to clean up the specific material spilled, then follow the general spill procedure found in the introduction section of this handbook.

Incompatibility: TEMODAR®101 (TEMOZOMIDE) is incompatible with oxidizers, strong acids, and bases. Avoid open flame and high temperatures.

TENIPOSIDE (ten-I-POE-side)
VM-26
EPT
VUMON®103

Chemical Abstracts Service (CAS) Registry Number: 29767-20-2 (Mixture)
Registry of Toxic Effects of Chemical Substance (RTECS): KC0180000
National Cancer Institute: NSC 122819
$C_{32}H_{32}O_{13}S$

Health & Safety Hazards/US Department of Transportation (DOT)/US Environmental Protection Agency (EPA)—Sources

Carcinogen G2A—International Agency for Research on Cancer, Possible Carcinogen—Material Safety Data Sheet, Sensitizer—Material Safety Data Sheet, Flammable—Material Safety Data Sheet, Cytotoxic—British Columbia Cancer Agency Canada, Irritant—British Columbia Cancer Agency Canada, Pregnancy Category (D)—US Food and Drug Administration, Developmental—US California Proposition 65.

TENIPOSIDE is available as an injection.

TENIPOSIDE may cause fetal harm; breastfeeding is discontinued because of potential for reproductive and developmental harm (*A Guide for Occupational Health Professionals Technical Manual*, Navy Environmental Health Center [NEHC-TM-OEM 6260.01a]).

First Aid/Medical Information/ Occupational Exposure Limits

First Aid Measures to include: Use general first aid measures except for the following:

Ingestion: Induction of vomiting is recommended if person is conscious, alert, and not experiencing convulsions.

Medical Information:

Caution and Warning Statements: Exposure to TENIPOSIDE may cause irritation of the skin and allergic reactions. Possible side effects may be myelosuppression, possible anaphylaxis, and GI effects. Contact with TENIPOSIDE can cause toxic effect of mitotic arrest. BC Cancer lists TENIPOSIDE as an irritant.

RTECS lists TENIPOSIDE as a suspected gastrointestinal or liver toxicant; as a neurotoxicant; and as a skin or sense organ toxicant (RTES).

Caution: Females and males planning to have a child, pregnant women, and nursing mothers should exercise caution regarding potential occupational exposure to this cytotoxic drug. No information or not enough information exists or was provided concerning occupational exposures that may potentially occur while handling this drug and its affects on reproductive systems, the fetus, and/or if it is secreted along with breast milk, which may harm nursing infants. Staff members should consult with the occupational health physician monitoring workers' health in your facility to be apprised of potential hazards and should be advised to avoid becoming pregnant and/or breastfeeding or should be transferred in accordance with policy/procedures to other duties that do not involve preparation, handling, and administering this drug.

TENIPOSIDE is in the Food and DA Pregnancy Category (D). This means that TENIPOSIDE is known to be harmful to an unborn baby.

Target Organs/Systems: Hematopoietic system, lymphatic system, skin, gastrointestinal system, and possibly fetus

Medical Conditions Generally Aggravated by Exposure:

- Systemic exposure to therapeutic doses of TENIPOSIDE may aggravate blood disorders, gastrointestinal disorders, cardiovascular disorders, and nervous system disorders.
- Reproductive and pregnancy issues.

Specific Medical Surveillance Information: Reproductive and pregnancy counseling.

Occupational Exposure Level/Limit (OEL) & Sampling Methods: Not otherwise specified

Environmental Sentinel Contamination Action Level (ESCAL): Not otherwise specified

Supplemental Response Information

Extinguishing Media: Use extinguishing agent which is the most appropriate to extinguish surrounding fire (carbon dioxide, foam, dry chemical or water fog as extinguishing media).

Solubility: TENIPOSIDE is insoluble in water and ether. It is slightly soluble in methanol and very soluble in acetone and dimethylformamide.

Chemical Degradation/Neutralization Method: Not otherwise specified

Note: If a specific degradation or neutralization method is not provided on this table and you do not have other specific information that will guide you on how to clean up the specific material spilled, then follow the general spill procedure found in the introduction section of this handbook.

Incompatibility: Not otherwise specified

THIOGUANINE (*thye-oh-GWON-een*)
6-THIOGUANINE

Chemical Abstracts Service (CAS) Registry
    Number: 154-42-7
Registry of Toxic Effects of Chemical Substance
    (RTECS): UP0740000
National Cancer Institute: NSC 752
$C_5H_5N_5S$

Health & Safety Hazards/US Department of Transportation (DOT)/US Environmental Protection Agency (EPA)—Sources

Acutely Toxic—US National Institute of Health (NIH) and Material Safety Data Sheet, Mutagen—University of Maryland at College Park, Teratogen—University of Maryland at College Park, Possible Teratogen—US National Institute of Health (NIH)—Material Safety Data Sheet, Chromosomal Aberrations—US National Institute of Health (NIH) and

Material Safety Data Sheet, Carcinogen—British Columbia Cancer Agency Canada, Mutagen—British Columbia Cancer Agency Canada, Pregnancy Category (D)—US Food and Drug Administration, Developmental—US California Proposition 65, National Fire Protection Association Health (2) Flammability (0) Instability (0)—Material Safety Data Sheet, Materials Identification System (R) and/or US Department of Defense System Health (2★) with additional chronic hazards present Fire Hazard (0) Reactivity (0) Personal Protection Code (-) (None stated)—Material Safety Data Sheet, UN 2811, CLASS 6.1.

THIOGUANNINE is available in 40 mg tablets, greenish-yellow.

THIOGUANINE may cause fetal harm; breastfeeding should be discontinued because of potential for reproductive and developmental harm (*A Guide for Occupational Health Professionals Technical Manual*, Navy Environmental Health Center [NEHC-TM-OEM 6260.01a]).

First Aid/Medical Information/ Occupational Exposure Limits

First Aid Measures to include: Use general first aid measures except for the following:

Ingestion: If swallowed, rinse out mouth with water and drink 2-4 cups of milk or water, provided person is conscious and alert. Do not induce vomiting.

Physician's note: Physicians treat symptomatically and supportively. Refer for gastric lavage.

Eye exposure: Immediately check for contact lenses and remove any contact lenses. Irrigate immediately with sodium bicarbonate solution, followed by copious quantities of running water for at least 15 minutes, occasionally lifting the upper and lower lids. Obtain ophthalmologic evaluation.

Inhalation: If inhaled, consider treatment for pulmonary irritation.

Dermal Contact: Avoid washing with solvents and exposure to UV light. Avoid rubbing of skin or increasing skin temperature.

Medical Information:

Caution and Warning Statements: 6-THIOGUANINE is acutely toxic and may cause cancer. **Caution**: This material's toxicological properties have not been fully investigated. Exposure may cause skin, eye, mucous membranes, and upper respiratory tract irritation. Possibly teratogenic and produces chromosomal aberrations. Avoid formation and breathing of aerosols. RTECS lists 6-THIOGUANINE as a suspected cardiovascular or blood toxicant and suspected gastrointes-

tinal or liver toxicant. 6-THIOGUANINE May cause congenital malformation in the fetus.

Caution: Females and males planning to have a child, pregnant women, and nursing mothers should exercise caution regarding potential occupational exposure to this cytotoxic drug. No information or not enough information exists or was provided concerning occupational exposures that may potentially occur while handling this drug and its affects on reproductive systems, the fetus, and/or if it is secreted along with breast milk, which may harm nursing infants. Staff members should consult with the occupational health physician monitoring workers' health in your facility to be apprised of potential hazards and should be advised to avoid becoming pregnant and/or breastfeeding or should be transferred in accordance with policy/procedures to other duties that do not involve preparation, handling, and administering this drug.

Therapeutic Levels: 6-THIOGUANINE is absorbed through the intestinal tract. Females and males planning to have a child, pregnant women, and nursing mothers should exercise caution regarding potential exposure to 6-thioguanine.

Target Organs/Systems: Bone marrow, fetus, skin, eyes, upper respiratory tract, mucous membranes, and fetus

Medical Conditions Generally Aggravated by Exposure:

- Hypersensitivity, prior resistance to THIOGUANINE or MERCAPTOPURINE (cross-resistance).
- Pregnancy.

Specific Medical Surveillance Information: Reproductive and pregnancy counseling.

Occupational Exposure Level/Limit (OEL) & Sampling Methods:

Environmental Sentinel Contamination Action Level (ESCAL): Not otherwise specified

Occupational Exposure Level (OEL) GSK: THIOGUANINE 10 μ/m3 Time-Weighted Average (8 hour TWA)

GSK Exposure Controls: An Exposure Control Approach (ECA) is established for operations involving this material based upon the OEL/ occupational hazard category and the outcome of a site- or operation-specific risk assessment. Refer to the exposure control matrix for more information about how ECA's are assigned and how to interpret them.

(Method not listed or specified)

Supplemental Response Information

Extinguishing Media: Use extinguishing agent which is the most appropriate to extinguish surrounding fire (foam, dry chemical or water fog as extinguishing media). Carbon dioxide extinguishers may be ineffective.

Solubility: 6-THIOGUANINE: No data provided except for the following note: By analogy with the closely related 6-mecaptopurine (6-mp), may be assumed to be practically water insoluble. Chemfinder reports a water solubility of <0.1 g/100 ml at 23 c.

Chemical Degradation/Neutralization Method: Not otherwise specified

Note: If a specific degradation or neutralization method is not provided on this table and you do not have other specific information that will guide you on how to clean up the specific material spilled, then follow the general spill procedure found in the introduction section of this handbook.

Incompatibility: 6-THIOGUANINE is incompatible with strong oxidizing agents.

THIOTEPA (1) *(thye-oh-TEP-a)*
THIOPLEX®104
TRIETHYLENE THIOPHSPHORAMIDE
TESPA
TRIS(1-AZIRIDNYL)-PHOSPHINE SULFIDE

Chemical Abstracts Service (CAS) Registry
Number: 52-24-4
Registry of Toxic Effects of Chemical Substance
(RTECS) SZ2975000
$C_6H_{12}N_3PS$
(Two Degradation Methods)

Health & Safety Hazards/US Department of Transportation (DOT)/US Environmental Protection Agency (EPA)—Sources

Carcinogen G1—International Agency for Research on Cancer, Carcinogen C2B—US National Toxicology Program, and US New Jersey State Department of Health and Senior Services Hazardous Substances Fact Sheet and Material Safety Data Sheet, Carcinogen—Berkeley University Hazardous Chemical List, Carcinogen—University of Maryland at College Park, Carcinogen—US Occupational Safety and Health Administration, Teratogen—University of Maryland at College Park, Tumorigenic—Material Safety Data Sheet, Mutagen—Material Safety Data Sheet, Reproductive Effector Tendencies—Material Safety Data Sheet, Sensitizer—Material Safety Data

Sheet, Cytotoxic—British Columbia Cancer Agency Canada, Cytotoxic—Material Safety Data Sheet, Irritant—ToxReport, Nonvesicant—British Columbia Cancer Agency Canada, Pregnancy Category (D)—US Food and Drug Administration, Highly Toxic—Material Safety Data Sheet, Poison B—Material Safety Data Sheet, Cytotoxic—Material Safety Data Sheet, Carcinogen—US California Proposition 65, National Fire Protection Association Health (3) Flammability (1) Instability (0)—Material Safety Data Sheet, National Fire Protection Association Health (3) Flammability (0) Instability (0)—Material Safety Data Sheet, Materials Identification System (R) and/or US Department of Defense System Health (3★) additional chronic hazard present Fire Hazard (0) Reactivity (0)—Material Safety Data Sheet Personal Protection Code (-) (None stated)—Material Safety Data Sheet, Materials Identification System (R) and/or US Department of Defense System Health (3) Fire Hazard (1) Reactivity (0) Personal Protective Code (X) (Ask Supervisor)—Material Safety Data Sheet, UN 2811, Class 6.1, or, UN 3249, Class 6.1, Group II.

THIOTEPA is colorless fluid from powder.

THIOTEPA is fine white crystalline flakes having a faint odor.

THIOTEPA can cause fetal harm; breastfeeding is discontinued because of potential for reproductive and developmental harm (*A Guide for Occupational Health Professionals Technical Manual*, Navy Environmental Health Center [NEHC TM OEM 6260.01a]).

First Aid/Medical Information/ Occupational Exposure Limits

First Aid Measures to include: Use general first aid measures except for the following:

Ingestion: Induce vomiting immediately as directed by medical personnel.

Physician's note: No specific antidote to THIOTEPA intoxication exists. Monitoring of hemograms and white blood cell counts may be helpful in assessing the level of overall toxicity to the hematopoietic system. Generally, induction of vomiting with ipecac procedures means a recovery of only 30% of the ingested dose. However, may still be useful in management of the poisoned patient. Save the initial emesis for analysis for THIOTEPA content.

Medical Information:

Caution and Warning Statements: THIOTEPA is highly toxic and may cause cancer and heritable genetic damage. May impair fertility and may cause harm to the unborn child. THIOTEPA can cause severe irritation with reversible opacity of the cornea. May cause skin irritation and can be absorbed through the skin in toxic amounts. Exposure to THIOTEPA can cause irritation and burning of the eyes, with possible eye damage. High exposure can cause nausea, vomiting, loss of appetite, and headache; repeat exposures can damage the bone marrow.

THIOTEPA is a cytotoxic agent. All work practices must be designed to reduce human exposure to the lowest level.

Caution: Females and males planning to have a child, pregnant women, and nursing mothers should exercise caution regarding potential occupational exposure to this cytotoxic drug. No information or not enough information exists or was provided concerning occupational exposures that may potentially occur while handling this drug and its affects on reproductive systems, the fetus, and/or if it is secreted along with breast milk, which may harm nursing infants. Staff members should consult with the occupational health physician monitoring workers' health in your facility to be apprised of potential hazards and should be advised to avoid becoming pregnant and/or breastfeeding or should be transferred in accordance with policy/procedures to other duties that do not involve preparation, handling, and administering this drug.

Therapeutic Levels: The Food and Drug Administration lists THIOTEPA as a Pregnancy Category (D). This means that THIOTEPA is known to be harmful to an unborn baby. It is not known whether THIOTEPA passes into breast milk.

Target Organs/Systems: Skin, eyes, bone marrow, kidneys, liver, spleen, lungs, blood system, gastrointestinal, heart, and reproductive systems

Medical Conditions Generally Aggravated by Exposure:

- Disorders involving the target organs of this compound can be aggravated by overexposures to this compound (especially in doses approaching therapeutic levels for this compound).
- In clinical-use—THIOTEPA is contraindicated in patients with a known hypersensitivity (allergy) to the preparation and history of liver, kidney or bone marrow damage.
- Reproductive and pregnancy issues.

Specific Medical Surveillance Information: Reproductive and pregnancy counseling.

A complete blood count is recommended if symptoms develop and /or overexposure is suspected.

Occupational Exposure Level/Limit (OEL) & Sampling Methods:

Environmental Sentinel Contamination Action Level (ESCAL): Not otherwise specified
Occupational Exposure Level (OEL) American Cyanamid:
0.0014 mg/m3
(Method not listed or specified)

Supplemental Response Information

Extinguishing Media: Use agent which is the most appropriate to extinguish surrounding fire (carbon dioxide, foam, dry chemical or water fog extinguishing media).

Solubility: THIOTEPA is soluble in water to about 19% (19 g/100 ml) @ 25°C; freely soluble in alcohol (pH range of 5.8–7.5). THIOTEPA is freely soluble in ethanol; soluble in ether, benzene, and chloroform.

Chemical Degradation/Neutralization Method: There are two or more recommended procedures for THIOTEPA. See below for additional method:

The International Agency for Research on Cancer (IARC) recommended degradation method for THIOTEPA:

The IARC recommends treating spill surfaces with a 5.25% sodium hypochlorite (bleach) solution after absorbing liquids with inert absorbent pads or removing any powder present: allow solution to stand for up to one hour, and then thoroughly wash spilled surfaces with soap and water; sample to determine if surface contamination is still present (if sampling method is available). If the drug is present, repeat above steps; dispose of wastes in accordance with your local procedures, state, and federal regulations.

Incompatibility: THIOTEPA is not compatible with acids and strong oxidizers.

THIOTEPA (2) *(thye-oh-TEP-a)*
THIOPLEX®104
TRIETHYLENE THIOPHSPHORAMIDE
TESPA
TRIS(1-AZIRIDNYL)-PHOSPHINE SULFIDE

Chemical Abstracts Service (CAS) Registry Number: 52-24-4
Registry of Toxic Effects of Chemical Substance (RTECS) SZ2975000
$C_6H_{12}N_3PS$
(Two Degradation Methods)

Health & Safety Hazards/US Department of Transportation (DOT)/US Environmental Protection Agency (EPA)—Sources

Carcinogen G1—International Agency for Research on Cancer, Carcinogen C2B—US National Toxicology Program and US New Jersey Department of Health and Senior Services Hazardous Substances Fact Sheet and Material Safety Data Sheet, Carcinogen—Berkeley University Hazardous Chemical List, Carcinogen—University of Maryland at College Park, Carcinogen—US Occupational Safety and Health Administration, Teratogen—University of Maryland at College Park, Tumorigenic—Material Safety Data Sheet, Mutagen—Material Safety Data Sheet, Reproductive Effector Tendencies—Material Safety Data Sheet, Sensitizer—Material Safety Data Sheet, Cytotoxic—British Columbia Cancer Agency Canada, Cytotoxic—Material Safety Data Sheet, Irritant—ToxReport, Nonvesicant—British Columbia Cancer Agency Canada, Pregnancy Category (D)—US Food and Drug Administration, Highly Toxic—Materials Safety Data Sheet, Poison B—Material Safety Data Sheet, Cytotoxic—Material Safety Data Sheet, Carcinogen—US California Proposition 65, National Fire Protection Association Health (3) Flammability (1) Instability (0)—Material Safety Data Sheet, National Fire Protection Association Health (3) Flammability (0) Instability (0)—Material Safety Data Sheet, Materials Identification System (R) and/or US Department of Defense System Health (3★) with additional chronic hazards present Fire Hazard (0) Reactivity (0) Personal Protection Code (-) (None stated)—Material Safety Data Sheet, Materials Identification System (R) and/or US Department of Defense System Health (3) Fire Hazard (1) Reactivity (0) Personal Protection Code (X) (Ask Supervisor)—Material Safety Data Sheet, UN 2811, Class 6.1, or, UN 3249, Class 6.1, Group II.

THIOTEPA is colorless fluid from powder.

THIOTEPA is fine white crystalline flakes having a faint odor.

THIOTEPA can cause fetal harm; breastfeeding should be discontinued because of the potential for reproductive and developmental harm (*A Guide for Occupational Health Professionals Technical Manual*, Navy Environmental Health Center [NEHC-TM-OEM 6260.01a]).

First Aid/Medical Information/ Occupational Exposure Limits

First Aid Measures to include: Use general first aid measures except for the following:

Ingestion: Induce vomiting immediately as directed by medical personnel.

Physician's note (A): No specific antidote to THIOTEPA intoxication exists. Monitoring of hemograms and white blood cell counts may be helpful in assessing the level of overall toxicity to the hematopoietic system. Generally, induction of vomiting with ipecac procedures means a recovery of only 30% of the ingested dose. However, may still be useful in management of the poisoned patient. Save the initial emesis for analysis for THIOTEPA content.

Physician's note (B): No specific antidote to THIOTEPA intoxication exists. Monitoring of hemograms and white blood cell counts may be helpful in assessing the level of overall toxicity to the hematopoietic system. Generally, induction of vomiting with syrup of ipecac produces a mean recovery of only 30% of the ingested dose, but may still be useful in management of the poisoned patient. Save the initial emesis for analysis of THIOTEPA.

Medical Information:

Caution and Warning Statements:

Warning: THIOTEPA is a human carcinogen. Highly toxic (poison B). THIOTEPA is highly toxic and may cause cancer and heritable genetic damage. May impair fertility and may cause harm to the unborn child. THIOTEPA can cause severe irritation with reversible opacity of the cornea. May cause skin irritation and can be absorbed through the skin in toxic amounts. Exposure to THIOTEPA can cause irritation and burning of the eyes, with possible eye damage. High exposure can cause nausea, vomiting, loss of appetite, and headache; repeat exposures can damage the bone marrow.

THIOTEPA is a cytotoxic agent. All work practices must be designed to reduce human exposure to the lowest level.

Caution: Females and males planning to have a child, pregnant women, and nursing mothers should exercise caution regarding potential occupational exposure to this cytotoxic drug. No information or not enough information exists or was provided concerning occupational exposures that may potentially occur while handling this drug and its affects on reproductive systems, the fetus, and/or if it is secreted along with breast milk, which may harm nursing infants. Staff members should consult with the occupational health physician monitoring workers' health in your facility to be apprised of potential hazards and should be advised to avoid becoming pregnant and/or breastfeeding or should be transferred in accordance with policy/procedures to other duties that do not involve preparation, handling, and administering this drug.

Therapeutic Levels: The Food and Drug Administration lists THIOTEPA as a Pregnancy Category (D). This means that THIOTEPA is known to be harmful to an unborn baby. It is not known whether THIOTEPA passes into breast milk.

Target Organs/Systems: Hematopoietic system, bone marrow, kidneys, liver, spleen, lungs, blood system, gastrointestinal, heart, eyes, and reproductive systems. This compound may cause allergic type reactions in sensitive individuals.

Medical Conditions Generally Aggravated by Exposure:

- Exposure to THIOTEPA may aggravate preexisting liver, kidney, or bone marrow damage. THIOTEPA will cause bone marrow depression (a decrease in the ability of the bone marrow to form mature blood cells). As a result, overexposure may cause leukopenia (a decrease in the number of circulating, formed white blood cells), thrombocytopenia (decrease in the number of platelets), and anemia (decrease in red blood cells). Clinically reported adverse reactions include nausea, vomiting, loss of appetite, dizziness, headache, amenorrhea (abnormal absence or suppression of the menstrual discharge), and interference with spermatogenesis. Death from septicemia (bacterial infection in the blood) and hemorrhage (bleeding) has occurred as a direct result of the depression of bone marrow caused by THIOTEPA.
- In clinical use—THIOTEPA is contraindicated in patients with a known hypersensitivity, allergy to the preparation, and history of liver, kidney, or bone marrow damage, recent chicken pox exposures, herpes zoster, and gout.
- Reproductive and pregnancy issues.

Specific Medical Surveillance Information: Reproductive and pregnancy counseling.

A complete blood count is recommended if symptoms develop and/or overexposure is suspected.

Occupational Exposure Level/Limit (OEL) & Sampling Methods:

Environmental Sentinel Contamination Action Level (ESCAL): Not otherwise specified
Occupational Exposure Level (OEL) American Cyanamid and Ben Venue Laboratories

THIOTEPA 0.0014 mg/m3
0.01 mg/m3 TWA
(Method not listed or specified)

Supplemental Response Information

Extinguishing Media: Use extinguishing agent which is the most appropriate to extinguish surrounding fire (carbon dioxide, foam, dry chemical or water fog extinguishing media).

Solubility: THIOTEPA is soluble in water to about 19% (19 g/100 ml) @ 25°C; freely soluble in alcohol. (pH range of 5.8–7.5) THIOTEPA is freely soluble in ethanol, soluble in ether, benzene, and chloroform.

Chemical Degradation/Neutralization Method: There are two or more recommended procedures for THIOTEPA. See below for an additional method:

A manufacturer's Material Safety Data Sheet (MSDS) recommends treating spill surfaces with a ~2 mol/liter (~8 g/100 ml), aqueous caustic soda (sodium hydroxide) solution after absorbing liquids with inert absorbent pads or removing any powder present: allow solution to stand for up to one hour, and then thoroughly wash spilled surfaces with soap and water; sample to determine if surface contamination is still present (if sampling method is available). If the drug is present, repeat above steps; dispose of wastes in accordance with your local procedures, state, and federal regulations.

Incompatibility: THIOTEPA (THIOPLEX®104) is incompatible with acids and strong oxidizers.

Note: Capable of explosive decomposition on contact with acidic substances or when heated above 40°C.

TOPOTECAN (*toe-poe-TEE-kan*)
HYCAMTIN®105

Chemical Abstracts Service (CAS) Registry Number: 123948-87-8

TOPOTECAN

Chemical Abstracts Service (CAS) Registry Number: 119413-54-6
$C_{23}H_{23}N_3O_5$

TOPOTECAN HCL

$C_{23}H_{24}ClN_3O_5$
(HYCAMTIN ®105 IS TOPOTECAN HCL)

Health & Safety Hazards/US Department of Transportation (DOT)/US Environmental Protection Agency (EPA)—Sources

Cytotoxic—Box Instruction, Cytotoxic—British Columbia Cancer Agency Canada, Cytotoxic—Material Safety Data Sheet, Carcinogen—Material Safety Data Sheet, Reproductive Effector—Material Safety Data Sheet, Fetotoxic—Material Safety Data Sheet, Mutagen—Material Safety Data Sheet, Human Mutagen—Material Safety Data Sheet, Nonvesicant—British Columbia Cancer Agency Canada, Pregnancy (D)—US Food and Drug Administration, Highly Potent—Material Safety Data Sheet, Material National Fire Protection Association Health (2) Flammability (1) Instability (0) Material Safety Data Sheet, Materials Identification System (R) and/or US Department of Defense System Health (2) Fire Hazard (1) Reactivity (0) Personal Protection Code (E) (Safety Glasses, Chemical Gloves, Dust Respirator)—Material Safety Data Sheet, UN 2811, Toxic, Class 6.1, Surface—UN 3249, Class 6.1 (TOPOTECAN Capsules), Group III, Toxic 6.

TOPOTECAN is a colorless fluid from powder.

TOPOTECAN 1%, consist of non-hazardous ingredients 99.0%.

(UV detection: 254 nm; color unknown, ~224 nm. Microgram levels of surface contamination can be visualized using ultraviolet light.)

First Aid/Medical Information/ Occupational Exposure Limits

First Aid Measures to include: Use general first aid measures except for the following:

Medical Information: Medical treatment in cases of overexposure should be treated as an overdose of a cytotoxic agent.

Caution and Warning Statements:

Warning: Manufacturer has designated this drug a carcinogen. May cause respiratory tract, eye and skin irritation. May cause heritable genetic effects based on animal data. Skin inflammation is characterized by itching, scaling, reddening, or occasionally blistering.

Overexposure in the workplace might have the following effects: reduced white blood cell count; nausea; diarrhea; vomiting and fatigue.

Caution: The toxicological properties of most cytotoxic drugs have not been fully investigated, particularly as it pertains to occupational exposure. TOPOTECAN is one of the drugs that has little occupational hazards information available. Therefore, therapeutic dose information was extrapolated below to assist in determining occupational toxicity, and signs and symptoms of overexposure. Therefore, it is prudent to minimize occupational exposure to TOPOTECAN.

Commonly reported side effects include suppression of bone marrow, nausea and vomiting, anorexia, diarrhea, constipation, headache, and alopecia (hair loss).

TOPOTECAN HCL (HYCAMTIN®105) may cause cancer and may produce adverse effects on the development of human offspring. Possible effects of overexposure in the workplace include nausea; vomiting; diarrhea; and bone marrow toxicity, reduced white blood cells.

Caution: Females and males planning to have a child, pregnant women, and nursing mothers should exercise caution regarding potential occupational exposure to this cytotoxic drug. No information or not enough information exists or was provided concerning occupational exposures that may potentially occur while handling this drug and its affects on reproductive systems, the fetus, and/or if it is secreted along with breast milk, which may harm nursing infants. Staff members should consult with the occupational health physician monitoring workers' health in your facility to be apprised of potential hazards and should be advised to avoid becoming pregnant and/or breastfeeding or should be transferred in accordance with policy/procedures to other duties that do not involve preparation, handling, and administering this drug.

Therapeutic Levels: The Food and Drug Administration lists this drug as a Pregnancy Code (D): HYCAMTIN®105 may cause fetal harm when administered to a pregnant woman. The effects of TOPOTECAN on pregnant women have not been studied; potentially hazardous to the fetus.

Target Organs/Systems: Respiratory tract, kidney, eyes, skin, reproductive, and possibly will harm the fetus

Medical Conditions Generally Aggravated by Exposure:

- If hypersensitivity to TOPOTECAN or to any of its ingredients; preexisting medical problems which causes bone marrow depression, kidney dysfunction, pregnancy, and infant nursing. (Healthline)
- Reproductive and pregnancy issues.

Specific Medical Surveillance Information: Reproductive and pregnancy counseling.

TOPOTECAN HCL (HYCAMTIN®105) medical surveillance—The need for pre-placement and periodic health surveillance must be determined by risk assessment. Following assessment, if the risk of exposure is considered significant then exposed individuals should undergo appropriate health surveillance that may include symptom enquiry, clinical examination, and monitoring of lead organ effects (e.g., full blood counts). In the event of overexposure, individuals should receive post exposure health surveillance focused on the most likely health effects (e.g., full blood counts).

Occupational Exposure Level/Limit (OEL) & Sampling Methods:

> *Environmental Sentinel Contamination Action Level (ESCAL)*: Visual
> *Occupational Exposure Level (OEL)* GSK Hazard Category 5:
> TOPOTECAN: 0.03 μ/m3 Time-Weighted Average (8 hour TWA)
> (Method not listed or specified)

Supplemental Response Information

Extinguishing Media: Use extinguishing agent which is the most appropriate to extinguish surrounding fire (carbon dioxide, foam, dry chemical or water fog as extinguishing media).

Solubility: TOPOTECAN is easily soluble in cold water. pH of aqueous solutions reported to be 3 (pH).

Chemical Degradation/Neutralization Method: A manufacturer's Material Safety Data Sheet (MSDS) recommends:

Cleaning spilled area by spreading an inert absorbent on the spill and place in a suitable, properly labeled container for disposal and treating collected wash water containing TOPOTECAN HCL (HY-CAMTIN®105) residual to a pH greater than 8 (pH); commercial bleach solution, containing approximately 5% hypochlorite, should then be added to the waste water (microgram levels of surface contamination can be visualized using ultraviolet light (UV) (GSK MSDS).

Furthermore, take wipe samples (if available at your facility) to determine if surface contamination is still present or use the above UV detection method. On spilled surfaces repeat above steps; dispose of wastes in accordance with your local procedures, state, and federal regulations.

Incompatibility: Not otherwise specified

TOSITUMOMAB (*toe-si-TYOO-mo-mab*)
BEXXAR®106
TOSITUMOMAB MONOCLONAL ANTIBODY

Chemical Abstracts Service (CAS) Registry Numbers: 208921-02-2, 192391-48-3
$C_{6416}H_{9874}N_{1688}O_{1987}S_{44}$

Health & Safety Hazards/US Department of Transportation (DOT)/US Environmental Protection Agency (EPA)—Sources

Pregnancy Category (X)—US Food and Drug Administration.

TOSITUMOMAB (BEXXAR®106) is available as an injection.

First Aid/Medical Information/ Occupational Exposure Limits

First Aid Measures to include: Use general first aid measures except for the following:

Ingestion: If victim is conscious and alert, wash out mouth with water. Give plenty of water to drink. Do not induce vomiting. Seek medical assistance.

Medical Information:

Caution and Warning Statements: BEXXAR®106 (TOSITUMOMAB) is not expected to be toxic following ingestion. Inhalation toxicity studies have not been conducted. Irritation is not expected from contact with eyes and/or skin.

Caution: The toxicological properties of most cytotoxic drugs have not been fully investigated, particularly as it pertains to occupational exposure. TOSITUMOMAB is one of the drugs that has little occupational hazards information available. Therefore, therapeutic dose information was extrapolated below to assist in determining occupational toxicity, and signs and symptoms of overexposure. Therefore, it is prudent to minimize occupational exposure to TOSITUMOMAB.

TOSITUMOMAB commonly reported side effects include mild to moderate "flu-like" symptoms with fever, nausea, and weakness; decreased white blood cell count with increased risk of infection; decreased platelet count with increased risk of bleeding; and decreased red blood cell count with increased risk of tiredness and anemia. Rare side effects are severe allergic reaction with flushing, hives, difficulty breathing, decreased blood pressure, loss of skin color, and loss of consciousness (ACS-cancer guide).

Caution: Females and males planning to have a child, pregnant women, and nursing mothers should exercise caution regarding potential occupational exposure to this cytotoxic drug. No information or not enough information exists or was provided concerning occupational exposures that may potentially occur while handling this drug and its affects on reproductive systems, the fetus, and/or if it is secreted along with breast milk, which may harm nursing infants. Staff members should consult with the occupational health physician monitoring workers' health in your facility to be apprised of potential hazards and should be advised to avoid becoming pregnant and/or breastfeeding or should be transferred in accordance with policy/procedures to other duties that do not involve preparation, handling, and administering this drug.

The Food and Drug Administration has assigned a Pregnancy Category (X) to TOSITUMOMAB.

Target Organs/Systems: Severe hypersensitivity reaction—immune system and possible fetus

Medical Conditions Generally Aggravated by Exposure:

- Any of the following medical problems: chickenpox or exposure to chickenpox, gout, heart disease, congestive heart failure, shingles, kidney stones, liver disease, or other forms of cancer.
- Pregnancy.

Specific Medical Surveillance Information: Reproductive and pregnancy counseling.

Occupational Exposure Level/Limit (OEL) & Sampling Methods: Not otherwise specified

Environmental Sentinel Contamination Action Level (ESCAL): Not otherwise specified

Supplemental Response Information

Extinguishing Media: Use extinguishing agent which is the most appropriate to extinguish surrounding fire (carbon dioxide, foam, dry chemical or water fog as extinguishing media).

Solubility: BEXXAR®106 is an aqueous solution. TOSITUMOMAB (BEXXAR®106) has a pH of approximately 7.2.

Chemical Degradation/Neutralization Method: A manufacturer's Material Safety Data Sheet (MSDS) recommends using alkaline soap/detergent and water to clean spill surfaces after absorbing liquids with inert absorbent pads or removing any powder present: repeat using soap and water; sample to determine if surface contamination is still present (if sampling method is available). If the drug is present, repeat above steps; dispose of wastes in accordance with your local procedures, state, and federal regulations.

Incompatibility: Not otherwise specified

TRIAZINATE

Chemical Abstracts Service (CAS) Registry
   Number: 31368-48-6
Registry of Toxic Effects of Chemical Substance
   (RTECS): XS3650000
$C_{23}H_{30}Cl_2FN_5O_5S_2$

Health & Safety Hazards/US Department of Transportation (DOT)/US Environmental Protection Agency (EPA)—Sources

Pregnancy Category (None)—US Food and Drug Administration.

First Aid/Medical Information/ Occupational Exposure Limits

First Aid Measures to include: Use general first aid measures.

Medical Information:

Caution and Warning Statements: Not otherwise specified

Target Organs/Systems: Not otherwise specified

Medical Conditions Generally Aggravated by Exposure: Not otherwise specified

Specific Medical Surveillance Information: Not otherwise specified

Occupational Exposure Level/Limit (OEL) & Sampling Methods: Not otherwise specified

Environmental Sentinel Contamination Action Level (ESCAL): Not otherwise specified

Supplemental Response Information

Extinguishing Media: Use extinguishing agent which is the most appropriate to extinguish surrounding fire (carbon dioxide, foam, dry chemical or water fog as extinguishing media).

Solubility: TRIAZINATE: Not otherwise specified

Chemical Degradation/Neutralization Method: Not otherwise specified

Note: If a specific degradation or neutralization method is not provided on this table and you do not have other specific information that will guide you on how to clean up the specific material spilled, then follow the general spill procedure found in the introduction section of this handbook

Incompatibility: Not otherwise specified

TRIMETREXATE GLUCURONATE

(tri-me-TREX-ate)
NEUTREXIN®107
TMQ
TMTX

$C_{25}H_{33}N_5O_{10}$

ADMINISTERED WITH CONCURRENT LEUCOVORIN (LCV) (ANHYDROUS)

Chemical Abstracts Service (CAS) Registry
   Number: 82952-64-5
$C_{19}-H_{23}-N_5-O_3$

TRIMETREXATE
NEUTREXIN®107

Chemical Abstracts Service (CAS) Registry
  Number: 52128-35-5
Registry of Toxic Effects of Chemical Substance
  (RTECS): LZ8945000
National Cancer Institute: NSC 352122
$C_{19}H_{23}N_5O_3 . C_6-H_{10}-O_7$
$C_{19}H_{23}N_5O_3$

Health & Safety Hazards/US Department of Transportation (DOT)/US Environmental Protection Agency (EPA)—Sources

Mutagen—Material Safety Data Sheet, Experimental Teratogen—Material Safety Data Sheet and US Food and Drug Administration Drug Label, Experimental Fetotoxic—Material Safety Data Sheet, Pregnancy Category (D)—US Food and Drug Administration, Developmental—US California Proposition 65, UN 2811.

(UV Detection: 254 nm; Color Unknown, 237 nm)

TRIMETREXATE can cause fetal harm; breast-feeding should be discontinued because of potential for reproductive and developmental harm (*A Guide for Occupational Health Professionals Technical Manual*, Navy Environmental Health Center [NEHC-TM-OEM 6260.01a]).

First Aid/Medical Information/ Occupational Exposure Limits

First Aid Measures to include: Use general first aid measures.

Medical Information:

Caution and Warning Statements: Patients receiving NEUTREXIN®107 (TRIMETREXATE GLUCURONATE for injection) may experience severe hematologic, hepatic, renal, and gastrointestinal toxicities. TRIMETREXATE GLUCURONATE is administered with concurrent leucovorin to avoid potentially serious or life-threatening toxicities to include bone marrow suppression, oral and gastrointestinal mucosal ulceration, and renal and hepatic dysfunction. Side effects of TRIMETREXATE GLUCURONATE therapy are nausea, loss of appetite or weight, mouth blistering, fatigue, diarrhea, fever, coughing, dizziness, chills, severe vomiting, and unusual bruising or bleeding.

Long term studies on TRIMETREXATE in animals to evaluate the carcinogenic potential have not been performed. Mutagenesis: TRIMETREXATE did induce an increase in the chromosomal aberration frequency in animal studies.

Impairment of fertility: no studies have been conducted to evaluate the potential of TRIMETREXATE to impair fertility. However, during toxicity studies with animals' degeneration of the tested and spermatocytes including the arrest of spermatogenesis was observed.

Caution: Females and males planning to have a child, pregnant women, and nursing mothers should exercise caution regarding potential occupational exposure to this cytotoxic drug. No information or not enough information exists or was provided concerning occupational exposures that may potentially occur while handling this drug and its affects on reproductive systems, the fetus, and/or if it is secreted along with breast milk, which may harm nursing infants. Staff members should consult with the occupational health physician monitoring workers' health in your facility to be apprised of potential hazards and should be advised to avoid becoming pregnant and/or breastfeeding or should be transferred in accordance with policy/procedures to other duties that do not involve preparation, handling, and administering this drug.

The Food and Drug Administration has assigned a Pregnancy Category (D) to NEUTREXIN®107. NEUTREXIN®107 can cause fetal harm when administered to a pregnant woman. TRIMETREXATE GLUCURONATE has been shown to be fetotoxic and teratogenic in rats and rabbits.

Target Organs/Systems: Bone marrow depression, GI tract, blood, liver, kidneys, and possible fetus

Medical Conditions Generally Aggravated by Exposure:

- Medical conditions that are aggravated by exposure to the material are any kind of bone marrow depression, hepatic function impairment, renal function impairment, or hypersensitivity to TRIMETREXATE, METHOTREXATE, or LEUCOVORIN. Others medical conditions are kidney or liver disease, stomach ulcers, or intestinal disease.
- It is not know if TRIMETREXATE is distributed into breast milk; breastfeeding in not recommended during therapy because of the potential for serious adverse effects in the nursing infant.

Specific Medical Surveillance Information: Reproductive and pregnancy counseling.

Recommended laboratory testing of patients receiving NEUTREXIN®107 with leucovorin protection consists of blood tests performed twice a week to assess the hematology (absolute neutrophil counts [ANC], platelets), renal function (serum creatinine, bun), and hepatic function (AST, ALT, alkaline phosphatase).

Occupational Exposure Level/Limit (OEL) & Sampling Methods: Not otherwise specified

Environmental Sentinel Contamination Action Level (ESCAL): Not otherwise specified

Supplemental Response Information

Extinguishing Media: Use extinguishing agent which is the most appropriate to extinguish surrounding fire (carbon dioxide, foam, dry chemical or water fog as extinguishing media).

Solubility: TRIMETREXATE GLUCURONATE: TRIMETREXATE Free base:

TRIMETREXATE GLUCURONATE is water soluble (>50 mg/ml), whereas TRIMETREXATE free base is practically water insoluble (<0.1 mg/ml). Methyl alcohol solubility is 0.6 mg/ml.

Chemical Degradation/Neutralization Method: Not otherwise specified

Note: If a specific degradation or neutralization method is not provided on this table and you do not have other specific information that will guide you on how to clean up the specific material spilled, then follow the general spill procedure found in the introduction section of this handbook.

Incompatibility: TRIMETREXATE is incompatible with oxidizing agents.

U

URAMUSTINE
URACIL MUSTARD
5-[(BIS(2-CHLOROETHYL)AMINO)] URACIL

Chemical Abstracts Service (CAS) Registry Number: 66-75-1
Registry of Toxic Effects of Chemical Substance (RTECS): YQ8925000
$C_8H_{11}Cl_2N_3O_2$

Health & Safety Hazards/US Department of Transportation (DOT)/US Environmental Protection Agency (EPA)—Sources

Carcinogen G2B—International Agency for Research on Cancer, Carcinogen—University of Maryland at College Park, Toxic—US National Institute of Health (NIH) and Material Safety Data Sheet, Carcinogen—US National Institute of Health (NIH) and Material Safety Data Sheet, Mutagen—US National Institute of Health (NIH) and Material Safety Data Sheet, Teratogen—US National Institute of Health (NIH) and Material Safety Data Sheet, Vesicant—Material Safety Data Sheet, Pregnancy Category (None)—US Food and Drug Administration, Carcinogen and Developmental Male and Female—US California Proposition 65, Oral Rate: Ld50: 3550 Micrograms/Kg; US California Environmental Protection Agency Listed, Title III, U237; UN 2811, Guide 154; MIDI: HW01—(http://usaphcapps.amedd.army.mil/midi/).

URAMUSTINE (URACIL MUSTARD)—Male: azoospermia; Female: amenorrhea; pregnancy: avoid breastfeeding; not recommended because of the risk of adverse effects, mutagenicity, carcinogenicity, reproductive, and developmental hazards (*A Guide for Occupational Health Professionals*, Navy Environmental Health Center, Technical Manual [NEHC-TM-OEM 6260.01a]).

URACIL MUSTARD is creamy white crystals or off-white powder.

First Aid/Medical Information/ Occupational Exposure Limits

First Aid Measures to include: Use general first aid measures except for the following:

Physician's note: Observe for delayed vesicant effects. Consider ophthalmological consultation.

Medical Information:

Caution and Warning Statements: This material may be absorbed through the intestinal tract. Exposure may cause tissue irritation. URAMUSTINE is listed as a toxic material with male and female reproductive toxicity characteristics.

Target Organs/Systems: Blood, liver, CNS, and male/female reproductive systems

Exposure to this drug can cause nausea, vomiting, diarrhea, abdominal pain; affecting the nervous system causing confusion, irritability, anxiety, depression, and muscle weakness. Exposure may cause damage to the bone marrow with low red and white blood cell count, causing anemia and reducing resistance to infections and damages the liver.

Medical Conditions Generally Aggravated by Exposure:

- Reproductive and pregnancy issues. Hypersensitivity to material, bone marrow depression, chickenpox (including recent exposure), herpes zoster, gout, infection, blood abnormalities, impaired lever or kidney function, and previous cytotoxic drug or radiation therapy.

Specific Medical Surveillance Information: Reproductive and pregnancy counseling.

If symptoms develop or overexposure is suspected, order a complete blood count; a liver function test should be performed along with an examination of the nervous system.

Occupational Exposure Level/Limit (OEL) & Sampling Methods: Not otherwise specified

V

VALRUBICIN (*val-ROO-bi-sin*)
VALSTAR®108

Chemical Abstracts Service (CAS) Registry
Number: 56124-62-0
Registry of Toxic Effects of Chemical Substance
(RTECS): AV9850000
$C_{34}H_{36}F_3NO_{13}$

Health & Safety Hazards/US Department of Transportation (DOT)/US Environmental Protection Agency (EPA)—Sources

Pregnancy Category (C)—US Food and Drug Administration, Mutagen—US Food and Drug Label.

VALRUBICIN is an orange to orange-red crystalline powder.

First Aid/Medical Information/ Occupational Exposure Limits

First Aid Measures to include: Use general first aid measures except for the following:

Ingestion: If victim is conscious and alert, rinse mouth out, give 2–3 glasses of water, and seek medical assistance.

Medical Information:

Caution and Warning Statements: Acute exposure: ingestion—moderate GI irritation, well known purga-

Environmental Sentinel Contamination Action Level (ESCAL): Not otherwise specified

Supplemental Response Information

Extinguishing Media: Use extinguishing agent which is the most appropriate to extinguish surrounding fire (carbon dioxide, foam, dry chemical or water fog as extinguishing media).

Solubility: URAMUSTINE is sparingly water soluble (<1 mg/ml at 68°F [NTP, 1992]).

Chemical Degradation/Neutralization Method: Not otherwise specified

Note: If a specific degradation or neutralization method is not provided on this table and you do not have other specific information that will guide you on how to clean up the specific material spilled, then follow the general spill procedure found in the introduction section of this handbook.

Incompatibility: Oxidizing agents and water. This material is unstable in the presence of water, high humidity, or aqueous vehicles.

tive; inhalation—upper respiratory tract irritation. This drug may cause headache, nausea, and eye and skin irritation.

Caution: Females and males planning to have a child, pregnant women, and nursing mothers should exercise caution regarding potential occupational exposure to this cytotoxic drug. No information or not enough information exists or was provided concerning occupational exposures that may potentially occur while handling this drug and its affects on reproductive systems, the fetus, and/or if it is secreted along with breast milk, which may harm nursing infants. Staff members should consult with the occupational health physician monitoring workers' health in your facility to be apprised of potential hazards and should be advised to avoid becoming pregnant and/or breastfeeding or should be transferred in accordance with policy/procedures to other duties that do not involve preparation, handling, and administering this drug.

VALRUBICIN is in the Food and Drug Administration Pregnancy Category (C). Systemic exposure to VALRUBICIN may result in harm to an unborn baby.

Target Organs/Systems: GI, upper respiratory tracts, skin, eyes, and possible fetus

Medical Conditions Generally Aggravated by:

- Pregnancy.

Specific Medical Surveillance Information: Reproductive and pregnancy counseling

Occupational Exposure Level/Limit (OEL) & Sampling Methods: Not otherwise specified

Environmental Sentinel Contamination Action Level (ESCAL): Not otherwise specified

Supplemental Response Information

Extinguishing Media: Use extinguishing agent which is the most appropriate to extinguish surrounding fire (carbon dioxide, foam, dry chemical or water fog as extinguishing media).

Solubility: VALRUBICIN (VALSTAR®108) is relatively water insoluble. VALRUBICIN (VAL-STAR®108) is soluble in dehydrated alcohol and in methyl alcohol.

Chemical Degradation/Neutralization Method: A manufacturer's Material Safety Data Sheet (MSDS) recommends treating spill surfaces with a 5–10% sodium hypochlorite (bleach) solution after absorbing liquids with inert absorbent pads or removing any powder present: allow solution to stand for up to one hour, and then thoroughly wash spilled surfaces with soap and water; sample to determine if surface contamination is still present (if sampling method is available). If the drug is present, repeat above steps, dispose of wastes in accordance with your local procedures, state, and federal regulations.

Incompatibility: Not otherwise specified

VELCADE®117

BORTEZOMIB (*bore-TEZ-oh-mib*)

$C_{19}H_{25}B-N_{4-}O_4$

PS341
MLN341
LDP341

Chemical Abstracts Service (CAS) Registry Number: 179324-69-7

Health & Safety Hazards/US Department of Transportation (DOT)/US Environmental Protection Agency (EPA)—Sources

Toxic—Material Safety Data Sheet, Reproductive Effector—Material Safety Data Sheet, Cytotoxic—British Columbia Cancer Agency Canada, Irritant—British Columbia Cancer Agency Canada, Nonvesicant—British Columbia Cancer Agency Canada, Pregnancy Category (D)—US Food and Drug Administration, UN 3249, Class 6.1.

VELCADE®117 (BORTEZOMIB) is available as an injection.

First Aid/Medical Information/ Occupational Exposure Limits

First Aid Measures to include: Use general first aid measures except for the following:

Ingestion: If victim is conscious and alert, rinse mouth out and give 2–4 cups of water. Seek medical assistance.

Medical Information:

Caution and Warning Statements: VELCADE®117 (BORTEZOMIB) is toxic, if inhaled or absorbed thorough the skin. This material is a skin and eye irritant. Repeated occupational overexposure may cause fatigue and fever, and effects on the hematological (decreases in hemoglobin/ anemia, blood counts and platelets), gastrointestinal (nausea, diarrhea, vomiting, abdominal), and nervous systems (headache, peripheral neuropathy). May affect fertility based on animal toxicity studies. Avoid skin contact, eye contact, and inhalation. Cancercare (CCC) lists BORTEZOMIB as an irritant.

Caution: Females and males planning to have a child, pregnant women, and nursing mothers should exercise caution regarding potential occupational exposure to this cytotoxic drug. No information or not enough information exists or was provided concerning occupational exposures that may potentially occur while handling this drug and its affects on reproductive systems, the fetus, and/or if it is secreted along with breast milk, which may harm nursing infants. Staff members should consult with the occupational health physician monitoring workers' health in your facility to be apprised of potential hazards and should be advised to avoid becoming pregnant and/or breastfeeding or should be transferred in accordance with policy/procedures to other duties that do not involve preparation, handling, and administering this drug.

Food and Drug Administration Pregnancy Category (D) women of childbearing potential should avoid becoming pregnant while being treated with VELCADE®117. It is not known whether BORTEZOMIB is excreted in human milk.

Target Organs/Systems: Blood, gastrointestinal, CNS, reproductive systems, and possible fetus

Medical Conditions Generally Aggravated by Exposure:

- Allergic reaction to BORTEZOMIB, boron or mannitol, heart disease, syncope, kidney disease, liver disease, peripheral neuropathy, tumor lysis syndrome, and medical problems which may cause dehydration.

- Reproductive and pregnancy issues.

Specific Medical Surveillance Information: Reproductive and pregnancy counseling.

Occupational Exposure Level/Limit (OEL) & Sampling Methods:

    Environmental Sentinel Contamination Action Level (ESCAL): Air, surface

Supplemental Response Information

Extinguishing Media: Use extinguishing agent which is the most appropriate to extinguish surrounding fire (carbon dioxide, foam, dry chemical or water fog as extinguishing media).

Solubility: VELCADE®117 is very water soluble with a pH range of 2 to 6.5.

Chemical Degradation/Neutralization Method: A manufacture's Material Safety Data Sheet (MSDS) for VELCADE®117 recommends washing spill area thoroughly with soap and water. Small quantities of 70% ethanol and 10% bleach may be used to clean work area or spill surfaces.

Incompatibility: Not otherwise specified

VINBLASTINE (1) (*vin-BLAST-een*)

$C_{46}H_{58}N_4O_9$

VINBLASTINE SULFATE

$C_{46}H_{60}N_4O_{13}S$

VELBAN®110
VLB
VINCALEUKOBLASTINE SULFATE

    Chemical Abstracts Service (CAS) Registry Number: 143-67-9

VINBLASTIN SULFATE

    Chemical Abstracts Service (CAS) Registry Number: 865-21-4 (mixture)

VINBLASTIN

    Registry of Toxic Effects of Chemical Substance (RTECS): YY8400000
    $C_{46}H_{58}N_4O_9$

$C_{46}-H_{58}-N_4-O_9 \cdot H_2O_4S$
(Two Degradation Methods)

Health & Safety Hazards/US Department of Transportation (DOT)/US Environmental Protection Agency (EPA)—Sources

Carcinogen G3—International Agency for Research on Cancer, Carcinogen—Berkeley University Hazardous Chemical List, Mutagen—Material Safety Data Sheet, Mutagen—University of Maryland at College Park, Teratogen—Material Safety Data Sheet, Teratogen—US National Institute of Health (NIH) and Material Safety Data Sheet, Teratogen—University of Maryland at College Park, Reproductive Effector—Material Safety Data Sheet, Highly Toxic—Material Safety Data Sheet, Toxic—US National Institute of Health (NIH) and Material Safety Data Sheet, Embryotoxic—US National Institute of Health (NIH) and Material Safety Data Sheet, Cytotoxic—Material Safety Data Sheet, Ototoxic—British Columbia Cancer Agency Canada, Vesicant—Material Safety Data Sheet, Vesicant—British Columbia Cancer Agency Canada, Cytotoxic—British Columbia Cancer Agency Canada, Lactation Avoid Breastfeeding (World Health Organization), Pregnancy Category (D)—US Food and Drug Administration, Developmental—US California Proposition 65, US California Environmental Protection Agency Listed—Chemfinder, National Fire Protection Association Health (2) Flammability (1) Instability (0)—Material Safety Data Sheet, National Fire Protection Association Health (2) Flammability (0) Instability (0)—Material Safety Data Sheet, National Fire Protection Association Health (2) Flammability (0) Instability (1)—Material Safety Data Sheet, National Fire Protection Association Health (3) Flammability (0) Instability (1)—Material Safety Data Sheet Health (3) Flammability (1) Instability (1)—Material Safety Data Sheet, National Fire Protection Association Health (3) Flammability (1) Instability (1) Special R = Reproductive, Hazardous Materials Identification System (R) and/or Department of Defense System Health (3★) with additional chronic hazards present Fire Hazard (1) Reactivity (0) Personal Protection Code (E) (Safety Glasses, Chemical Gloves, Dust Respirator)—Material Safety Data Sheet, Materials Identification System (R) and/or US Department of Defense System Health (2★) with additional chronic hazards present Fire Hazard (0) Reactivity (0) Personal Protection Code (–) (None stated), Materials Identification System (R) and/or US Department of Defense System Health

(2★) with additional chronic hazards present Fire Hazard (1) Reactivity (0) Personal Protection Code (-) (None stated)—Material Safety Data Sheet, UN 3249, Class 6.1, Group II; ALKALOID SALTS, SOLID, Not otherwise specified (VINBLASTINE SULFATE), UN1544, Class 6.1, Group II.

VINBLASTINE is a colorless fluid from powder.

VINBLASTINE SULPHATE is a white or slightly yellowish, very hygroscopic, amorphous or crystalline powder.

VINBLASTINE SULFATE can cause fetal harm; breastfeeding should be discontinued because of potential for reproductive and developmental hazards (*A Guide for Occupational Health Professionals Technical Manual*, Navy Environmental Health Center [NEHC-TM-OEM 6260.01a]).

VINBLASTINE SULFATE is the sulfate of an alkaloid, VINCALEUKOBLASTINE, extracted from catharanthus roseus (vinca rosea) (apocynaceae).

First Aid/Medical Information/ Occupational Exposure Limits

First Aid Measures to include: Use general first aid measures except for the following:

Ingestion:

Physician's note (A): Should ingestion occur the stomach should be evacuated. Evacuation should be followed by oral administration of activated charcoal and a cathartic.

Eye Contact:

Physician's note (B): VINCA alkaloids do not cause direct chemical burns of eye tissue, but interfere with the reproduction of the eye epithelium, which occurs continuously. The result is a delayed burn and subsequent scarring. While very painful, all cases have recovered completely without any loss of eye function. A steroid eye ointment or drops serve to minimize inflammation.

Dermal Contact: Avoid rubbing of skin or increasing its temp (since VLB acts as a vesicant on skin exposure).

Physician's note (C) (VINBLASTINE SULFATE): There is no specific antidote for VINBLASTINE SULFATE. Overdose treatment is supportive and may include the following:

1. Administration of activated charcoal slurry along with a cathartic is preferred over induced vomiting or gastric lavage, if orally ingested;
2. Restriction of the volume of daily fluid intake and perhaps the administration of a diuretic affecting the function of the loop of henle and the distal tubule;
3. Administration of an anticonvulsant if needed;
4. Prevention of ileus and monitoring the cardiovascular system;
5. Determination of daily blood counts for guidance in transfusion requirements and assessing the risk of infection due to myelosuppression.

Medical Information:

Caution and Warning Statements: Harmful—Toxic, VINBLASTINE SULFATE can cause birth defects. Direct contact with VINBLASTINE SULFATE may interfere with the reproduction of the corneal epithelium. Some patients treated have developed second malignancies and decrease in fertility. Inhalation of powder may cause local irritation of the nose and throat, tearing pain, blurred vision, delayed burn and scaring. May irritate the skin and cause sensitivity. Avoid rubbing skin or increasing its temperature (since VINBLASTINE SULFATE acts as a vesicant on skin exposure). Inhalation of powder may cause local irritation of the nose and throat, tearing pain blurred vision, delayed burn and scaring. National Institute of Health (NIH) Material Safety Data Sheet (MSDS) states the following: may irritate the skin and cause sensitivity.

Caution: Females and males planning to have a child, pregnant women, and nursing mothers should exercise caution regarding potential occupational exposure to this cytotoxic drug. No information or not enough information exists or was provided concerning occupational exposures that may potentially occur while handling this drug and its affects on reproductive systems, the fetus, and/or if it is secreted along with breast milk, which may harm nursing infants. Staff members should consult with the occupational health physician monitoring workers' health in your facility to be apprised of potential hazards and should be advised to avoid becoming pregnant and/or breastfeeding or should be transferred in accordance with policy/procedures to other duties that do not involve preparation, handling, and administering this drug.

VINBLASTINE is in the Food and Drug Administration Pregnancy Category D. This means that VINBLASTINE is known to be harmful to an unborn baby. It is not known whether VINBLASTINE passes into breast milk. Breastfeeding should be avoided during treatment with VINBLASTINE.

Target Organs/Systems: Eyes (corneal), heart, skin, autonomic nervous system, respiratory system, blood, bone marrow, and possibly fetus

Medical Conditions Generally Aggravated by Exposure:

- Preexisting skin and respiratory conditions.
- Individuals with significant granulocytopenia, unless this is a result of the disease being treated, or individuals with bacterial infections.
- Reproductive and pregnancy issues.

Specific Medical Surveillance Information: Reproductive and pregnancy counseling.

Occupational Exposure Level/Limit (OEL) & Sampling Methods:

Environmental Sentinel Contamination Action Level (ESCAL): Surface

Occupational Exposure Level (OEL)

LEG 0.47 µg/m3 Time-Weighted Average (TWA) for 12 hours

Excursion limit: 5.64 mg/m3 for no more than a total of 30 minutes.

"Worse case" computer aided prediction of spray/mist or fume/dust components and concentration:

Composite exposure standard for mixture (TWA): 3.0000 mg/m3. Operations, which produce a spray/mist or fume/dust, introduce particulates to the breathing zone. If the breathing zone concentration of any of the components listed below is exceeded, "worst case" considerations deem the individual to be over-exposed.

Breathing Component Conc. %	Zone mg/m3	Mixture (%)
VINBLASTINE SULFATE	3.0000	0.7

(Method not listed or specified)

Supplemental Response Information

Extinguishing Media: Use extinguishing agent which is the most appropriate to extinguish surrounding fire (carbon dioxide, foam, dry chemical or water fog as extinguishing media).

Solubility: VINBLASTINE:

VINBLASTINE SULFATE:

VINBLASTINE is completely water soluble with a pH range of 3.5–5.5 (0.15% AQ. Sol). Furthermore, it is easily soluble in methanol.

VINBLASTINE SULFATE solubility is negligible to soluble in water with a pH range of 3.5–5.0. A 0.1% in 0.9% sodium chloride solution is practically insoluble in alcohol.

Chemical Degradation/Neutralization Method: Two or more degradation/neutralization procedures exist for this drug. See below for additional method.

A manufacturer's Material Safety Data Sheet (MSDS) recommends treating spill surfaces with basic (pH of approximately 10) sodium hypochlorite solution, after absorbing liquids with inert absorbent pads or removing any powder present: allow solution to stand for up to one hour, and then thoroughly wash spilled surfaces with soap and water; sample to determine if surface contamination is still present (if sampling method is available). If the drug is present, repeat above steps; dispose of wastes in accordance with your local procedures, state, and federal regulations.

Incompatibility: VINBLASTINE SULFATE is incompatible with strong oxidizing agents, peroxides, permanganates, amino-acids, aminophylline, ascorbic acid, dexamethasone, frusemide, riboflavine, sulfhydryl-containing reagents, nitric acid, and strong bases. Avoid exposure to light and protect from moisture.

VINBLASTINE (2) (*vin-BLAST-een*)

$C_{46}H_{58}N_4O_9$

VINBLASTINE SULFATE

$C_{46}H_{60}N_4O_{13}Sw$

VINCALEUKOBLASTINE SULFATE
VELBAN®110
VLB

Chemical Abstracts Service (CAS) Registry Number: 143-67-9

VINBLASTIN SULFATE

Chemical Abstracts Service (CAS) Registry Number: 865-21-4 (mixture)

VINBLASTIN

$C_{46}H_{58}N_4O_9$
$C_{46}-H_{58}-N_4-O_9 \cdot H_2O_4S$
Registry of Toxic Effects of Chemical Substance (RTECS): YY8400000

(Two Degradation Methods)

Health & Safety Hazards/US Department of Transportation (DOT)/US Environmental Protection Agency (EPA)—Sources

Carcinogen G3—International Agency for Research on Cancer, Carcinogen—Berkeley University Hazardous Chemical List, Mutagen—Material Safety Data Sheet, Mutagen—University of Maryland at College Park, Teratogen—Material Safety Data Sheet, Teratogen—US National Institute of Health (NIH) and Material Safety Data Sheet, Teratogen—University of Maryland at College Park, Reproductive Effector—Material Safety Data Sheet, Highly Toxic—Material Safety Data Sheet, Toxic—US National Institute of Health (NIH) and Material Safety Data Sheet, Embryotoxic—US National Institute of Health (NIH) and Material Safety Data Sheet, Cytotoxic—Material Safety Data Sheet, Ototoxic—British Columbia Cancer Agency Canada, Vesicant—Material Safety Data Sheet, Vesicant—British Columbia Cancer Agency Canada, Cytotoxic—British Columbia Cancer Agency Canada, Lactation Avoid Breastfeeding (World Health Organization), Pregnancy D—US Food and Drug Administration, Developmental—US California Proposition 65, US California Environmental Protection Agency Listed—Chemfinder, National Fire Protection Association Health (2) Flammability (1) Instability (0)—Material Safety Data Sheet, National Fire Protection Association Health (2) Flammability (0) Instability (0)—Material Safety Data Sheet, National Fire Protection Association Health (2) Flammability (0) Instability (1)—Material Safety Data Sheet, National Fire Protection Association Health (3) Flammability (0) Instability (1)—Material Safety Data Sheet, National Fire Protection Association Health (3) Flammability (1) Instability (1)—Material Safety Data Sheet, National Fire Protection Association Health (3) Flammability (1) Instability (1) R = Reproductive- Material Safety Data Sheet, Materials Identification System (R) and/or US Department of Defense System Health (3★) with additional chronic hazards present Fire Hazard (1) Reactivity (0) Personal Protective Code (E) (Safety Glasses, Chemical Gloves, Dust Respirator)—Material Safety Data Sheet, Materials Identification System (R) and/or US Department of Defense System Health (2★) with additional chronic hazards present Fire Hazard (0) Reactivity (0) Personal Protection Code (-) (None stated)—Material Safety Data Sheet, Materials Identification System (R) and/or US Department of Defense System Health (2★) with additional chronic hazards present Fire Hazard (1) Reactivity (0) Personal Protection Code (-)(None stated)—Material Safety Data Sheet, UN 3249, Class 6.1, Group II.

VINBLASTINE is a colorless fluid from powder.

VINBLASTINE SULPHATE is a white or slightly yellowish, very hygroscopic, amorphous or crystalline powder.

VINBLASTINE SULFATE can cause fetal harm; breastfeeding should be discontinued because of potential for reproductive and developmental harm (A Guide for Occupational Health Professionals Technical Manual, Navy Environmental Health Center [NEHC-TM-OEM 6260.01a]).

VINBLASTINE SULFATE is the sulfate of an alkaloid, VINCALEUKOBLASTINE, extracted from catharanthus roseus (vinca rosea) (apocynaceae).

First Aid/Medical Information/ Occupational Exposure Limits

First Aid Measures to include: Use general first aid measures except for the following:

Ingestion:

Physician's note (A): Should ingestion occur the stomach should be evacuated. Evacuation should be followed by oral administration of activated charcoal and a cathartic.

Eye Contact:

Physician's note (B): VINCA alkaloids do not cause a direct chemical burn of eye tissue, but interfere with the reproduction of the eye epithelium, which occurs continuously. The result is a delayed burn and subsequent scarring. While very painful, all cases have recovered completely without any loss of eye function. A steroid eye ointment or drops serve to minimize inflammation.

Dermal Contact: Avoid rubbing of skin or increasing its temp (since VLB acts as a vesicant on skin exposure)

Physician's note (C): (VINBLASTINE SULFATE)—There is no specific antidote for VINBLASTINE SULFATE. Overdose treatment is supportive and may include the following:

1. Administration of activated charcoal slurry along with a cathartic is preferred over induced vomiting or gastric lavage, if orally ingested;
2. Restriction of the volume of daily fluid intake and perhaps the administration of a diuretic

affecting the function of the loop of henle and the distal tubule;

3. Administration of an anticonvulsant if needed;
4. Prevention of ileus and monitoring the cardiovascular system;
5. Determination of daily blood counts for guidance in transfusion requirements and assessing the risk of infection due to myelosuppression.

Medical Information:

Caution and Warning Statements: Harmful—Toxic, VINBLASTINE SULFATE can cause birth defects. Direct contact with VINBLASTINE SULFATE may interfere with the reproduction of the corneal epithelium. Some patients treated have developed second malignancies and decrease in fertility. Inhalation of powder may cause local irritation of the nose and throat, tearing pain, blurred vision, delayed burn and scarring. May irritate the skin and cause sensitivity. Avoid rubbing skin or increasing its temperature (since VINBLASTINE SULFATE acts as a vesicant on skin exposure). Inhalation of powder may cause local irritation of the nose and throat, tearing pain, blurred vision, delayed burn and scarring. National Institute of Health (NIH) Material Safety Data Sheet (MSDS) lists VINBLASTINE SULFATE as a skin irritate that causes sensitivity.

Caution: Females and males planning to have a child, pregnant women, and nursing mothers should exercise caution regarding potential occupational exposure to this cytotoxic drug. No information or not enough information exists or was provided concerning occupational exposures that may potentially occur while handling this drug and its affects on reproductive systems, the fetus, and/or if it is secreted along with breast milk, which may harm nursing infants. Staff members should consult with the occupational health physician monitoring workers' health in your facility to be apprised of potential hazards and should be advised to avoid becoming pregnant and/or breastfeeding or should be transferred in accordance with policy/procedures to other duties that do not involve preparation, handling, and administering this drug.

VINBLASTINE is in the Food and Drug Administration Pregnancy Category (D). This means that VINBLASTINE is known to be harmful to an unborn baby. It is not known whether VINBLASTINE passes into breast milk.

Target Organs/Systems: Eyes (corneal), heart, skin, autonomic nervous system, respiratory system, blood, bone marrow, and possible fetus

Medical Conditions Generally Aggravated by Exposure:

- Preexisting skin and respiratory conditions.
- Individuals with significant granulocytopenia, unless this is a result of the disease being treated, or individuals with bacterial infections.
- Reproductive and pregnancy issues.

Specific Medical Surveillance Information: Reproductive and pregnancy counseling.

Occupational Exposure Level/Limit (OEL) & Sampling Methods:

Environmental Sentinel Contamination Action Level (ESCAL): Surface

Occupational Exposure Level (OEL):
LEG 0.47 µg/m3 Time-Weighted Average (TWA) *for* 12 hours

Excursion limit: 5.64 mg/m3 for no more than a total of 30 minutes.

"Worse case" computer aided prediction of spray/mist or fume/dust components and concentration: composite exposure standard for mixture (TWA): 3.0000 mg/m3. Operations, which produce a spray/mist or fume/dust, introduce particulates to the breathing zone. If the breathing zone concentration of any of the components listed below is exceeded, "worst case" considerations deem the individual to be overexposed.

Breathing Component Conc. %	Zone mg/m3	Mixture (%)
VINBLASTINE SULFATE	3.0000	0.7

(Method not listed or specified)

Supplemental Response Information

Extinguishing Media: Use extinguishing agent which is the most appropriate to extinguish surrounding fire (carbon dioxide, foam, dry chemical or water fog as extinguishing media).

Solubility: VINBLASTINE:
VINBLASTINE SULFATE:
VINBLASTINE is completely water soluble with a pH range of 3.5–5.5 (0.15% AQ. Sol). Furthermore, it is easily soluble in methanol.

VINBLASTINE SULFATE solubility is negligible to soluble in water with a pH range of 3.5–5.0. A 0.1% in 0.9% sodium chloride solution is a practically insoluble in alcohol.

Chemical Degradation/Neutralization Method: Two or more degradation/neutralization procedure exists for this drug.

A manufacturer's Material Safety Data Sheet (MSDS) recommends treating spill surfaces with a 5–10% sodium hypochlorite (bleach) solution after absorbing liquids with inert absorbent pads or removing any powder present: allow solution to stand for up to one hour, and then thoroughly wash spilled surfaces with soap and water; sample to determine if surface contamination is still present (if sampling method is available). If the drug is present, repeat above steps; dispose of wastes in accordance with your local procedures, state, and federal regulations.

Incompatibility: VINBLASTINE SULFATE is incompatible with strong oxidizing agents, peroxides, permanganates, amino-acids, aminophylline, ascorbic acid, dexamethasone, frusemide, riboflavine, sulfhydryl-containing reagents, nitric acid, and strong bases. Avoid exposure to light and protect form moisture.

VINCRISTINE (*vin-KRIS-teen*)

(*vin-chris-teen*)

$C_{46}H_{58}N_4O_{14}S$

VINCRISTINE SULFATE

Chemical Abstracts Service (CAS) Registry Number: 2068-78-2 (mixture)
Registry of Toxic Effects of Chemical Substance (RTECS): OH6340000
$C_{46}H_{56}N_4O_{10}$

VINCRISTINE

$C_{46}H_{56}N_4O_{10}$

LEUROCRISTINE

Chemical Abstracts Service (CAS) Registry Number: 57-22-7 (mixture)
Registry of Toxic Effects of Chemical Substance (RTECS): OH6300000

VCR
ONCOVIN®103

VINCASAR PFS®112

Chemical Abstracts Service (CAS) Registry Number: 2068-78-2

VINCRISTINE SULFATE

Chemical Abstracts Service (CAS) Registry Number: 57-22-7
$C_{46}H_{58}N_4O_{14}S$

VINCRISTINE

$C_{46}H_{56}N_4O_{10}$

Health & Safety Hazards/US Department of Transportation (DOT)/US Environmental Protection Agency (EPA)—Sources

Carcinogen—Material Safety Data Sheet, Carcinogen G3—International Agency for Research on Cancer, Mutagen—University of Maryland at College Park, Teratogen—University of Maryland at College Park, Reproductive Effector—Material Safety Data Sheet, Toxic—Material Safety Data Sheet, Extremely Toxic—Material Safety Data Sheet, Cytotoxic—Material Safety Data Sheet, Cytotoxic—British Columbia Cancer Agency Canada, Ototoxic—Drugs.com, Vesicant—British Columbia Cancer Agency Canada, Lactation Avoid Breastfeeding (World Health Organization), Pregnancy Category (D)—US Food and Drug Administration, Developmental—US California Proposition 65, National Fire Protection Association Health (2) Flammability (0) Instability (0)—Material Safety Data Sheet, National Fire Protection Association Health (1) Flammability (0) Instability (1)—Material Safety Data Sheet, National Fire Protection Health (2) Flammability (1) Instability (0)—Material Safety Data Sheet, National Fire Protection Association Health (4) Flammability (1) Instability (0)—Material Safety Data Sheet, National Fire Protection Association Health (2) Flammability (0) Instability (0) Reproductive and Blood and Bone Marrow Effect—Material Safety Data Sheet, Materials Identification System (R) and/or US Department of Defense System Health (1★) with additional chronic hazards present Fire Hazard (0) Reactivity (1) Personal Protection Code (-) (None stated)—Material Safety Data Sheet, Materials Identification System (R) and/or US Department of Defense System Health (4) Fire Hazard (1) Reactivity (0) Personal Protection Code (E) (Safety Glasses, Chemical Gloves, Dust Respirator)—Material

Safety Data Sheet, Materials Identification System (R) and/or US Department of Defense System Health (3) Fire Hazard (0) Reactivity (0) Personal Protection Code (X) (Ask Supervisor)—Material Safety Data Sheet, Materials Identification System (R) and/or US Department of Defense System Health (2★) with additional chronic hazards present Fire Hazard (1) Reactivity (0) Personal Protection Code (E) (Safety Glasses, Chemical Gloves, Dust Respirator)—Material Safety Data Sheet, UN 2811, UN 1544, Class 6.1.

VINCRISTINE (ONCOVIN®113) is available as an injection.

VINCRISTINE SULFATE is a white solid.

VINCRISTINE SULFATE can cause fetal harm; breastfeeding should be discontinued because of potential for reproductive and developmental harm (*A Guide for Occupational Health Professionals Technical Manual*, Navy Environmental Health Center [NEHC-TM-OEM 6260.01a]).

VINCRISTINE is a colorless fluid from powder.

First Aid/Medical Information/ Occupational Exposure Limits

First Aid Measures to include: Use general first aid measures except for the following:

Eye Contact:

Physician's note (A): VINCA alkaloids do not cause a direct chemical burn of eye tissue, but interfere with the reproduction of the eye epithelium, which occurs continuously. The result is a delayed burn and subsequent scarring. While very painful, all cases have recovered completely without any loss of eye function.

Physician's note (B): VINCRISTINE SULPHATE should be treated as potentially carcinogenic, and may be mutagenic, teratogenic, or allergenic. Diazepam or phenobarbitone may be used to control seizures should they occur. If respiratory distress occurs after inhalation of airborne droplets, administer emergency airway support and 100% humidified supplemental oxygen with assisted ventilation if needed. If coughing or difficulty in breathing develops, evacuating for respiratory tract irritation, bronchitis or pneumonitis. Because of the potentially hazardous nature of VINCRISTINE SULPHATE, if the solution is swallowed, gets in eyes or in contact with the skin, medical attention should be sought immediately after the preceding first aid measures are taken.

Ingestion: Do not induce vomiting. If conscious and alert, rinse mouth and drink 2–4 cups of milk or water. Seek medical attention.

Medical Information:

Caution and Warning Statements: VINCRISTINE SULFATE is a cytotoxic agent. All work practices must be designed to reduce human exposure to the lowest level. VINCRISTINE SULFATE is extremely hazardous in case of ingestion or inhalation.

VINCRISTINE SULFATE is extremely hazardous in case of ingestion or inhalation. VINCRISTINE SULFATE is very hazardous in case of eye contact (irritant). Furthermore, this drug is hazardous in case of skin contact (irritant and permeator). This drug is listed as a birth defect hazard. There is a possible risk of impaired fertility, possible risk of harm to unborn child, and a possible risk of irreversible effects if swallowed. Repeated exposure to a highly toxic material may produce general deterioration of health by an accumulation in one or more human organs. Exposure may cause liver and kidney damage.

Caution: Females and males planning to have a child, pregnant women, and nursing mothers should exercise caution regarding potential occupational exposure to this cytotoxic drug. No information or not enough information exists or was provided concerning occupational exposures that may potentially occur while handling this drug and its affects on reproductive systems, the fetus, and/or if it is secreted along with breast milk, which may harm nursing infants. Staff members should consult with the occupational health physician monitoring workers' health in your facility to be apprised of potential hazards and should be advised to avoid becoming pregnant and/or breastfeeding or should be transferred in accordance with policy/procedures to other duties that do not involve preparation, handling, and administering this drug.

VINCRISTINE is in the Food and Drug Administration Pregnancy Category (D). This means that VINCRISTINE is known to be harmful to an unborn baby. It is not known whether VINCRISTINE passes into breast milk. It is recommended that personnel with preexisting dermatitis as well as women during the first three months of pregnancy not be exposed to VINCRISTINE (VCR).

Target Organs/Systems: Kidneys, blood, liver, bone marrow, bladder, GI tract, cardiovascular system, eyes, head, muscle tissue, central nervous, peripheral nervous, fetus, and autonomic nervous systems

Medical Conditions Generally Aggravated by Exposure:

- Workers with neuromuscular dysfunction or sensitivity to VINCRISTINE SULFATE should not be exposed to VINCRISTINE SULFATE. It is recommended that personnel with preexisting dermatitis as well as women during the first three months of pregnancy not be exposed to VINCRISTINE (VCR).

- Reproductive and pregnancy issues.

Specific Medical Surveillance Information: Reproductive and pregnancy counseling.

Medical surveillance should include liver and kidney function tests, hematological workup, and cardiovascular examination. It is recommended that personnel with preexisting dermatitis, as well as women during the first three months of pregnancy, not be exposed to VINCRISTINE (VCR).

Occupational Exposure Level/Limit (OEL) & Sampling Methods:

Environmental Sentinel Contamination Action Level (ESCAL): Not otherwise specified
Occupational Exposure Level (OEL) Lilly: 0.14 g/m3 per 12 hours
Excursion Limit: 1.68 µg/m3 (30 minutes) (Method not listed or specified)

Supplemental Response Information

Extinguishing Media: Use extinguishing agent which is the most appropriate to extinguish surrounding fire (carbon dioxide, foam, dry chemical or water fog as extinguishing media).

Solubility: VINCRISTINE is easily soluble in cold water with a pH range of 3.5 to 5.5; methanol solubility.

Chemical Degradation/Neutralization Method: A manufacturer's Material Safety Data Sheet (MSDS) recommends treating spill surfaces with a 5–10% sodium hypochlorite (bleach) solution with a pH of approximately 10 after absorbing liquids with inert absorbent pads or removing any powder present: allow solution to stand for up to one hour, and then thoroughly wash spilled surfaces with soap and water; sample to determine if surface contamination is still present (if sampling method is available). If the drug is present, repeat above steps; dispose of wastes in accordance with your local procedures, state, and federal regulations.

Incompatibility: VINCRISTINE SULFATE is incompatible with strong oxidizing agents, heat, moisture, heavy metal salts, and direct sunlight.

Warning: Aluminum needles or intravenous sets should not be used for preparation or administration of VINCRISTINE SULFATE.

VINDESINE (*VIN-de-seen*)
ELDISINE®114

Registry of Toxic Effects of Chemical Substance (RTECS): YY8080000
$C_{43}H_{55}N_5O_7$

VINDESINE SULFATE

Chemical Abstracts Service (CAS) Registry Numbers: 53643-48-4, 59917-39-4
Registry of Toxic Effects of Chemical Substance (RTECS): YY8090000
$C_{49}H_{71}N_5O_{17}S$

Health & Safety Hazards/US Department of Transportation (DOT)/US Environmental Protection Agency (EPA)—Sources

Mutagen—Material Safety Data Sheet, Teratogen—Material Safety Data Sheet, Reproductive Effector—Material Safety Data Sheet, Tumorigenic—RTECS Yy8080000, Sensitizer—Material Safety Data Sheet, Carcinogen—Material Safety Data Sheet, Pregnancy Category (None)—US Food and Drug Administration, Vesicant—British Columbia Cancer Agency Canada.

VINDESINE is a clear fluid dissolved from powder.

VINDESINE SULPHATE is a white or almost white, hydroscopic amorphous substance.

First Aid/Medical Information/ Occupational Exposure Limits

First Aid Measures to include: Use general first aid measures except for the following:

Eye Contact:

Physician's note: VINCA alkaloids do not cause a direct chemical burn of eye tissue, but interfere with the reproduction of the eye epithelium, which occurs continuously. The result is a delayed burn and subsequent scarring. While very painful, all cases have recovered completely without any loss of eye function.

Ingestion: Do not induce vomiting. If conscious and alert, rinse mouth and drink 2–4 cups of milk or water. Seek medical attention.

Medical Information:

Caution and Warning Statements: There is little information concerning the chemical, physical, and biological properties of VINDESINE. VINDESINE toxicity and side effects are similar to those of VINBLASTINE. VENDESINE is a cytotoxic agent. All work practices must be designed to reduce human exposure to the lowest level.

VINCRISTINE SULFATE is a cytotoxic agent. All work practices must be designed to reduce human exposure to the lowest level. VINCRISTINE SULFATE is extremely hazardous in cause of ingestion or inhalation. VINCRISTINE SULFATE is very hazardous in case of eye contact (irritant). This drug is listed as hazardous in case of skin contact (irritant and permeator) and as a birth defect hazard. There is a possible risk of impaired fertility, possible risk of harm to unborn child, and a possible risk of irreversible effects if swallowed. Repeated exposure to a highly toxic material may produce general deterioration of health by an accumulation in one or more human organs. Exposure may cause liver and kidney damage. BC Cancer Agency lists VINDESINE as a vesicant.

Caution: Females and males planning to have a child, pregnant women, and nursing mothers should exercise caution regarding potential occupational exposure to this cytotoxic drug. No information or not enough information exists or was provided concerning occupational exposures that may potentially occur while handling this drug and its affects on reproductive systems, the fetus, and/or if it is secreted along with breast milk, which may harm nursing infants. Staff members should consult with the occupational health physician monitoring workers' health in your facility to be apprised of potential hazards and should be advised to avoid becoming pregnant and/or breastfeeding or should be transferred in accordance with policy/procedures to other duties that do not involve preparation, handling, and administering this drug.

VINCRISTINE is in the Food and Drug Administration Pregnancy Category (D). This means that VINCRISTINE is known to be harmful to an unborn baby. It is not known whether VINCRISTINE passes into breast milk. It is recommended that personnel with preexisting dermatitis as well as women during the first three months of pregnancy not be exposed to VINCRISTINE (VCR).

Target Organs/Systems: Nerves, kidneys, blood, liver, bone marrow, bladder, GI tract, cardiovascular system, eyes, head, muscle tissue, central nervous, peripheral nervous, autonomic nervous systems, and possibly fetus

Medical Conditions Generally Aggravated by Exposure:

- Workers with neuromuscular dysfunction or sensitivity to VINCRISTINE SULFATE should not be exposed to VINCRISTINE SULFATE. It is recommended that personnel with preexisting dermatitis as well as women during the first three months of pregnancy not be exposed to VINCRISTINE (VCR).
- Reproductive and pregnancy issues.

Specific Medical Surveillance Information: Reproductive and pregnancy counseling.

Medical surveillance should include liver and kidney function tests, hematological workup, and cardiovascular examination. It is recommended that personnel with preexisting dermatitis, as well as women during the first three months of pregnancy, not be exposed to VINCRISTINE (VCR).

Occupational Exposure Level/Limit (OEL) & Sampling Methods:

Environmental Sentinel Contamination Action Level (ESCAL): Not otherwise specified
Occupational Exposure Level (OEL) Lilly: 0.14 µg/m3 per 12 hours
Excursion Limit: 1.68 µg/m3 (30 mins)
(Method not listed or specified)

Supplemental Response Information

Extinguishing Media: Use extinguishing agent which is the most appropriate to extinguish surrounding fire (carbon dioxide, foam, dry chemical or water fog as extinguishing media).

Solubility: VINDESINE: The aqueous solubility for VINDESINE is >1,000 mg/ml in distilled water with a ~3.5 pH. VINDESINE is freely soluble in water and in methyl alcohol; insoluble in cyclohexane.

Chemical Degradation/Neutralization Method: A manufacturer's Material Safety Data Sheet (MSDS) recommends treating spill surfaces with a ~2 mol/liter (~8 g/100 ml), aqueous caustic soda (sodium hydroxide) solution after absorbing liquids with inert absorbent pads or removing any powder present: allow solution to stand for up to one hour, and then thoroughly wash spilled surfaces with soap and water; sample to determine if surface contamination is still present (if sampling method is available). If the drug is present, repeat above steps; dispose of wastes in accordance with your local procedures, state, and federal regulations.

Incompatibility: VINDESINE SULFATE is incompatible with strong oxidizing agents.

VINORELBINE TARTRATE
(*vi-NOR-el-been*)
NAVELBINE®116

Chemical Abstracts Service (CAS) Registry
Number: 125317-39-7

$C_{44}H_{52}N_4O_8$

$C_{44}-H_{54}-N_4-O_8.2C_4-H_6-O_6$

VINORELBINE TARTRATE)

Chemical Abstracts Service (CAS) Registry
Number: 71486-22-1

VINORELBINE

Registry of Toxic Effects of Chemical Substance
(RTECS): RD2535000

Health & Safety Hazards/US Department of Transportation (DOT)/US Environmental Protection Agency (EPA)—Sources

Cytotoxic—Box Instruction, Cytotoxic—Material Safety Data Sheet, Cytotoxic—British Columbia Cancer Agency Canada, Experimental Embryotoxic—Material Safety Data Sheet, Experimental Fetotoxic—Material Safety Data Sheet, Suspect Carcinogen—Material Safety Data Sheet, Mutagen—Material Safety Data Sheet, Reproductive Effector—Material Safety Data Sheet, Vesicant—British Columbia Cancer Agency Canada, Pregnancy Category (D)—US Food and Drug Administration, National Fire Protection Association Health (2) Flammability (0) Instability (0)—Material Safety Data Sheet, National Fire Protection Association Health (3) Flammability (0) Instability (0)—Material Safety Data Sheet, Materials Identification System (R) and/or US Department of Defense System Health (2) Fire Hazard (0) Reactivity (0) Personal Protection Code (X) (Ask Supervisor)—Material Safety Data Sheet, Materials Identification System (R) and/or Department of Defense System Health (3★) with additional chronic hazards present Fire Hazard (0) Reactivity (0) Personal Protection Code (-) (None stated)—Material Safety Data Sheet, TSCA LISTED; LD50 RAT, ORAL =26/MG/KG; LD50 MALE MICE, ORAL 77MG/KG.

VINORELBINE (NAVELBINE®116) is a colorless fluid or available as 20 mg and 30 mg capsules.

VINORELBINE TARTRATE is a white or almost white or yellow to light brown, hygroscopic, amporphous powder.

First Aid/Medical Information/ Occupational Exposure Limits

First Aid Measures to include: Use general first aid measures except for the following:

Physician's note: Medical treatment in causes of overexposure should be treated as an overdose of a cytotoxic agent. Treat according to locally accepted protocols. For additional guidance, consult the local poison control information center. No specific antidotes are recommended.

Medical Information:

Caution and Warning Statements: May cause sensitization by skin contact.

Caution: There is limited but increasing evidence that personnel involved in the preparation and administration of parenteral antineoplastics may be at some risk due to potential mutagenicity, teratogenicity, and/or carcinogenicity of these agents. All work practices must be designed to reduce human exposure to the lowest level possible. BC Cancer Agency lists VINORELBINE as a vesicant.

Danger! VINORELBINE may cause cancer (suspect) and may be fatal if swallowed. Avoid skin and eye contact. There is an irritation potential to skin, eyes, and mucous membranes; and may initiate allergic reactions. This drug may produce adverse effects on human fertility and may impair the quality or quantity of human milk production.

Sign and symptoms of exposure/overexposure are myelosuppression, bone marrow aplasia, sepsis, granulocytopenia, paralytic ileus, stomatitis, esophagitis, asthenia, nausea, vomiting, constipation, diarrhea, peripheral neuropathy, dyspnea, fatigue, and alopecia (hair loss).

Immediate effects are eye, skin, and respiratory irritation, bone marrow toxicity, increase susceptibility to infection, shortness of breath, coughing, abdominal pain, and constipation may occur. Delay effects are hypersensitivity, may occur ranging from mild to severe. VINORELBINE may cause fetal harm if administered to a pregnant woman.

Caution: Females and males planning to have a child, pregnant women, and nursing mothers should exercise caution regarding potential occupational exposure to this cytotoxic drug. No information or not enough information exists or was provided concerning occupational exposures that may potentially occur while handling this drug and its affects on reproductive systems, the fetus, and/or if it is secreted along with breast milk, which may harm nursing infants. Staff members should consult with the occupational health physician monitoring workers' health in your facility to be apprised of potential hazards and should be advised to avoid becoming pregnant and/or breastfeeding or should be transferred in accordance with policy/procedures to other duties that do not involve preparation, handling, and administering this drug.

Food and Drug Administration listed as a Pregnancy Category (D); NAVELBINE®116 may cause fetal harm if administered to a pregnant woman. A single dose of VINORELBINE has been shown to be embryo- and/or fetotoxic in mice and rabbits at doses of 9 mg/m² and 5.5 mg/m², respectively (one third and one sixth the human dose). At nonmaternotoxic doses, fetal weight was reduced and ossification was delayed. There are no studies in pregnant women. If NAVELBINE®116 is used during pregnancy, or if the patient becomes pregnant while receiving this drug, the patient should be apprised of the potential hazards to the fetus. It is not known whether the drug is excreted in human milk.

Target Organs/Systems: Skin, eyes, blood, reproductive, bone marrow, liver, nerve damage (neuropathy), rapidly dividing cells, and possibly fetus

Medical Conditions Generally Aggravated by Exposure:

- New or expecting mothers might be at greater risk from overexposure.
- Disorders involving the target organs of this product can be aggravated by exposures to this product (especially in doses approaching therapeutic levels for this product). Bone marrow toxicity specifically granulocytopenia, with increased susceptibility to infection.
- Reproductive and pregnancy issues.

Specific Medical Surveillance Information: Reproductive and pregnancy counseling.

Occupational Exposure Level/Limit (OEL) & Sampling Methods:

Environmental Sentinel Contamination Action Level (ESCAL): Not otherwise specified

Occupational Exposure Level/Limit (OEL) US American Conference of Governmental Industrial Hygienist (ACGIH): STEL 0.5 mg/m3

Occupational Exposure Level (OEL) GSK 0.5 µ/m3 Time-Weighted Average (8 hr TWA)

Occupational exposure Level (OEL) Bedfird (Ben Venue Lab Inc.) Laboratories: 0.5 mcg/m3 Time-Weighted Average (8-hr TWA) (Method not listed or specified)

Supplemental Response Information

Extinguishing Media: Use extinguishing agent which is the most appropriate to extinguish surrounding fire (i.e., water or foam extinguishers are recommended).

Warning: Carbon dioxide and dry chemical may be ineffective.

Solubility: VINORELBINE TARTRATE: The aqueous solubility for VINORELBINE TARTRATE is >1,000 mg/ml in distilled water. pH for NAVELBINE®116 injection solution is ~3.5. (Soluble in water.) VINORELBINE TARTRATE is freely soluble in water and in methyl alcohol.

Chemical Degradation/Neutralization Method: A manufacturer's Material Safety Data Sheet (MSDS) recommends using alkaline soap/detergent and water to clean spill surfaces after absorbing liquids with inert absorbent pads or removing any powder present: repeat using soap and water; sample to determine if surface contamination is still present (if sampling method is available). If drug is still present, repeat above steps; dispose of wastes in accordance with your local procedures, state, and federal regulations.

Incompatibility: VINORELBINE TARTRATE is incompatible with oxidizing agents; water-reactive materials.

Trademark Citations Sorted by Assigned Numbers

2.2

®#	Trademarks	Trademark Owner(s)	Owner's Address
01	ORENCIA®1	Bristo-Myers Squibb	345 Park Avenue New York, NY 10154
02	PROLEUKIN®2	Novartis Pharmaceuticals Ag.	4560 Horton Street Emeryville, CA 94608
03	CAMPATH®3	Genzyme Oncology Corp.	Cambridge, MA 02142
		Ilex Pharmaceuticals, L.P.	4545 Horizon Hill Blvd. San Antonio, TX 78229
04	ALIMTA®4	Eli Lilly and Company	Indianapolis, IN 46285
05	HEXALEN®5	Mgi Pharma, Inc.Eisai Medical Res	Bloomington, MN 55437
		Medimmune Oncology, Inc.	100 Front Street, Suite 400 West Conshohocken, PA 19428
06	CYTADREN®6	Novartis Pharmaceuticals Corp.	East Hanover, NJ 07936
		Novartis Pharmaceuticals Canada, Inc.	385 Bouchard Boulevard Dorval, H9R 4P5 Quebec
07	AMSA P-D®7	Erfa Sciences, Inc.Erfa Sciences Canada, Inc.	8250 Décarie Suite #110 Montréal, (QC) H4p 2p5 Canada
08	AMIMIDEX®8	Astrazeneca Pharmaceuticals L.P.	Wilmington, DE 19850-5437
09	TRISENOX®9	Cephalon, Inc.	41 Moores Road Frazer, PA 19355
10	ELSPAR®10	Merck & Co., Inc.	126 E. Lincoln Avenue Rahway, NJ 07065
11	LEUNASE®11	Sanofi-Aventis, Australia Pty, Ltd.	Macquarie Park NSW 2113, Australia
12	AVASTIN®12	Genentech, Inc.	1 DNA Way South San Francisco, CA 94080-4990
13	VIDAZA®13	Celgene Corp	86 Morris Avenue Summit, NJ 07901

®#	Trademarks	Trademark Owner(s)	Owner's Address
14	IMURAN®14	GlaxoSmithKline	Uxbridge, Middlesex UB11 1BT, UK
		GlaxoSmithKline	Research Triangle Park, NJ 27709
		GlaxoSmithKline Inc. Canada	7333 Mississauga Road North Mississauga L5N 6l4 Ontario
15	TARGRETIN®15	Eisai Corp of North America	Woodcliff Lake, NJ
		Elisai R&D Management Co., Ltd.	6-10 Koishikawa 4-Chome Bunkyo-Ku, Tokyo 112-8088 Japan
16	CASODEX®16	Astrazeneca Pharmaceuticals L.P.	Wilmington, DE 19850-5437
		Astrazeneca Uk, Ltd.	15 Stanhope Gate London, W1Y 6LN United Kingdom
17	BLENOXANE®17	Bristol-Myers Squibb Company	345 Park Avenue New York, NY 10022
18	CAMPTOSAR®18	Licensed From Yakult Honsha Co., Ltd., Japan, and	13-5 Shinbashi 5-Chome, Minatoku, Tokyo 105-0004 Japan
		Daiichi Sankyo, Inc. (US), Daiichi Pharmaceutical Co., Ltd., Japan	Parsippany, NJ
19	XELODA®19	F. Hoffman-La Roche Laboratories Inc.	340 Kingland Street Nutley, NJ 07110
		F. Hoffmann-La Roche Ag.	Grenzacherstrasse 124 4002, Basel Switzerland
20	PARAPLATIN®20	Bristol-Myers Squibb Company	345 Park Avenue New York, NY 10154
21	BICNU®21	Bristol-Myers Squibb Company	345 Park Avenue New York, NY 10022
22	LEUKERAN®22	GlaxoSmithKline/ SmithKline Beecham	Research Triangle Park, NJ 27709
		GlaxoSmithKline Inc. Canada	7333 Mississauga Road North Mississauga L5N 6l4 Ontario
25	VISTIDE®25	Gilead Sciences, Inc.	353 Lakeside Drive Foster City, CA 94404
26	PLATINOL®26 (AQ) BMS)	Bristol-Myers Squibb Company	345 Park Avenue New York, NY 10154
27	LEUSTATIN®27 (ORTHO BIO TECH)	Ortho Biotech Products L.P.	Raritan, NJ 08869
		Johnson & Johnson	One Johnson & Johnson Plaza New Brunswick, NJ 08933-7001

®#	Trademarks	Trademark Owner(s)	Owner's Address
28	CLABRIBINE NOVAPLUS®28	Novation, L.L.C.	Irving, TX 75014
31	CYTOSAR-U®31	Pfizer Pharm Products	New York, NY
		Pfizer Enterprises	Sarl Rond-Point Du Kirchberg 51, Avenue J.F. Kennedy L-1855 Luxembourg Luxembourg
32	TARABINE PFS®32	Pharmacia & Upjohn	235 East 42nd Street New York, NY 10017
		Pfizer Enterprises Canada	Sarl Rond-Point Du Kirchberg 51, Avenue J.F. Kennedy L-1855 Luxembourg Luxembourg
33	ALEXAN®33	Ebewe	Hong Kong
		Pfizer Intramed	Mondseestrasse 11, Austria
34	ACLACINOMYCINE®34	Sanofi-Aventis Laboratories	Bridgewater, NJ 08807
		Sanofi Winthrop	France
35	DTIC-DOME®35	Bayer Pharmaceuticals Corp.	400 Morgan Lane West Haven, CT 06516-4175
37	PROCYTOX®37	Baxter International Inc.	One Baxter Parkway Deerfield, IL 60015
38	DTIC®38	Schering Corp	Kenilworth, NJ 07033
39	ACTINOMYCIN D®39	Merck	Whitehouse Station, NJ 08889
40	COMEGEN LYOVAC®40	Merck Fosst	16711 Transcanada Hwy, Kirkland, Quebec H9H 3I1
41	CERUBIDINE®41	Aventis Pharma, S.A.	20, Avenue Raymond Aron, 92160 Antony, France
42	DAUNOXOME®42	Gilead Sciences, Inc.	333 Lakeside Drive Foster City, CA 94404
44	ZANOSAR®44	Teva Pharm, U.S.A. Parenteral Medicines, Inc.	Irvine CA 92618
		Pharmacia & Upjohn Company, L.L.C.	100 Route 206 North Peapack, NJ 07977
45	PHARMORUBICI®45	Sicor Inc.	19 Hughes Irvine, CA 92618
46	ELLENCE®46	Pfizer Pharm Products	235 East 42nd Street New York, NY 10017
47	ERBITUX®47	Imclone LLC	180 Varick Street, 6th Floor New York, NY 10014

®#	Trademarks	Trademark Owner(s)	Owner's Address
48	EMCYT®48	Pfizer-Pharmacia & Upjohn Company	235 East 42nd Street New York, NY 10017
		Pfizer Health AB Canada	112 87 Stockholm Sweden
49	VEPESID®49	Bristol-Myers Squibb Company	345 Park Avenue New York, NY 10022
50	PROSCAR®50	Merck & Co., Inc.	126 East Lincoln Avenue Rahway, NJ
51	PROPECIA®51	Merck & Co, Inc.	One Merck Drive P.O. Box 100, Whitehouse Station, NJ 16711
52	FUDR®52	Hospira, Inc.	Lake Forest, IL
53	ADRUCIL®53	Pharmacia, Inc.	P.O. Box 16529 Columbus, OH 43216-6529
54	HALOTESTIN®54	Pharmacia & Upjohn Company	235 East 42nd Street New York, NY 10017
		Pfizer Enterprises Canada	Sarl Rond-Point Du Kirchberg 51, Avenue J.F. Kennedy L-1855 Luxembourg Luxembourg
55	EULEXIN®55	Schering	Kenilworth, NJ 07033
56	CYTOVENE®56	F. Hoffmann-La Roche, Inc.	Mississauga, Ontario, Canada
		F. Hoffmann-La Roche, Inc.	340 Kingsland Street Nutley, NJ 07110
		F. Hoffmann-La Roche, Ag.	4070 Basel Switzerland
57	VITRASERT®57	Bausch & Lomb Inc.	One Bausch & Lomb Place Rochester, NY 14604
58	VALCYTE®58	F. Hoffmann-La Roche Ag.	340 Kingland Street Nutley, NJ 07110
		F. Hoffmann-La Roche, Ag.	Grenzacherstrasse 124 4002, Basel Switzerland
59	CYMEVENE®59	F. Hoffmann-La Roche Inc.	340 Kingland Street Nutley, NJ 07110
		F. Hoffmann-La Roche, Ag. Canada	Grenzacherstrasse 124 4002 Basel, Switzerland
60	MYLOTARG®60	Wyeth	Five Giralda Farms Madison, NJ, 07940-0874

®#	Trademarks	Trademark Owner(s)	Owner's Address
61	GEMZAR®61	Eli Lilly and Co	Lilly Corporate Center Indianapolis, IN 46285
62	GEMCIN®62	Eli Lilly and Co	Lilly Corporate Center Indianapolis, IN 46285
63	GEMTRO®63	Eli Lilly and Co	Lilly Corporate Center Indianapolis, IN 46285
64	ZOLADEX®64	Astrazeneca Pharmaceuticals, L.P.	Wilmington, DE 19850-5437
		Astrazeneca UK LTD Canada	15 Stanhope Gate London W1Y 6LN United Kingdom
65	HYDREA®65	Bristol-Myers Squibb	Princeton, NJ
		Bristol-Myers Squibb Canada Co./La Société Bristol-Myers Squibb Canada	2344 Alfred-Nobel Boulevard Suite 300 Montreal H4S 0A4 Quebec
66	DROXIA®66	Bristol-Myers Squibb	Princeton, NJ
67	ZEVALIN®67	Idec Pharmaceuticals Corp.	11011 Torreyana Road San Diego, CA 92121
68	IDAMYCIN PFS®68	Pfizer Pharmacia & Upjohn Company	235 East 42nd Street New York, NY 10017
		Pharmacia & UpJohn, S.P.A. Canada	Via Robert Koch No.1.2. Milan Italy
69	IFOSPHAMIDE®69	Bristol-Myers Squibb	Princeton, NJ
70	IFEX®70	Bristol-Myers Squibb Company	345 Park Avenue New York, NY 10154
71	GLEEVEC®71	Novartis Pharmaceuticals Corp.	East Hanover, NJ 07936
		Novartis, Ag. Canada	4002 Basel Switzerland
72	LUPRON®72	Abbott Endocrine Inc.	100 Abbott Park Road Abbott Park, IL 60064
73	LUPRON®73	Tap Pharmaceutical Products, Inc. (Joint V. Abbott and Takeda)	Deerfield, IL 60015
74	ERGAMISOL®74	Janssen Pharm (part of Johnson and Johnson)	Netherlands
		Johnson & Johnson	One Johnson & Johnson Place New Brunswick, NJ
75	CEENU®75	Bristol-Myers Squibb Company	345 Park Avenue New York, NY 10022

®#	Trademarks	Trademark Owner(s)	Owner's Address
76	MUSTARGEN®76	Ovation Pharmaceuticals, Inc.	Four Parkway North Suite 200 Deerfield, IL 60015
77	MEGACE ES®77	Bristol-Myers Squibb	Princeton, NJ
78	MYLERAN®78	GlaxoSmithKline	Research Triangle Park, NJ 27709
		GlaxoSmithKline Inc. Canada	7333 Mississauga Road North Mississauga L5N 6l4 Ontario
79	ALKERAN®79	GlaxoSmithKline	Research Triangle Park, NJ 27709
		GlaxoSmithKline, Inc. Canada	7333 Mississauga Road North Mississauga L5N 6l4 Ontario
80	PURINETHOL®80	GlaxoSmithKline	Research Triangle Park, NJ 27709
		Biogal Pharmaceutical Works, Ltd. Canada	Pallagi Ut 13 H–4042 Debrecen Hungary
81	RHEUMATREX®81	Wyeth Holdings Corp	Five Giralda Farms Madison, NJ 07940
82	METHYL-GAG®82	Dakota Pharma, Ltd.	Dracut, MA 01826
84	MUTAMYCIN®84	Bristol-Myers Squibb Company	345 Park Avenue New York, NY 10022
85	LYSODREN®85	Bristol-Myers Squibb Company	345 Park Avenue New York, NY 10154
86	NOVANTRONE®86	Emd Serono Inc./OSI Oncology	Melville, NY 11747
		Wyeth Holdings Corp Canada	Five Giralda Farms Madison, NJ 07940
87	NILANDRON®87	Sanofi-Aventis, L.L.C.	Bridgewater, NJ 08807
88	ELOXATIN®88	Sanofi-Aventis, L.L.C.	Bridgewater, NJ 08807
		Sanofi-Aventis Une Société Anonyme Canada	174, Avenue De France 75635 Paris Cedex 13 France
89	ONCASPAR®89	Enzon Pharmaceuticals, Inc.	685 Route 202/206 Bridgewater, NJ 08807
90	NIPENT®90	Hospira Boulder, Inc.	650 From Road Mack–Cali Centre II Second Floor Paramus, NJ 07652
91	MITHRACIN®91	Bayer Corp	West Haven, CT
		Pfizer Products, Inc. Canada	Eastern Point Road Groton, CT 06340

®#	Trademarks	Trademark Owner(s)	Owner's Address
92	DELTASONE®92	Pfizer Enterprises Canada	Sarl Rond-Point Du Kirchberg 51, Avenue J.F. Kennedy L 1855 Luxembourg Luxembourg
93	MATULANE®93	Sigma-Tau Pharmacuetical, Inc.	Gaithersburg, MD 20878
94	ZINECARD®94	Pfizer-Pharmacia & Upjohn Company	235 East 42nd Street New York, NY 10017
		Pharmacia, Inc. Canada	P.O. Box 16529 Columbus, OH 43216-6529
95	REMICADE®95	Centocor Ortho Biotech, Inc.	Horsham, PA 19044
		Centocor Ortho Biotech, Inc. Canada	800 Ridgeview Drive Horsham, PA 19044
96	RITUXAN®96	Biogen Ibec Inc./Genentech Inc.	Cambridge, MA; San Francisco, CA
		Idec Pharmaceuticals Corp. Canada	3030 Callan Road San Diego, CA 92121
98	NOLVADEX®98	Astrazeneca Pharmaceuticals LP	Wilmington, DE 19850-5437
		Astrazeneca UK, Ltd. Canada	15 Stanhope Gate, London, W1Y 6LN United Kingdom
99	TAXOL®99	Bristol-Myers-Squibb	Princeton, NJ
		Bristol-Myers Squibb Company Canada	345 Park Avenue New York, NY 10154
100	TAXOTERE® 100	Sanofi-Aventis, L.L.C.	Bridgewater, NJ 08807
		Aventis Pharma, S.A. Canada	20, Avenue Raymond Aron 92160 Antony, France
101	TEMODAR®101	Schering-Plough	Kenilworth, NJ 07033
		Schering Canada, Inc.	3535 Trans-Canada Highway Pointe Claire, H9R 1B4 Quebec
102	METHAZOLASTONE®102	Schering-Plough	Kenilworth, NJ 07033
103	VUMON®103	Bristol-Myers-Squibb	Princeton, NJ
		Bristol-Myers Squibb Company Canada	345 Park Avenue New York, NY 10154
104	THIOPLEX®104	Immunex	Seattle, WA 98101
105	HYCAMTIN®105	GlaxoSmithKline	Franklin Plaza, Philadelphia, PA
		SmithKline Beecham, P.L.C. Canada	980 Great West Road Brentford Middlesex TW8 9GS England

®#	Trademarks	Trademark Owner(s)	Owner's Address
106	BEXXAR®106	GlaxoSmithKline	Franklin Plaza, Philadelphia, PA
		SmithKline Beecham Corp. Canada	One Franklin Plaza 200 North 16th Street Philadelphia, PA 19102
107	NEUTREXIN®107	Medimmune Inc.	Gaithersburg, MD
		Medimmune Oncology, Inc. Canada	100 Front Street, Suite 400 West Conshohocken, PA 19428
108	VALSTAR®108	Endo Pharm	Chadds Ford, PA 19317
		Anthra Pharmaceuticals, Inc. Canada	103 Carnegie Center, Suite 102 Princeton, NJ 08540
110	VELBAN®110	Eli Lilly And Co	Lilly Corporate Center Indianapolis, IN 46285
111	ALKABAN AQ®111	Quad Pharm (Par Pharmaceuticals)	Spring Valley, NY
112	VINCASAR PFS(@112	Pharmacia & Upjohn	235 East 42nd Street New York, NY 10017
		Pfizer Enterprises Canada	Sarl Rond-Point Du Kirchberg 51, Avenue J.F. Kennedy L-1855 Luxembourg Luxembourg
113	ONCOVIN(@113	Eli Lilly	Lilly Corporate Center Indianapolis, IN 46285
		Eli Lilly and Co. Canada	307 East Mccarty Street Indianapolis, IN 46285
114	ELDISINE®114	Eli Lilly and Co.	Lilly Corporate Center Indianapolis, IN 46285
		Eli Lilly and Co. Canada	307 East Mccarty St. Indianapolis, In 46206
116	NAVELBINE®116	GlaxoSmithKline	Research Triangle Park, NJ 27709
117	VELCADE®117	Millennium Pharm Inc.	Cambridge, MA 02139
		Millennium Pharmaceuticals, Inc. Canada	40 Landsdowne Street Cambridge, MA 02139

®#	Trademarks	Trademark Owner(s)	Owner's Address
34	ACLACINOMYCINE®34	Sanofi-Aventis Laboratories	Bridgewater, NJ 08807
		Sanofi Winthrop	France
39	ACTINOMYCIN D®39	Merck	Whitehouse Station, NJ 08889
53	ADRUCIL®53	Pharmacia Inc.	P.O. Box 16529 Columbus, OH 43216-6529
33	ALEXAN®33	Ebewe	Hong Kong
		Pfizer Intramed	Mondseestrasse 11 Austria
04	ALIMTA®4	Eli Lilly and Company	Indianapolis, IN 46285
111	ALKABAN AQ®111	Quad Pharm (Par Pharmaceuticals)	Spring Valley, NY
79	ALKERAN®79	GlaxoSmithKline	Research Triangle Park, NJ 27709
		GlaxoSmithKline, Inc. Canada	7333 Mississauga Road North Mississauga L5N 6l4 Ontario
08	AMIMIDEX®8	Astrazeneca Pharmaceuticals, L.P.	Wilmington, DE 19850-5437
07	AMSA P-D®7	Erfa Sciences, Inc. Erfa Sciences Canada, Inc.	8250 Décarie Suite #110 Montréal, (QC) H4p 2p5 Canada
12	AVASTIN®12	Genentech, Inc.	1 DNA Way South San Francisco, CA 94080-4990
106	BEXXAR®106	GlaxoSmithKline	Franklin Plaza, Philadelphia, PA
		SmithKline Beecham Corp. Canada	One Franklin Plaza 200 North 16th Street Philadelphia, PA 19102
21	BICNU®21	Bristol-Myers Squibb Company	345 Park Avenue New York, NY 10022
17	BLENOXANE®17	Bristol-Myers Squibb Company	345 Park Avenue New York, NY 10022

®#	Trademarks	Trademark Owner(s)	Owner's Address
03	CAMPATH®3	Genzyme Oncology Corp.	Cambridge, MA 02142
		Ilex Pharmaceuticals, L.P.	4545 Horizon Hill Blvd. San Antonio, Texas 78229
18	CAMPTOSAR®18	Licensed From Yakult Honsha Co., Ltd, Japan, and	13-5 Shinbashi 5-Chome,Minatoku,Tokyo 105-0004 Japan
		Daiichi Sankyo, Inc. (US), Daiichi Pharmaceutical Co., Ltd., Japan	Parsippany, NJ
16	CASODEX®16	Astrazeneca Pharmaceuticals, L.P.	Wilmington, DE 19850-5437
		Astrazeneca Uk Ltd	15 Stanhope Gate, London, W1Y 6LN United Kingdom
75	CEENU®75	Bristol-Myers Squibb Company	345 Park Avenue New York, NY 10022
41	CERUBIDINE®41	Aventis Pharma S.A.	20, Avenue Raymond Aron, 92160 Antony, France
28	CLABRIBINE NOVAPLUS®28	Novation, L.L.C.	Irving, TX 75014
40	COMEGEN LYOVAC®40	Merck Fosst	16711 Transcanada Hwy, Kirkland, Quebec H9H 3l1
59	CYMEVENE®59	F. Hoffmann-La Roche, Inc.	340 Kingland Street Nutley, NJ 07110
		F. Hoffmann-La Roche, Ag. Canada	Grenzacherstrasse 124 4002 Basel, Switzerland
06	CYTADREN®6	Novartis Pharmaceuticals Corp.	East Hanover, NJ 07936
		Novartis Pharmaceuticals Canada, Inc.	385 Bouchard Boulevard Dorval, H9R 4P5 Quebec
31	CYTOSAR-U®31	Pfizer Pharm Products	New York, NY
		Pfizer Enterprises	Sarl Rond-Point Du Kirchberg 51, Avenue J. F. Kennedy L-1855 Luxembourg Luxembourg
56	CYTOVENE®56	F. Hoffmann-La Roche, Inc.	Mississauga, Ontario, Canada
		F. Hoffmann-La Roche, Inc.	340 Kingsland Street Nutley, NJ 07110
		F. Hoffmann-La Roche, Ag.	4070 Basel Switzerland
42	DAUNOXOME®42	Gilead Sciences, Inc.	333 Lakeside Drive Foster City, CA 94404

®#	Trademarks	Trademark Owner(s)	Owner's Address
92	DELTASONE®92	Pfizer Enterprises Canada	Sarl Rond-Point Du Kirchberg 51, Avenue J. F. Kennedy L-1855 Luxembourg Luxembourg
66	DROXIA®66	Bristol-Myers Squibb	Princeton, NJ
38	DTIC®38	Schering Corp.	Kenilworth, NJ 07033
35	DTIC-DOME®35	Bayer Pharmaceuticals Corp.	400 Morgan Lane West Haven, CT 06516-4175
114	ELDISINE®114	Eli Lilly and Co.	Lilly Corporate Center Indianapolis, IN 46285
		Eli Lilly and Co. Canada	307 East Mccarty St. Indianapolis, In 46206
46	ELLENCE®46	Pfizer Pharm Products	235 East 42nd Street New York, NY 10017
88	ELOXATIN®88	Sanofi-Aventis, L.L.C.	Bridgewater, NJ 08807
		Sanofi-Aventis Une Société Anonyme Canada	174, Avenue De France 75635 Paris Cedex 13 France
10	ELSPAR®10	Merck & Co., Inc.	126 E. Lincoln Avenue Rahway, NJ 07065
48	EMCYT®48	Pfizer-Pharmacia & Upjohn Company	235 East 42nd Street New York, NY 10017
		Pfizer Health AB Canada	112 87 Stockholm Sweden
47	ERBITUX®47	Imclone, L.L.C.	180 Varick Street, 6th Floor New York, NY 10014
74	ERGAMISOL®74	Janssen Pharm (part of Johnson and Johnson)	Netherlands
		Johnson & Johnson	One Johnson & Johnson Place New Brunswick, NJ
55	EULEXIN®55	Schering	Kenilworth, NJ 07033
52	FUDR®52	Hospira, Inc.	Lake Forest, IL
62	GEMCIN®62	Eli Lilly and Co.	Lilly Corporate Center Indianapolis, IN 46285
63	GEMTRO®63	Eli Lilly and Co.	Lilly Corporate Center Indianapolis, IN 46285
61	GEMZAR®61	Eli Lilly and Co.	Lilly Corporate Center Indianapolis, IN 46285

®#	Trademarks	Trademark Owner(s)	Owner's Address
71	GLEEVEC®71	Novartis Pharmaceuticals Corp	East Hanover, NJ 07936
		Novartis, Ag. Canada	4002 Basel Switzerland
54	HALOTESTIN®54	Pharmacia & Upjohn Company	235 East 42nd Street New York, NY 10017
		Pfizer Enterprises Canada	Sarl Rond-Point Du Kirchberg 51, Avenue J.F. Kennedy L-1855 Luxembourg Luxembourg
05	HEXALEN®5	Mgi Pharma, Inc. Eisai Medical Res.	Bloomington, MN 55437
		Medimmune Oncology, Inc.	100 Front Street, Suite 400 West Conshohocken, PA 19428
105	HYCAMTIN®105	GlaxoSmithKline	Franklin Plaza, Philadelphia, PA
		SmithKline Beecham P.L.C. Canada	980 Great West Road Brentford Middlesex TW8 9GS England
65	HYDREA®65	Bristol-Myers Squibb	Princeton, NJ
		Bristol-Myers Squibb Canada Co./ La Société Bristol-Myers Squibb Canada	2344 Alfred-Nobel Boulevard Suite 300, Montreal H4S 0A4 Quebec
68	IDAMYCIN PFS®68	Pfizer Pharmacia & Upjohn Company	235 East 42nd Street New York, NY 10017
		Pharmacia & UpJohn, S.P.A. Canada	Via Robert Koch No.1.2. Milan, Italy
70	IFEX®70	Bristol-Myers Squibb Company	345 Park Avenue New York, NY 10154
69	IFOSPHAMIDE®69	Bristol-Myers Squibb	Princeton, NJ
14	IMURAN®14	GlaxoSmithKline	Uxbridge, Middlesex UB11 1BT, UK
		GlaxoSmithKline	Research Triangle Park, NJ 27709
		GlaxoSmithKline Inc. Canada	7333 Mississauga Road North Mississauga L5N 6l4 Ontario
22	LEUKERAN®22	GlaxoSmithKline/ SmithKline Beecham	Research Triangle Park, NJ 27709
		GlaxoSmithKline, Inc. Canada	7333 Mississauga Road North Mississauga L5N 6l4 Ontario
11	LEUNASE®11	Sanofi-Aventis, Australia Pty, Ltd.	Macquarie Park NSW 2113, Australia

®#	Trademarks	Trademark Owner(s)	Owner's Address
27	LEUSTATIN®27 (ORTHO BIO TECH)	Ortho Biotech Products, L.P.	Raritan, NJ 08869
		Johnson & Johnson	One Johnson & Johnson Plaza New Brunswick, NJ 08933-7001
72	LUPRON®72	Abbott Endocrine, Inc.	100 Abbott Park Road Abbott Park, IL 60064
73	LUPRON®73	Tap Pharmaceutical Products, Inc. (Joint V. Abbott and Takeda)	Deerfield, IL 60015
85	LYSODREN®85	Bristol-Myers Squibb Company	345 Park Avenue New York, NY 10154
93	MATULANE®93	Sigma-Tau Pharmacuetical, Inc.	Gaithersburg, MD 20878
77	MEGACE ES®77	Bristol-Myers Squibb	Princeton, NJ
102	METHAZOLASTONE®102	Schering-Plough	Kenilworth, NJ 07033
82	METHYL-GAG®82	Dakota Pharma, Ltd.	Dracut, MA 01826
91	MITHRACIN®91	Bayer Corp.	West Haven, CT
		Pfizer Products, Inc. Canada	Eastern Point Road Groton, CT 06340
76	MUSTARGEN®76	Ovation Pharmaceuticals, Inc.	Four Parkway North Suite 200 Deerfield, IL 60015
84	MUTAMYCIN®84	Bristol Myers Squibb Company	345 Park Avenue New York, NY 10022
78	MYLERAN®78	GlaxoSmithKline	Research Triangle Park, NJ 27709
		GlaxoSmithKline Inc. Canada	7333 Mississauga Road North Mississauga L5N 6l4 Ontario
60	MYLOTARG®60	Wyeth	Five Giralda Farms Madison, NJ 07940-0874
116	NAVELBINE®116	GlaxoSmithKline	Research Triangle Park, NJ 27709
107	NEUTREXIN®107	Medimmune, Inc.	Gaithersburg, MD
		Medimmune Oncology, Inc. Canada	100 Front Street, Suite 400 West Conshohocken, PA 19428
87	NILANDRON®87	Sanofi-Aventis, L.L.C.	Bridgewater, NJ 08807
90	NIPENT®90	Hospira Boulder, Inc.	650 From Road Mack-Cali Centre II, Second Floor Paramus, NJ 07652
98	NOLVADEX®98	Astrazeneca Pharmaceuticals, L.P.	Wilmington, DE 19850-5437
		Astrazeneca UK, Ltd. Canada	15 Stanhope Gate London, W1Y 6LN United Kingdom

®#	Trademarks	Trademark Owner(s)	Owner's Address
86	NOVANTRONE®86	Emd Serono Inc./OSI Oncology	Melville, NY 11747
		Wyeth Holdings Corp. Canada	Five Giralda Farms Madison, NJ 07940
89	ONCASPAR®89	Enzon Pharmaceuticals, Inc.	685 Route 202/206 Bridgewater, NJ 08807
113	ONCOVIN(@113	Eli Lilly	Lilly Corporate Center Indianapolis, IN 46285
		Eli Lilly and Co. Canada	307 East Mccarty Street Indianapolis, IN 46285
01	ORENCIA®1	Bristo-Myers Squibb	345 Park Avenue New York, NY 10154
20	PARAPLATIN®20	Bristol-Myers Squibb Company	345 Park Avenue New York, NY 10154
45	PHARMORUBICI®45	Sicor, Inc.	19 Hughes Irvine, CA 92618
26	PLATINOL®26 (AQ) BMS)	Bristol-Myers Squibb Company	345 Park Avenue New York, NY 10154
37	PROCYTOX®37	Baxter International, Inc.	One Baxter Parkway Deerfield, IL 60015
02	PROLEUKIN®2	Novartis Pharmaceuticals, Ag.	4560 Horton Street Emeryville, CA 94608
51	PROPECIA®51	Merck and Co, Inc. Merck & Co., Inc.	One Merck Drive P.O. Box 100 Whitehouse Station, NJ 16711
50	PROSCAR®50	Merck & Co., Inc.	126 East Lincoln Avenue Rahway, NJ 07065
80	PURINETHOL®80	GlaxoSmithKline	Research Triangle Park, NJ 27709
		Biogal Pharmaceutical Works, Ltd. Canada	Pallagi Ut 13 H-4042 Debrecen Hungary
95	REMICADE®95	Centocor Ortho Biotech Inc.	Horsham, PA 19044
		Centocor Ortho Biotech Inc. Canada	800 Ridgeview Drive Horsham, PA 19044
81	RHEUMATREX®81	Wyeth Holdings Corp.	Five Giralda Farms Madison, NJ 07940
96	RITUXAN®96	Biogen Ibec Inc./ Genentech Inc.	Cambridge, MA; San Francisco, CA
		Idec Pharmaceuticals Corp. Canada	3030 Callan Road San Diego, CA 92121

®#	Trademarks	Trademark Owner(s)	Owner's Address
32	TARABINE PFS®32	Pharmacia & Upjohn	235 East 42nd Street New York, NY 10017
		Pfizer Enterprises Canada	Sarl Rond-Point Du Kirchberg 51, Avenue J.F. Kennedy L-1855 Luxembourg Luxembourg
15	TARGRETIN®15	Eisai Corp. of North America	Woodcliff Lake, NJ
		Elisai R&D Management Co., Ltd.	6-10 Koishikawa 4-Chome Bunkyo-Ku, Tokyo 112-8088 Japan
99	TAXOL®99	Bristol-Myers-Squibb	Princeton, NJ
		Bristol-Myers Squibb Company Canada	345 Park Avenue New York, NY 10154
100	TAXOTERE® 100	Sanofi-Aventis, L.L.C.	Bridgewater, NJ 08807
		Aventis Pharma, S.A. Canada	20, Avenue Raymond Aron 92160 Antony, France
101	TEMODAR®101	Schering-Plough	Kenilworth, NJ 07033
		Schering Canada, Inc.	3535 Trans-Canada Highway Pointe Claire, H9R 1B4 Quebec
104	THIOPLEX®104	Immunex	Seattle, WA 98101
09	TRISENOX®9	Cephalon, Inc.	41 Moores Road Frazer, PA 19355
58	VALCYTE®58	F. Hoffmann-La Roche, Ag.	340 Kingland Street Nutley, NJ 07110
		F. Hoffmann-La Roche, Ag.	Grenzacherstrasse 124 4002, Basel Switzerland
108	VALSTAR®108	Endo Pharm Anthra Pharmaceuticals, Inc. Canada	Chadds Ford, PA 19317 103 Carnegie Center, Suite 102 Princeton, NJ 08540
110	VELBAN®110	Eli Lilly and Co.	Lilly Corporate Center Indianapolis, IN 46285
117	VELCADE®117	Millennium Pharm, Inc.	Cambridge, MA 02139
		Millennium Pharmaceuticals, Inc. Canada	40 Landsdowne Street Cambridge, MA 02139

®#	Trademarks	Trademark Owner(s)	Owner's Address
49	VEPESID®49	Bristol-Myers Squibb Company	345 Park Avenue New York, NY 10022
13	VIDAZA®13	Celgene Corp.	86 Morris Avenue Summit, NJ 07901
112	VINCASAR PFS(@112	Pharmacia & Upjohn	235 East 42nd Street New York, NY 10017
		Pfizer Enterprises Canada	Sarl Rond-Point Du Kirchberg 51, Avenue J. F. Kennedy L–1855 Luxembourg Luxembourg
25	VISTIDE®25	Gilead Sciences, Inc.	353 Lakeside Drive Foster City, CA 94404
57	VITRASERT®57	Bausch & Lomb, Inc.	One Bausch & Lomb Place Rochester, NY 14604
103	VUMON®103	Bristol-Myers-Squibb	Princeton, NJ
		Bristol-Myers Squibb Company Canada	345 Park Avenue New York, NY 10154
19	XELODA®19	F. Hoffman-La Roche Laboratories, Inc.	340 Kingland Street Nutley, NJ 07110
		F. Hoffmann-La Roche, Ag.	Grenzacherstrasse 124 4002, Basel Switzerland
44	ZANOSAR®44	Teva Pharm U.S.A. Parenteral Medicines, Inc.	Irvine, CA 92618
		Pharmacia & Upjohn Company, L.L.C.	100 Route 206 North Peapack, NJ 07977
67	ZEVALIN®67	Idec Pharmaceuticals, Corp.	11011 Torreyana Road San Diego, CA 92121
94	ZINECARD®94	Pfizer-Pharmacia & Upjohn Company	235 East 42nd Street New York, NY 10017
		Pharmacia, Inc. Canada	P.O. Box 16529 Columbus, OH 43216-6529
64	ZOLADEX®64	Astrazeneca Pharmaceuticals, L.P.	Wilmington, DE 19850-5437
		Astrazeneca UK, Ltd. Canada	15 Stanhope Gate London W1Y 6LN United Kingdom

APPENDIXES

3

—	No data/information was listed or specified
??	Source information was not specific
AAP	The American Academy of Pediatrics
ACGIH	American Conference of Governmental Industrial Hygienists
Action Level	Action levels are used by OSHA and NIOSH to express a health or physical hazard. They indicate the level of a harmful or toxic substance/activity that requires medical surveillance, increased industrial hygiene monitoring, or biological monitoring. Action levels are generally set at one half of the permissible exposure limit (PEL), but the actual level may vary from standard to standard. The intent is to identify a level at which the vast majority of randomly sampled exposures will be below the PEL.
AEGL	U.S. Environmental Protection Agency definition—AEGL(s) represent threshold exposure limits for the general public and are applicable to emergency exposure periods ranging from 10 minutes to 8 hours. AEGL-2 and AEGL-3, and AEGL-1 values as appropriate, will be developed for each of five exposure periods (10 and 30 minutes, 1 hour, 4 hours, and 8 hours) and will be distinguished by varying degrees of severity of toxic effects. It is believed that the recommended exposure levels are applicable to the general population including infants and children, and other individuals who may be susceptible. The three AEGL(s) have been defined as follows:

AEGL-1 is the airborne concentration, expressed as parts per million or milligrams per cubic meter (ppm or mg/m3) of a substance above which it is predicted that the general population, including susceptible individuals, could experience notable discomfort, irritation, or certain asymptomatic nonsensory effects. However, the effects are not disabling and are transient and reversible upon cessation of exposure.

AEGL-2 is the airborne concentration (expressed as ppm or mg/m3) of a substance above which it is predicted that the general population, including susceptible individuals, could experience irreversible or other serious, long-lasting adverse health effects or an impaired ability to escape.

AEGL-3 is the airborne concentration (expressed as ppm or mg/m3) of a substance above which it is predicted that the general population, including susceptible individuals, could experience life-threatening health effects or death.

Airborne concentrations below the AEGL-1 represent exposure levels that can produce mild and progressively increasing but transient and nondisabling odor, taste, and sensory irritation or certain asymptomatic, nonsensory effects. With increasing airborne concentrations above each AEGL, there is a progressive increase in the likelihood of occurrence and the severity of effects described for each corresponding AEGL. Although the AEGL values represent threshold levels for the general public, including susceptible subpopulations, such as infants, children, the elderly, persons with asthma, and those with other illnesses, it is recognized that individuals, subject to unique or idiosyncratic responses, could experience the effects described at concentrations below the corresponding AEGL.

ALARA	ALARA is an acronym for the phrase as low as reasonably achievable. It is most often used in reference to chemical or radiation exposure levels.
	ALARA is a work principle, a mindset that will result in low exposures. In an ideal world, one could reduce his or her exposure to hazardous drugs to zero. In reality, reducing an exposure to zero is not always possible; certain social, technical, economic, practical, or public policy considerations will result in a small but acceptable level of risk. The best way to prevent this risk from increasing is to keep one's exposure ALARA.
AND	Antineoplastic and cytotoxic are interchangeable as used in this handbook; antineoplastic drugs make up the majority of the cytotoxic drugs.
ASHP	American Society of Health-System Pharmacists
BAL	BAL is shorthand for the drug dimercaprol.
BEI	Biological exposure indices—American Conference of Governmental Industrial Hygienist (ACGIH)
BERK	Berkeley University hazardous chemical lists
BF	Breastfeeding
BOX INST	Information that accompanies prescription drugs or information found on the prescription drug label
CA	Carcinogen—a substance that causes cancer
CAL EPA	State of California Environmental Protection Agency–maintained list of hazardous chemicals
CAL PROP 65	California State Proposition 65 maintains a list of carcinogens, and developmental and reproductive effects; may require special product labeling
CA–Minnesota	Listed by individual state government
CAS # or CAS NO	CAS#—CAS registry number—a unique number assigned to a substance or mixture by the American Chemical Society Abstract Service
CD	Cytotoxic drugs
CEILING	Ceiling (OSHA) (ACGIH)—this refers to concentrations that must not be exceeded during any part of the working exposure. As such, ceiling TLV(s) take precedent over all TWA(s) and STEL(s)
Centre College List	Centre College maintains a list of hazardous chemicals
CHROM Aberrations	Chromosomal aberrations
CYTO	Cytotoxic—relating to substances that are toxic to cells; i.e., cell-killing
DEV	Developmental
Dose-Response Relationship	The relationship between the amount of exposure (dose) to a substance and the resulting changes in body function or health (response)
EMB	Embryotoxic—this describes any chemical that is harmful to an embryo
ESCAL	Environmental Sentinel Contamination Action Level—an established organizational administrative level used to initiate corrective actions to reduce environmental contaminate levels as part of the facility's chemical-ALARA program as set forth in the facility's hazardous drugs safety and health plan
EU	European Union
EXP	Experimental studies on animals; not human exposure based
FDA	Food and Drug Administration

FDA-C	Food and Drug Administration pregnancy category "C" drug; category "C" medicines have no evidence of human safety, and might have evidence of reproductive harm in animals
FDA-D	Food and Drug Administration pregnancy category "D" drug; category "D" medicines are known to be dangerous to babies, but might have enough of a benefit to mothers that their use may be justified during chemotherapy (limited medical benefit)
FDA-X	Food and Drug Administration pregnancy category "X" drug; category "X" medicines are known to be dangerous, with risks that outweigh any possible medical benefit. They should not be used during pregnancy.
FETO	Fetotoxic—toxic to the fetus
FLAM	Flammable—author stated that the substance/drug was flammable
FS	Fact sheet, New Jersey Department of Health and Senior Services, hazardous substance fact sheet
Full Facepiece Respirator	Covers from roughly the hairline to below the chin. On the average provides the greatest protection, usually seal most reliably, and provides some eye protection as well.
Half Mask Respirator	Fits over the nose, mouth, and under the chin
HD	Hazardous drugs
HMIS	DOD hazardous material information system (refer to 3.14)
IARC	International Agency for Research on Cancer—the authority on designating substances as carcinogen
IDLH	The OSHA regulation (1910.134[b]) defines the term as "an atmosphere that poses an immediate threat to life, would cause irreversible adverse health effects, or would impair an individual's ability to escape from a dangerous atmosphere." IDLH values are often used to guide the selection of breathing apparatus that are made available to workers or firefighters in specific situations.
IOELV	Indicative occupational exposure limit values (IOELV) are human exposure limits to hazardous substances specified by the council of the European Union. They are not binding on member states but must be taken into consideration in setting national occupational exposure limits. Indicative occupational exposure limit value is defined as "the limit of the time-weighted average of the concentration of a chemical agent in the air within the breathing zone of a worker over a specified reference period.
Isolator Barrier 100% Vented Outside	Compounding isolator is generally defined as a class of isolator designed for use during pharmacy drug compounding. Compounding isolators utilize an airtight glove/glove port design that allows the user to perform hands-on tasks inside the isolator without compromising the intended performance of the isolator. Isolator barrier are 100% vented for hazardous drugs applications.
JCAHO	Joint Commission on Accreditation of Healthcare Organizations—founded in 1951 and is dedicated to improve the safety and quality of healthcare organizations with voluntary accreditation
JHA/JSA	Job hazard analysis (interchangeable with job safety analysis)—a job hazard analysis or job safety analysis (JHA/JSA) process is the breaking down into its component parts of any method or procedure to determine the hazards connected with each key step and the requirements for performing it safely. It is a good tool to assist in determining personal protection equipment.
JSA/JHA	Job safety analysis (interchangeable with job hazard analysis)—a job hazard analysis or job safety analysis (JHA/JSA) process is the breaking down into its component parts of any method or procedure to determine the hazards connected with each key step and the requirements for performing it safely. It is a good tool to assist in determining personal protection equipment.

M&F	Male and female
MAKS (DFG)	MAK—a population-based threshold limit value (the MAK value) is defined as the maximum value on the exposure scale below which a constant baseline risk is observed
Metabolite, Metabolism	Metabolism—the conversion or breakdown or a substance from one form to another by a living organism. A metabolite is any product of metabolism.
MCEF	Mixed cellulose ester filter (MCEF) 0.8 micron; air sampling filter
MCG	MCG is the symbol for the microgram (μ)
MEL	Maximum Exposure Limit (MEL) is the highest allowable concentration of a chemical to which a worker may be exposed over a period. MEL is expressed usually in parts per-million (ppm) for an 8-hour reference period though some chemicals may require shorter reference periods. (UK)
MIDI-	The military item disposal instructions (midi) system is a database application designed to provide instructions and methods of destruction for the disposal of hazardous and nonhazardous items. Midi information can be found at http://chppm-www .apgea.army.mil/hmwp/ or http://chppm-www.apgea.army.mil/hmwp/midi.aspx.
Mitosis	Mitosis—cell division in which the nucleus divides into nuclei containing the same number of chromosomes
MOD	Moderate
MSDS	Material safety data sheet
MUT	Mutagen (mutagenic)—causing mitosis or transformation to occur
N.O.S.	Not otherwise specified
N100 or P100	Particulate filter (99.97% filter efficiency level) effective against particulate aerosols free from oil; time use restrictions may apply
NAERG# (YEAR)	North American Emergency Response Guide number (date of publication)
NFPA	National fire protection association (NFPA) 704 hazard diamond (refer to 3.15)
NIEHS	National Institute of Environmental Health Sciences
NIH	National Institute of Health
NIOSH	National Institute for Occupational Safety and Health
NTP	National Toxicology Program is part of the Department of Health and Human Services. NTP develops and carries out tests to predict whether a chemical will cause harm to humans.
OEL	Occupational Exposure Level/Limit
OES	OES—Occupational Exposure Standard
OSHA	Occupational Safety and Health Administration or Act
OTO	Ototoxic
P100	Particulate filter (99.97% filter efficiency level) effective against all particulate aerosols
PEL	Permissible Exposure Limit
PI	Product information
PO	Potential human carcinogen
POS	Possible
Powdered Air-Purifying Respirator (PAPR)	A device equipped with a facepiece, hood, or helmet, breathing tube, canister, cartridge, filter, canister with filter, or cartridge with filter, and a blower
PROB	Probable
Product Label	Food and drug administration product label information
R100	Particulate filter (99.97% filter efficiency level) effective against all particulate aerosols, time use restrictions may apply
REL	Recommended exposure limit

REP	Reproductive effectors
Risk And Risk Reduction	Risk is the probability that something will cause injury or harm. Risk reduction is actions that can decrease the likelihood those individuals, groups, or communities will experience disease or other health conditions.
Risk Communication	Risk communication is the exchange of information to increase understanding of health risks
RTECS	Registry of Toxic Effects of Chemical Substances—maintained by National Institute of Occupational Safety and Health (NIOSH)
SAX	N. Irving Sax and Richard J. Lewis, *Dangerous Properties of Industrial Materials*, 7th ed.
SKI PERM	Skin permeable—danger of cutaneous (skin) absorption
STEL	Short Term Exposure Limit—ACGIH
SUSP	Suspect
TBA	To be determine later
TEEL	Temporary emergency exposure limits (TEEL) (U.S. Department of Energy)
	TEEL-0 = the threshold concentration below which most people will experience no appreciable risk of health effects.
	TEEL-1= the maximum concentration in air below which it is believed nearly all individuals could be exposed without experiencing other than mild transient adverse health effects or perceiving a clearly defined objectionable odor.
	TEEL-2 = the maximum concentration in air below which it is believed nearly all individuals could be exposed without experiencing or developing irreversible or other serious health effects or symptoms that could impair their abilities to take protective action.
	TEEL-3 = the maximum concentration in air below which it is believed nearly all individuals could be exposed without experiencing or developing life-threatening health effects. Note: *it is recommended that for application of TEELS, the concentration at the receptor point of interest be calculated as the peak 15-minute time-weighted average concentration.*
TER	Teratogen—a substance that causes defects in development between conception and birth. Teratogen is a substance that causes a structural or functional birth defect.
TITLE 111	SARA TITLE III consolidated list of lists—chemicals subject to the emergency planning and community right-to-know act and section 112(r) of CAA
TLV	Threshold Limit Values—ACGIH
TOX	Listed by the author as being a toxic substance
TOX-Florida	Listed by individual state government
TUM	Tumorigenic—tumor—an abnormal mass of tissue that results from excessive cell division that is uncontrolled and progressive. Tumors can be either benign (not cancer) or malignant (cancer).
TWA	Time-Weighted Average
UMCP	University of Maryland, College Park—maintains lists of hazardous chemicals
UN or NA	United Nations or North America
USP	United States Pharmacopoeia (USP) is the official public standards-setting authority for all prescription and over-the-counter medicines, dietary supplements, and other healthcare products manufactured and sold in the United States
WEEL	Workplace Environmental Exposure Level (WEEL)—two types:
	Long-term exposure limit (8-hours time weighted average [TWA] reference period); units are ppm and mg.m-3. Short-term exposure limit (has a 15-minute reference period)
WHO	World Health Organization—working group on human lactation

Chemical Abstract Service (CAS) Number Index 3.2

CAS Number	Drug Name (Nomenclature)	Page	Page
N.O.S.	Abatacept	15	15
57576-44-0	Aclarubicin (Aclacinomycin) (57576-44-0) (75443-99-1)	15	17
75443-99-1	Aclarubicin (Aclacinomycin) (57576-44-0) (75443-99-1)	15	17
25316-40-9	Adriamycin With Hydrochloride (Doxorubicin For Free Base) (23214-92-8) (25316-40-9)	17	18
23214-92-8	Adriamycin With Hydrochloride (Doxorubicin For Free Base) (23214-92-8) (25316-40-9)	17	18
110942-02-4	Aldesleukin (Proleukin) (L2-7001) (110942-02-4)	18	20
216503-57-0	Alemtuzumab (Campath) (216503-57-0)	20	21
645-05-6	Altretamine (Hexalen) (Hemel) (645-05-6)	21	22
150399-23-8	Alimta (Pemetrexed)(150399-23-8)	22	24
125-84-8	Aminoglutethimide (Cytadren) (125-84-8)	24	24
51264-14-3	Amsacrine (Amsacrine Hcl) (M-Amsa) (Amsa P-D) (Acridinylanisidide) (54301-15-4) (51264-14-3)	25	26
54301-15-4	Amsacrine (Amsacrine Hcl) (M-Amsa) (Amsa P-D) (Acridinylanisidide) (54301-15-4) (54301-15-4)	25	26
120511-73-1	Anastrozole (Arimidex) (120511-73-1)	26	27
1327-53-3	Arsenic Trioxide (Trisenox)(1327-53-3)	27	30
9015-68-3	Asparaginase (L-Asparaginase)(Elspar) (Leunase)(Leucogen) (Crisantaspare) (9015-68-3)	30	33
216974-75-3	Avastin (Bevacizumab) (Bevacizumabum) (216974-75-3)	33	34
320-67-2	Azacytidine (5-Azacytidine) (320-67-2)	34	35
446-86-6	Azathioprine (Imuran) (Tabthioprine) (Azanin) (Imurel) (C9-H7-N702-S) (446-86-6)	35	38
153559-49-0	Bexarotenum (Bexarotene) (Targretin) (153559-49-0)	38	39
90357-06-5	Bicalutamide (Casodex) (90357-06-5)	39	40

CAS Number	Drug Name (Nomenclature)	Page	Page
71439-68-4	Bisantrene Hydrochloride (CL 216942) (NSC 337766) (ADAH) (71439-68-4) (78186-34-2)	40	41
78186-34-2	Bisantrene Hydrochloride (CL 216942) (NSC 337766) (ADAH) (71439-68-4) (78186-34-2)	40	41
67763-87-5	Bleomycin (Blenoxane) (Bleocin) (9041-93-4) (11056-06-7) (67763-87-5)	41	43
11056-06-7	Bleomycin (Blenoxane) (Bleocin) (9041-93-4) (11056-06-7) (67763-87-5)	41	43
9041-93-4	Bleomycin (Blenoxane) (Bleocin) (9041-93-4) (11056-06-7) (67763-87-5)	41	43
55-98-1	Busulfan (Myleran) (55-98-1)	43	44
97682-44-5	Camptosar (Irinotecan HCL) (Camptothecin) (CPT) (CPT-11) (C33H38N4O6) (97682-44-5) (7689-03-4) (100286-90-6) (111348-33-5) (136572-09-3)	44	46
100286-90-6	Camptosar (Irinotecan HCL) (Camptothecin) (CPT) (CPT-11) (C33H38N4O6) (97682-44-5) (7689-03-4) (100286-90-6) (111348-33-5) (136572-09-3)	44	46
111348-33-5	Camptosar (Irinotecan HCL) (Camptothecin) (CPT) (CPT-11) (C33H38N4O6) (97682-44-5) (7689-03-4) (100286-90-6) (111348-33-5) (136572-09-3)	44	46
136572-09-3	Camptosar (Irinotecan Hcl) (Camptothecin) (CPT) (CPT-11) (C33H38N4O6) (97682-44-5) (7689-03-4) (100286-90-6) (111348-33-5) (136572-09-3)	44	46
7689-03-4	Camptosar (Irinotecan Hcl) (Camptothecin) (CPT) (CPT-11) (C33H38N4O6) (97682-44-5) (7689-03-4) (100286-90-6) (111348-33-5) (136572-09-3)	44	46
154361-50-9	Capecitabine (Xeloda) (5'-Deoxy-5-Fluorocytisine) (154361-50-9) (158798-73-3)	46	47
158798-73-3	Capecitabine (Xeloda) (5'-Deoxy-5-Fluorocytisine) (154361-50-9) (158798-73-3)	46	47
41575-94-4	Carboplatin (Paraplatin) (Diammine) (C6h12n2o4pt) (41575-94-4) (7440-06-4)	47	51
7440-06-4	Carboplatin (Paraplatin) (Diammine) (C6h12n2o4pt) (41575-94-4) (7440-06-4)	47	51
154-93-8	Carmustine (BCNU) (BICNU) (Bischloroethyl Nitrosourea) (154-93-8)	51	52
305-03-3	Chlorambucil (CCNU) (Leukeran) (Ambochlorin) (305-03-3)	52	54
51-75-2	Chlormethine (Mechlorethanmine) (Nitrogen Mustard) (51-75-2)	54	57
54749-90-5	Chlorozotocin (DCNU) (54749-90-5)	57	58
149394-66-1	Cidofovir (Vistide) (149394-66-1) (113852-37-2)	58	59
113852-37-2	Cidofovir (Vistide) (149394-66-1) (113852-37-2)	58	59
15663-27-1	Cisplatin (Cis-Platin) (Platinol AQ) (15663-27-1)	59	61
4291-63-8	Cladribine (Leustatin) (2-Chloro-2'-Deoxyadeno-Sine) (2-CDA) (RWJ26251) (4291-63-8)	61	62
147-94-4	Cytarabine (Udicil) (Cytosar-U) (ARA-C) (147-94-4)	62	64

CAS Number	Drug Name (Nomenclature)	Page	Page
69-74-9	Cytosine Arabinoside (Alexan) (Same As Cytostatic) (69-74-9)	66	67
50-18-0	Cytoxan Anhydrous (Cyclophosphamide Hydrate/Monohydrate) (Cycolophosphamide) (Neosar) (50-18-0) (6055-19-2) (60007-96-7) (60030-72-0) (6007-95-6)	62	64
6055-19-2	Cytoxan Anhydrous (Cyclophosphamide Hydrate/Monohydrate) (Cycolophosphamide) (Neosar)(50-18-0) (6055-19-2) (60007-96-7) (60030-72-0) (6007-95-6)	62	64
60007-96-7	Cytoxan Anhydrous (Cyclophosphamide Hydrate/Monohydrate) (Cycolophosphamide) (Neosar) (50-18-0) (6055-19-2) (60007-96-7) (60030-72-0) (6007-95-6)	62	64
60030-72-0	Cytoxan Anhydrous (Cyclophosphamide Hydrate/Monohydrate) (Cycolophosphamide) (Neosar) (50-18-0) (6055 19 2) (60007 96-7) (60030-72-0) (6007-95-6)	62	64
6007-95-6	Cytoxan Anhydrous (Cyclophosphamide Hydrate/Monohydrate) (Cycolophosphamide)(Neosar)(50-18-0)(6055-19-2)(60007-96-7) (60030-72-0) (6007-95-6)	62	64
4342-03-4	Dacarbazine (DTIC-DOME) (4342-03-4) (55390-090-10) (37626-23-6)	69	70
55390-090-10	Dacarbazine (DTIC-DOME) (4342-03-4) (55390-090-10) (37626-23-6)	69	70
37626-23-6	Dacarbazine (DTIC-DOME) (4342-03-4) (55390-090-10) (37626-23-6)	69	70
50-76-0	Dactinomycin (Actinomycin D) (Cosmegen) (50-76-0)	70	72
23541-50-6	Daunorubicin Hcl (Cerubidine) (Daunoxome) (Liposoma) (23541-50-6) (20830-81-3)	72	79
20830-81-3	Daunorubicin Hcl (Cerubidine) (Daunoxome) (Liposoma) (23541-50-6) (20830-81-3)	79	79
21436-03-3	Diaminocyclohexane (Oxalatoplatinum) (C8H14N2O4Pt) (Eloxatin) ((+)-(S,S)-1,2-DIAMINOCYCLOHEXANE) (21436-03-3) (61825-94-3)	79	80
61825-94-3	Diaminocyclohexane (Oxalatoplatinum) (C8H14N2O4Pt) (Eloxatin) ((+)-(S,S)-1,2-DIAMINOCYCLOHEXANE) (21436-03-3) (61825-94-3)	79	80
23261-20-3	Dianhydrogalactitol (DAD) (DAG)(DULCITOL DIEPOXIDE) (NSC-132313) (23261-20-3)	80	80
57998-68-2	Diaziquone (AZQ) (C16H20N406) (57998-68-2)	80	81
528-74-5	Dichloromethotrexate (NCI-CO 4875) (NSC29630) (C20-H20-CL2-N8-O5) (528-74-5) (88442-77-7)	81	82
88442-77-7	Dichloromethotrexate (NCI-CO 4875) (NSC29630) (C20-H20-CL2-N8-O5) (528-74-5) (88442-77-7)	81	82
18883-66-4	Diethylstilbestrol Tozocin (Zanosar) (STN) (STRZ) (Streptozocin) (18883-66-4) (66395-18-4) (66395-17-3)	82	83
66395-18-4	Diethylstilbestrol Tozocin (Zanosar) (STN) (STRZ) (Streptozocin) (18883-66-4) (66395-18-4) (66395-17-3)	82	83
66395-17-3	Diethylstilbestrol Tozocin (Zanosar) (STN) (STRZ) (Streptozocin) (18883-66-4) (66395-18-4) (66395-17-3)	82	83

CAS Number	Drug Name (Nomenclature)	Page	Page
19767-45-4	Ifosfamide (Ifex) (Iphospamide) (3778-73-2) (66849-33-0) (66849-34-1) (84711-20-6) (19767-45-4)	118	120
152459-95-5	Imatinib Mesylate (Gleevec) (Sti-571) (152459-95-5) (220127-57-1)	120	121
220127-57-1	Imatinib Mesylate (Gleevec) (Sti-571) (152459-95-5) (220127-57-1)	120	121
9015-68-3	L-Asparaginase (Elspar) (Leunase) (Leucogen) (9015-68-3)	30	33
53714-56-0	Leuprorelin (Leuprolide) (Leuprolide Acetate) (NSC377526) (53714-56-0)	2-453	2-461
14769-73-4	Levamisole (Ergamisol) (Levamisole Hydrochloride) (C11H12N2-S,HCL) (14769-73-4) (16595-80-5)	2-462	2-469
16595-80-5	Levamisole (Ergamisol) (Levamisole Hydrochloride) (C11H12N2-S,HCL) (14769-73-4) (16595-80-5)	2-462	2-469
13010-47-4	Lomustine (CCNU) (CECENU) (CEENU) (1-(2-CHLOROETHYL)-3-CYCLO-HEXYL-1-NITROSOUREA) (13010-47-4)	2-469	2-473
55-86-7	Mechlorethamine HCL (Nitrogen Mustard) (Mustargen) (55-86-7)	2-473	2-480
595-33-5	Megestrol Acetate (Megestrol) (Megace) (595-33-5) (3562-63-8)	2-480	2-485
3562-63-8	Megestrol Acetate (Megestrol) (Megace) (595-33-5) (3562-63-8)	2-480	2-485
8057-25-8	Melphalan (Phenylalanine Mustard) (Alkeran) (148-82-3) (8057-25-8)	2-485	2-501
148-82-3	Melphalan (Phenylalanine Mustard) (Alkeran) (148-82-3) (8057-25-8)	2-485	2-501
71628-96-1	Menogaril (7-O-Methylnogarol) (NSC269148) (71628-96-1) (69256-91-3) (74202-31-6)	2-501	2-506
69256-91-3	Menogaril (7-O-Methylnogarol) (NSC269148) (71628-96-1) (69256-91-3) (74202-31-6)	2-501	2-506
74202-31-6	Menogaril (7-O-Methylnogarol) (NSC269148) (71628-96-1) (69256-91-3) (74202-31-6)	2-501	2-506
50-44-2	Mercaptopurine (6-Mercaptopurin) (6MP) (Mercapurin) (C5H4N4S) (6112-76-1) (50-44-2)	2-506	2-512
6112-76-1	Mercaptopurine (6-Mercaptopurin) (6MP) (Mercapurin) (C5H4N4S) (50-44-2) (6112-76-1)	2-506	2-512
59-05-2	Methotrexate (MTX) (Amethopterin) (Methotrex) (Rheumatrex) (59-05-2)	2-513	2-537
459-86-9	Methyl-Gag (Mitoguazone) (MGBG) (459-86-9) (7059-23-6) (75020-13-2)	121	122
7059-23-6	Methyl-Gag (Mitoguazone) (MGBG) (459-86-9) (7059-23-6) (75020-13-2)	121	122
75020-13-2	Methyl-Gag (Mitoguazone) (MGBG) (459-86-9) (7059-23-6) (75020-13-2)	121	122
50-07-7	Mitomycin C (Mutamycin) (C15H18N405) (50-07-7)	122	126
53-19-0	Mitotane (Lysodren) (MJ7236) (0,P-DDD) (53-19-0)	126	127
70476-82-3	Mitoxantrone Hydrochloride (Novantrone) (DHAD) (70476-82-3) (65271-80-9)	127	130
65271-80-9	Mitoxantrone Hydrochloride (Novantrone) (DHAD) (70476-82-3) (65271-80-9)	127	130
63612-50-0	Nilutamide (Nilandron) (RU23908) (Anandron) (63612-50-0)	130	131

CAS Number	Drug Name (Nomenclature)	Page	Page
61825-94-3	Oxaliplatin (Eloxatin) (Dacplat) (Trans-I-Diaminocyclohexane Oxalatoplatinum) (C8H14N2O4Pt) (61825-94-3)	130	131
13909-02-9	PCNU (1-(2-CHLOROETHYL)-3-(2,6-DIOXO-3-PIPERIDYL)-1-NITROSOUREA)(Urea)(NSC-95466) (13909-02-9)	133	133
130167-69-0	Peg-Aspargase (Oncaspar) (130167-69-0)	133	134
150399-23-8	Pemetrexed (Alimta) (150399-23-8)	21	22
140-64-7	Pentamidine (Pentamindine Isethionate) (Ebupent) (140-64-7)	134	135
53910-25-1	Pentostatin (Pd-Adi) (Nipent) (53910-25-1)	135	136
18378-89-7	Plicamycin (Mithramycin) (Mithracin) (18378-89-7)	137	138
53-03-2	Prednisone	138	139
366-70-1	Procarbazine (Matulane) (Procarbazine Hydrochloride) (366-70-1)	139	141
21416-67-1	Razoxane (Zinecard) (ICRF-187) (Dexrazoxane) (21416-67-1) (24584-09-6)	141	142
24584-09-6	Razoxane (Zinecard) (ICRF-187) (Dexrazoxane) (21416-67-1) (24584-09-6)	141	142
331731-18-1	Remicade (CHIMERIC ANT-TNF MONOCLONAL ANTIBODY) (Inflixnab) (170277-31-3) (331731-18-1)	142	143
170277-31-3	Remicade (CHIMERIC ANT-TNF MONOCLONAL ANTIBODY) (Inflixnab) (170277-31-3) (331731-18-1)	142	143
174722-31-7	Rituxan (Rituximab) (Mobthera) (IDEC-CB8) (174722-31-7)	143	144
13909-09-6	Semustine (METHYL-CCNU) (ME-CCNU) (13909-09-6) (33073-59-5) (33185-87-4) (56748-54-0)	144	145
33073-59-5	Semustine (METHYL-CCNU) (ME-CCNU) (13909-09-6) (33073-59-5) (33185-87-4) (56748-54-0)	144	145
33185-87-4	Semustine (METHYL-CCNU) (ME-CCNU) (13909-09-6) (33073-59-5) (33185-87-4) (56748-54-0)	144	145
56748-54-0	Semustine (METHYL-CCNU) (ME-CCNU) (13909-09-6) (33073-59-5) (33185-87-4) (56748-54-0)	144	145
56605-16-4	Spiromustine (Spirohydantoin Mustard) (56605-16-4)	145	146
10540-29-1	Tamoxifen Citrate (Nolvadex) (10540-29-1) (54965-24-1)	146	147
54965-24-1	Tamoxifen Citrate (Nolvadex) (10540-29-1) (54965-24-1)	146	147
33069-62-4	Taxol 0.6 Wt % (Paclitaxel) (Tax) (C47h51no14) (33069-62-4)	147	151
114977-28-5	Taxotere (Docetaxel) (C43H53NO14) (114977-28-5)	151	152
37076-68-9	Tegafur (Ftorafur) (37076-68-9) (17902-23-7)	153	153
17902-23-7	Tegafur (Ftorafur) (37076-68-9) (17902-23-7)	153	153
85622-93-1	Temozolomide (Temodar) (Methazolastone) (C6H6N6O2) (85622-93-1)	153	154
29767-20-2	Teniposide (VM-26) (29767-20-2)	154	155
154-42-7	Thioguanine (6-Thioguanine) (154-42-7)	155	157
52-24-4	Thiotepa (Thioplex) (TRIETHYLENE THIOPHSPHORAMIDE) (TESPA) (TRIS(1-AZIRIDNYL)-PHOSPHINE SULFIDE) (52-24-4)	157	160

CAS Number	Drug Name (Nomenclature)	Page	Page
123948-87-8	Topotecan (Hycamtin) (123948-87-8)	160	162
208921-02-2	Tositumomab (Bexxar) (208921-02-2) (192391-48-3)	162	163
192391-48-3	Tositumomab (Bexxar) (208921-02-2) (192391-48-3)	162	163
31368-48-6	Triazinate (C26H30CLFN5O5S2) (NSC 139105) (31368-48-6)(41191-04-2)	163	163
41191-04-2	Triazinate (C26H30CLFN5O5S2) (NSC 139105) (31368-48-6)(41191-04-2)	163	163
82952-64-5	Trimetrexate (Neutrexin) (Trimetrexate Glucuronate) (TMQ) (82952-64-5)	163	165
66-75-1	Uramustine (Uracil Mustard) (5-[(BIS(2-CHLOROETHYL)AMINO)] URACIL) (66-75-1)	165	166
56124-62-0	Valrubicin (Valstar) (56124-62-0)	166	167
179324-69-7	Velcade (Bortezomib) (PS341)(MLN341) (LDP341) (179324-69-7)	167	168
143-67-9	Vinblastine (Vinblastine Sulfate) (VLB) (Velsar) (VLB) (143-67-9) (865-21-4)	168	173
865-21-4	Vinblastine (Vinblastine Sulfate) (VLB) (Velsar) (VLB) (143-67-9) (865-21-4)	168	173
2068-78-2	Vincristine (Vincristine Sulfate) (VCR) (Leurocristine) (2068-78-2) (57-22-7)	173	175
57-22-7	Vincristine (Vincristine Sulfate) (VCR) (Leurocristine) (2068-78-2) (57-22-7)	173	175
53643-48-4	Vindesine (Eldisine) (Fildesin) (Vincaleukoblastine) (53643-48-4)	175	176
125317-39-7	Vinorelbine Tartrate (Navelbine) (C44H52N4O8) (71486-22-2) (125317-39-7)	176	178
71486-22-2	Vinorelbine Tartrate (Navelbine) (C44H52N4O8) (71486-22-2) (125317-39-7)	176	178

Introduction to Personal Protective Equipment

Personal Protective Equipment (PPE)

The PPE must be used in conjunction with engineering and administrative controls and safe work practices whenever work exposures cannot be reduced to acceptable limits. Examples of PPE include safety glasses or goggles, face shields, gloves, gowns, and respirators.

Respirators

Dusts and aerosols—Where a BSC is not currently available, and whenever sprays, splashes, or aerosols of cytotoxic drugs may be generated, worker should wear either a NIOSH-approved full face piece, air-purifying, particulate respirator; or a less than full face piece, air-purifying, particulate respirator, provided the employee wears a face shield and splash goggles complying with ANSI Z87.1 1989. Air-purifying, particulate respirators should have a filter designated equal to or greater than N100, P100 or R100 rating (previously HEPA filter).

Vapors or unknowns—Where a NIOSH-approved airline or self-contained breathing apparatus (SCBA). An example where vapors may be present is in a large spill scenario with a cytotoxic drug known to produce vapors or spills of unknown cytotoxic drugs. It is suggested that the local emergency response team be activated to handle these situations.

Use respirators in accordance with local respiratory protection program and OSHA (29 CFR 1910.134) and NIOSH recommendations. Select particulate respirator filters in accordance with NIOSH (42 CFR 84).

Never wear surgical masks in place of respirators, since surgical masks *do not* protect against breathing aerosols.

Clean reusable respirators with mild detergent and clean water after use.

Respirator Storage

After inspection, cleaning, and any necessary minor repairs, store respirators to protect against sunlight, heat, extreme cold, excessive moisture, damaging chemicals, or other contaminants. Respirators placed at stations and work areas for emergency use shall be stored in compartments built for that purpose, shall be quickly accessible at all times, and will be clearly marked. Routinely used respirators, such as half-mask or full-face air-purifying respirators, shall be placed in sealable plastic bags. Respirators may be stored in such places as lockers or toolboxes only if they are first placed in carrying cases or cartons. Respirators shall be packed or stored so that the face piece and exhalation valves will rest in a normal position and not be crushed. Emergency use respirators shall be stored in a sturdy compartment that is quickly accessible and clearly marked.

Respirator Fit Checking

Each time a respirator is donned, the user will perform positive and negative pressure fit checks. These checks are not a substitute for fit testing. Respirators users must be properly trained in the performance of these checks and understand their limitations.

A. Negative Pressure Check

Applicability/Limitations: This test cannot be carried out on all respirators; however, it can be used on face pieces of air purifying respirators equipped with tight-fitting respirator inlet covers and on atmosphere supplying respirators equipped with breathing tubes, which can be squeezed or blocked at the inlet to prevent the passage of air.

Procedure: Close off the inlet opening of the respirator's canister(s), cartridge(s), or filter(s) with the palm of the hand, or squeeze the breathing air tube or block its inlet so that it will not allow the passage of air. Inhale gently and hold for at least 10 seconds. If the face piece collapses slightly and no inward leakage of air into the face piece is detected, it can be reasonably assumed that the respirator has been properly positioned and the exhalation valve and face piece are not leaking.

B. Positive Pressure Check

Applicability/Limitations: This test cannot be carried out on all respirators; however, respirators equipped with exhalation valves can be tested.

Procedure: Close off the exhalation valve or the breathing tube with the palm of the hand. Exhale gently. If the respirator has been properly positioned, a slight positive pressure will build up inside the face piece without detection of any outward air leak between the sealing surface of the face piece and the face.

C. Federal Regulations

Federal regulations (29 CFR 1910.134 appendix A) require qualitative fit tests of respirators and describe systematic procedures. This test checks the subject's response to a chemical introduced outside the respirator face piece. This response is either voluntary or involuntary depending on the chemical used. Several methods may be used. The two most common are the irritant smoke test and the odorous vapor test.

1. Irritant Smoke

The irritant smoke test is an involuntary response test. Air purifying respirators must be equipped with a high efficiency particulate air (HEPA) filter for this test. An irritant smoke, usually either stannic chloride or titanium tetrachloride, is directed from a smoke tube toward the respirator. If the test subject does not respond to the irritant smoke, a satisfactory fit is assumed to be achieved. Any response to the smoke indicates an unsatisfactory fit.

The irritant smoke is an irritant to the eyes, skin, and mucous membranes. It should not be introduced directly onto the skin. The test subject must keep his or her eyes closed during the testing if a full face piece mask is not used.

2. Odorous Vapor (not to be used with the N100, P100, or R100 Canister/Respirator Mask)

The odorous vapor test is a voluntary response test. It relies on the subject's ability to detect an odorous chemical while wearing the respirator. Air purifying respirators must be equipped with an organic cartridge or canister for this test. Isoamyl acetate (banana oil) is the usual test. An Isoamyl acetate-saturated gauze pad is placed near the face piece-to-face seal of the respirator of the test subject's skin. If the test subject is unable to smell the chemical, than a satisfactory fit is assumed to be achieved, if the subject smells the chemical, the fit is unsatisfactory.

If the subject cannot smell the chemical, the respirator will be momentarily pulled away from the subject's face. If the subject is then able to smell the chemical, a satisfactory fit is assumed. If the subject cannot smell the chemical with the respirator pulled away from the face, this test is inappropriate for this subject, and a different test will be used.

This test is limited by the wide variation of odor thresholds among individuals and the possibility of olfactory fatigue. Since it is a voluntary response test, it depends upon an honest response.

N, P, and R Category Filters Respirator (N100, P100, and R100 Respirator)

For air purifying respirators (APRs) there are nine classes of particulates filters (three levels of filter efficiency, each with three categories of resistance to filter efficiency degradation). The most common commercially available cartridges are the "N-95" (not oil resistant and 95% efficient) and "P-100" (oil-proof and 100% efficient).

The three levels of filter efficiency are 95%, 99%, and 99.97% and are labeled as either 95, 99, or 100. Higher filter efficiency means lower leakage, hence greater protection. Since there are no safe or threshold levels where exposure to a biological agent (bacteria, virus, or spore) is considered safe, the particulate filter that offers the highest level of protection must be used. The 99.97% (100) filter efficiency recommendation is consistent with OSHA/NIOSH recommendations for use with cytotoxic drugs in the healthcare workplace.

The three categories of resistance to filter efficiency degradation relate to the presence or absence of oil particles in the work environment and are labeled as either N- (non-oil resistant), R- (oil resistant), or P- (oil proof). NIOSH generally recommends the following in choosing an N, R, or P category filter:

- If no oil particles are present in the work environment, use a filter of any series (i.e., N-, R-, or P-series filter).
- If oil particles (e.g., lubricants, cutting fluids, glycerine, etc.) are present, use an R- or P-series filter.
- If oil particles are present and the filter is to be used for more than one work shift, use only a P-series filter.
- If it is unknown whether oil particles are present, use only a P-series filter.

Based on the above considerations, fire fighters and emergency medical personnel shall use as a minimum, a P-100 APR or a HEPA filter PAPR respirator for protection against respiratory exposure to cytotoxic drugs. Consequently, the widely distributed N-95 respirator is not appropriate for use and is inconsistent with current guidelines. Powered air-purifying respirators (PAPRs) require high-efficiency particulate air (HEPA) filters. Such filters are equivalent to a P-100. Furthermore, disposable respirators shall not be reused. If PAPRs are used, the filters shall not be reused and the respirator must be sterilized in accordance with manufacturers' instructions and local hazardous waste procedures.

Eye and Face Protection

Face shields and splash goggles complying with ANSI Z87.1-1989 whenever splash, sprays, or aerosols of cytotoxic drugs may be generated. A workplace hazard analysis should be initiated to determine workplace hazards and appropriate PPE for tasks conducted with handling of cytotoxic drugs.

Clean reusable face shields and splash goggles with mild detergent and clean water after each use.

Disposable Gowns and Shoe Covers

Wear protective, disposable gown and shoe covers that are made of lint free, low-permeability fabric or preferably use a gown made out of material that was tested against specific cytotoxic drugs you are using and reported as manufacturer's breakthrough times. Laboratory coats and other cloth fabrics absorb fluids, so they provide an inadequate barrier to hazardous drugs and are not recommended. The existing guidelines do not contain a recommendation for the maximum length of time that a gown should be worn. Because no recommendations are stated in the literature, at a minimum, change the gown every time it is contaminated or gloves are changed.

Furthermore, gowns and shoe covers should always be worn during chemotherapy preparation and when administering intravenous (IV) chemotherapy. Gowns also should be used during the administration of hazardous drugs by any other route, especially if splashing is possible. Gowns worn while preparing hazardous drugs should be removed before leaving the immediate BSC area, before the inner gloves are removed. Gowns worn while administering hazardous drugs should be changed when leaving the patient care area or immediately if contaminated. The practice of hanging up a gown between uses may lead to surface contamination and should be discontinued. Gowns are intended to be single use and should not be worn more than once.

Gowns should have a solid front with back closure, long sleeves with elastic or closed-knit cuffs. Remember to *never* wear contaminated gowns outside the preparation area.

Many of the manufacturers have package sets/kits of PPE for various tasks performed routinely in areas using cytotoxic drugs to include spill kits. Examples of some of the CD kits are shown below.

You should request and use permeation data from the manufacturer in selection of personal protective equipment (PPE). Select your PPE based on how long it takes for a cytotoxic drug to permeate through the glove, gown, apron, etc. Using prudent industrial hygiene principle Choose the manufacturer's product that has the longest permeation time for the cytotoxic drug or drugs being used in your facility. Currently only a few CDs (~13) have permeation data for glove and outer garments, it is better to use PPE with limited permeation data (breakthrough times) than using one that has no permeation data available (examples of some gloves breakthrough data, refer to 3.4).

Chemotherapy Gloves

Chemotherapy Gloves: Gloves are the first line of defense, since the hands provide the greatest potential for exposure. Wear two pairs of disposable chemotherapy gloves that are tested against cytotoxic drugs of interest for examples of chemotherapy gloves.

Change gloves at least hourly (depending on manufacturer's breakthrough time) and immediately if they are torn, punctured, or become overly contaminated.

Wash hands before and after removing gloves. Remember *never* wear contaminated gloves outside the immediate preparation area.

Examples of Available Chemotherapy Gloves with Manufacturers' Breakthrough Times

3.4

Manufacturer	Best				Kimberly-Clark		Micro-fex	Intacta	
Brand or/and Model	N-dex® 9905pf	N-dex® S9905pf	N-dex® 6005pf (14 mil)	Nitri care® 3305pf	Pfe-xtra®	Purple nitrile-xtra®	Neopro ec® (astm F739)	Polyurethane gloves made with intacta® (ASTM f739:99)	Polyurethane gloves made with intacta® (en 374-3)
Drug name									
	Manufacturer breakthrough times (in minutes)								
Carmustine (154-93-8)	>480	>480	>480	>480	60	180	96	10	<10
Cisplatin aq (15663-27-1)	>480	>480	>480	>480	480	480	240	—	—
Cytoxan (50-18-0) (6055-19-2) (60007-96-7) (60030-72-0) (6007-95-6)	—	—	—	—	480	480	240	—	—
Dacarbazine (4342-03-4) (55390-090-10) (37626-23-6)	>480	>480	>480	>480	480	480	240	10	>480
Doxorubicin hcl (25316-40-9) (23214-92-8) (22314-92-8)	>480	>480	>480	>480	480	480	240	—	—
Etoposide (33419-42-0)	>480	>480	>480	>480	480	480	240	—	—
Fluorouracil (51-21-8)	>480	>480	>480	>480	480	480	240	—	—
Ifosfamide (3778-73-2) (66849-33-0) (66849-34-1) (84711-20-6) (19767-45-4)	>480	>480	>480	>480	—	—	—	—	—
Methotrexate (59-05-2)	>480	>480	>480	>480	—	—	—	—	—
Methotrexate (amethopterine hydrate) (59-05-2)	—	—	—	—	—	—	240	—	—
Mitomycin (50-07-7)	>480	>480	>480	>480	—	—	—	—	—
Mitoxantrone hcl (70476-82-3) (65271-80-9)	>480	>480	>480	>480	—	—	—	10	>480
Paclitaxel (33069-62-4)	—	—	—	—	480	480	240	—	—
Thio-tepa (thiotepa) (52-24-4)	—	—	—	—	—	—	240	—	—
Vincristine sulfate (2068-78-2) (57-22-7)	>480	>480	>480	>480	480	480	240	—	—

Suppliers of Chemotherapy Protection and Safety Products (not a comprehensive list)

Chemo Gloves	Internet Contact Information
Regent Medical	www.regentmedical.com
Kendall LTP (now part of Covidien)	www.kendall–ltp.com
Ansell	www.ansellhealthcare.com
Best Manufacturing	www.bestglove.com
Safeskin Corporation	www.safeskin.com
Digitcare (HaloKote Chemotherapy™ gloves)	www.digitcare.net/faq.htm

Protective Apparel	Internet Contact Information
Kendall	www.kendall–ltp.com
Safeskin Corporation	www.safeskin.com

Respiratory Protection and Safety Protection Products	Internet Contact Information
Masksnmore (P100)	www.masksnmore.com/3mfica.html
Biosword Protection Systems (P100 & N100)	www.biosword.com/products/8233.htm
Ansell	www.ansellhealthcare.com/
Safeskin Corporation	www.safeskin.com
Carmel Pharma, Inc.	www.carmelpharma.se/
Newsagesafety (P100)	www.newagesafety.com/dust-masks.php?pg=2
Cooper Safety (P100) (N100)	www.coopersafety.com/shop/respirators/3mp100.cfm

Sample Job Hazard Analysis Form Example Based on OSHA★

Position/Job Title:	Job Location:	Analyst Name:	Date:	File Control #

Task #	Task Description:			
Hazard Type:	Hazard Description:			
Consequence:	Hazard Controls:			

Rational or Comments:		Safety Review By:	Date of Review

★OSHA form example was modified. Refer to the Job Hazard Analysis, OSHA Booklet # 3071, 2002 (Revised).

List of PPE and Engineering Controls for Use with Cytotoxic Drug Hazard Task Risk Analysis/Signs

PPE and Engineering Symbols	Description	PPE and Engineering Symbols	Description
	Gown, impervious to cytotoxic drugs of interest		Disposable n100 or p100 half-face NIOSH approved respirator complying with NIOSH (standard 29 CFR 1910.134, "respiratory protection")(OSHA standard 29 CFR 1910.132, "general requirements")
	Shoe, covers		Half-face NIOSH approved respirator with n/p100 cartridges complying with NIOSH (standard 29 CFR 1910.134, "respiratory protection") (OSHA standard 29 CFR 1910.132, "general requirements")
	Apron, impervious to cytotoxic drugs		Encapsulated chemical suite impervious to cytotoxic drugs with boots
	Chemotherapy gloves, impervious to cytotoxic drugs (tested against cytotoxic drugs, with manufacturer's breakthrough data available) (OSHA standard 29 CFR 1910.138, "Hand Protection") (OSHA standard 29 CFR 1910.132, "General Requirements")		Airline with escape bottle or SCBA, demand positive pressure (standard 29 CFR 1910.134, "respiratory protection") (OSHA standard 29 CFR 1910.132, "general requirements")
	Splash goggles (complying with ANSI z87.1-1989) (OSHA standard 29 CFR 1910.133, "Eye And Face Protection")		Absorbent pads
	Face shield (complying with ansi z87.1-1989) (OSHA standard 29 CFR 1910.133, "Eye And Face Protection")(OSHA standard 29 CFR 1910.132, "General Requirements")		Secondary containment
	Luer-lock@ fittings or similar device is preferred over using push connections on syringes, tubing and iv sets. Luer-lok@ fittings should always be used during drug transfers from vials to syringes or from syringes to intravenous sets. These devices should be implemented as an engineering control under your chemical ALARA program to meet OSHA guidelines and other regulatory guidelines.		Closed system—a closed system is defined as a device that does not exchange unfiltered air or contaminants with the adjacent environment. A closed system should be implemented as an engineering control under the chemical ALARA program to meet OSHA guidelines and other guidelines.
	Barrier isolator		Biological safety cabinet (BSC) class ii or class iii 100% exhausted outside of the work environment) is the primary control measure used to reduce or eliminate potential exposure to cytotoxic drugs. BSCs should be serviced and certified by a qualified technician at least every six months. In addition, a technician should check the BSC any time the cabinet is repaired or moved.

Date: _____   Location: _____

_____

Assessment Conducted By:

_____

_____

Specific Tasks Performed at This Location:

_____

_____

_____

_____

Hazard Assessment and Selection of Personal Protective Equipment

I. Overhead Hazards

Hazards to consider include:

Suspended loads that could fall
Overhead beams or loads that could be hit against
Energized wires or equipment that could be hit against
Employees work at elevated site that could drop objects on others below
Sharp objects or corners at head level

Hazards Identified:

_____

_____

_____

Head Protection

Hard Hat:	Yes	No
If yes, type:		
Type A (impact and penetration resistance, plus low-voltage electrical insulation)		
Type B (impact and penetration resistance, plus high-voltage electrical insulation)		
Type C (impact and penetration resistance)		

II. Eye and Face Hazards

Hazards to consider include:

Chemical splashes
Dust
Smoke and fumes
Welding operations
Lasers/optical radiation
Bioaerosols
Projectiles

Hazards Identified:

_____

_____

_____

Eye Protection

Safety glasses or goggles   Yes   No
Face shield   Yes   No

III. Hand Hazards

Hazards to consider include:

Chemicals
Sharp edges, splinters, etc.
Temperature extremes
Biological agents
Exposed electrical wires
Sharp tools, machine parts, etc.
Material handling

Hazards Identified:

_____

_____

_____

Hand Protection

Gloves	Yes	No
Chemical resistant (Chemotherapy)		
Temperature resistant		
Abrasion resistant		
Other (Explain)		

IV. Foot Hazards

Hazards to consider include:

Heavy materials handled by employees
Sharp edges or points (puncture risk)
Exposed electrical wires
Unusually slippery conditions
Contamination hazard
Wet conditions
Construction/demolition

Hazards Identified:

_____

_____

_____

Foot Protection

Safety shoes	Yes	No
Types:		
Toe protection		
Metatarsal protection		
Puncture resistant		
Electrical insulation		
Other (Explain)		

V. Other Identified Safety and/or Health Hazards

I certify that the above inspection was performed to the best of my knowledge and ability, based on the hazards present on _____.

_____   _____

(Signature)   (Date)

Rationale for Adopting the Environmental Sentinel Contamination Action Level (ESCAL) Concept

Current regulatory guidelines (OSHA Hazardous Drugs Guidelines, USACHPPM TG 149, Preventing Occupational Exposure to Antineoplastic and Other Hazardous Drugs in Health Care Settings [NIH Publication 2004], ASHP Guidelines for Handling Hazardous Drugs and Prudent Industrial Hygiene Practice) recommends for occupational exposures to hazardous drugs especially cytotoxic investigational drugs be eliminated or reduce to a lowest level possible. The implementation of the Environmental Sentinel Contamination Action Level (ESCAL) concept will ensure occupational exposures to hazardous (cytotoxic) drugs are decreased in accordance with previously cited references. The ESCAL process couples a proactive ALARA★ program with a quantitative analytical monitoring to ascertain how successful safe work practices, engineering and administrative controls are being administered by supervisors and overseen by the local Hazardous Drug Committee Furthermore, implementation of the ESCAL program will ensure due diligence is achieved in preventing or reducing occupational exposure by using a systematic approach in applying hierarchical control measures (engineering controls and personal protective equipment) and procedures are formalized in the local Hazardous Drug Safety and Health Plan. Refer to the Hierarchical Control Measures—Logic Sequence Diagram below.

Hierarchical Control Measures – Logic Sequence

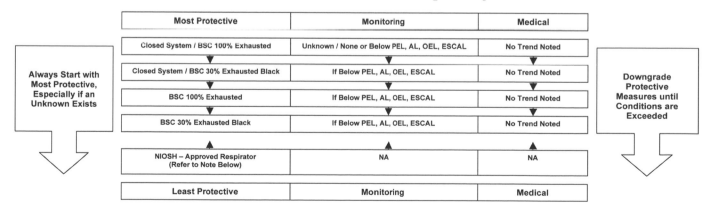

Note: Usually PPE (i.e., respirators) are used in conjunction with safe work practices, engineering, and administrative controls whenever work exposures cannot be reduced to acceptable limits without using the approved PPE (i.e., respirators).

★ The "ALARA" term may need to be changed to "ALAP" (As Low as Practical) if this term is used in the new TB MED (ALAP is considered an obsolete term). Australia and Great Britain uses "As Low as Reasonable Practical" (ALARP). The two terms mean essentially the same thing and their core is the concept of "reasonable practicable"; that involves weighing a risk against the trouble, time, and money needed to control it. Therefore, ALARA and ALARP describe the level to which we realistically expect to see workplace risks controlled.

There is limited but increasing scientific evidence that personnel involved in the preparation and administration of parenteral cytotoxic (antineoplastic) drugs may be at some risk due to potential mutangenicity, teratogenicity, and/or carcinogenicity of these agents. Some cytotoxic drugs toxicological properties have not been fully investigated while others are considered investigational drugs. By definition investigational drugs are drugs whereby toxicological properties have not been fully investigated, *particularly* as it pertains to occupational exposure of workers. In most cases, there are no known safe established occupational exposure levels (OEL) to cytotoxic drugs. Therefore, safe work practices, engineering and administrative controls, personal protective equipment, occupational and environmental monitoring are used to reduce contamination levels to as low as reasonably achievable (ALARA).

The Environmental Sentinel Contamination Action Level (ESCAL) is defined as the lowest feasible detection concentration of a drug based on the selected analytical method. The ESCAL is use to determine the effectiveness of safe work practices and engineering controls, unless there is an established OSHA PEL or ACGIH TLV whereby both (ESCAL and PEL or/and TLV) would be used to determine compliance and effectiveness of work practices and engineering controls. Here is an example of how ESCAL is systematically applied: if ESCAL concentration are detected for selected hazardous (cytotoxic) drugs, than a revaluation of existing engineering controls, safe work practices, and personal protective equipment (PPE) must be performed; and corrective action must be implemented to eliminate or reduce the environmental surface contamination levels. Engineering controls (BSC class 2 with 100% exhaust, barrier chambers with 100% exhaust, closed systems, etc.), safe work practices should be implemented prior to requiring staff to wear PPE. If after implementation of all feasible corrective actions, an ESCAL concentration is still present, continued emphases must be maintained on environmental contamination reduction to achieve levels to As Low as Reasonably Achievable (ALARA) or they are below detectable limits, using selected analytical methods. The local Hazardous Drug Committee maintains documentations in accordance with the local Hazardous Drug Safety and Health Plan.

Potential regulatory compliance implications may come from the Occupational Safety and Health Administration (OSHA), which has not set specific permissible exposure limits (PELs) for most cytotoxic drugs but has issued guidelines urging employers to set up a Hazardous Drugs Safety and Health Plan, which incorporates the use of engineering controls, personal protective equipment, and safe work practices that assist in keeping occupational exposures as low as possible. A gross violation of such guidelines or equivalent procedures or lack of exposure data could result in a citation under the General Duty Clause of the Occupational Safety and Health Act (Public Law 91-596).

United States Pharmacopoeia (USP) is the official public standards-setting authority for all prescription and over-the-counter medicines, dietary supplements, and other healthcare products manufactured and sold in the United States. USP has recently released a new standard entitled USP Chapter 797. The purpose of USP Chapter 797 is to describe conditions and practices to prevent harm, including death, to patients that could result from the following: (1) microbial contamination (non-sterility); (2) excessive bacterial endotoxins; (3) variability in the intended strength of correct ingredients that exceeds either monograph limits for official articles (see "official" and "article" in the General Notices and Requirements) or 10 percent for nonofficial articles; (4) unintended chemical and physical contaminants; and (5) incorrect types and qualities of ingredients in Compounded Sterile Preparations (CSPs). Nonsterile CSPs are potentially most hazardous to patients when administered into body cavities, central nervous and vascular systems, eyes, and joints; and when used as baths for live organs and tissues.

As stated above, patient safety is the primary emphasis of USP Chapter 797, not employee safety. However, several areas of USP Chapter 797 can be used to augment Hazardous Drugs safety and health guidance set forth by OSHA, NIOSH, ASHP, and USACHPPM TG 149. Under the USP Chapter 797 Hazardous Drugs states:

- Hazardous drugs shall only be prepared for administration under conditions that protect the healthcare workers and other personnel in the preparation and administration.
- Hazardous drugs shall be stored separately from other inventory in a manner to prevent contamination and personnel exposure. Such storage is preferably within a containment area such as a negative pressure room. The storage area must have sufficient general exhaust ventilation, at least 12 air exchanges per hour (ACPH) to dilute and remove any airborne contaminants.
- Hazardous drugs shall be handled with caution using appropriate chemotherapy gloves during distribution, receiving, stocking, inventorying, preparing for administration, and disposal.
- Hazardous drugs shall be prepared in an ISO Class 5 environment with protective engineering controls in place, and following aseptic practices specified for the appropriate contamination risk levels defined in this chapter.
- Access shall be limited to areas where drugs are stored and prepared to protect persons not involved in drug preparation.
- All hazardous drugs shall be prepared in a Class II or III biological safety cabinet (BSC), or a compounding aseptic isolator (CAI) that meets or exceeds the standards for CAI in this chapter.
- Covers other primary engineering controls—refer to USP Chapter 797 for details. (Other references: Medical Air Solutions, LLC discussion concerning USP 797 http://medicalairsolutions.com/usp797.htm.)
- Appropriate personnel protective equipment (PPE) shall be worn when compounding in a BSC or CAI, and when using CSTD (closed-system vial transfer device). Appropriate PPE may include gowns, facemasks, eye protection, hair covers, shoe covers or dedicated shoes, double gloving, and complying with manufacturers' recommendations when using CAI (www.cdc.gov/niosh/docs/2004-165/).
- All personnel who compound hazardous drugs shall be fully trained in the storage, handling, and disposal of these drugs. This training shall occur prior to preparing or handling hazardous CSPs, and its effectiveness shall be verified by testing specific hazardous drugs preparation techniques; such verification shall be documented

for each person at least annually. This training must include didactic overview of hazardous drugs including mutagenic, teratogenic, and carcinogenic properties, and it shall include ongoing training for each new hazardous drug that enters the marketplace. Compounding personnel of reproductive capability must confirm in writing that they understand the risks of handling hazardous drugs. The training shall include at least the following: (1) safe aseptic manipulation practices; (2) negative pressure techniques when utilizing BSC or CAI; (3) correct use of CSTD devices; (4) containment, cleanup, and disposal procedures for breakages and spills; and (5) treatment of personnel contact and inhalation exposure.

- Because standards of assay and unacceptable quantities of contamination of each drug have not been established in the literature, the following paragraph is a recommendation only. Future standards will be adopted as these assay methods are developed and proven. Ongoing quality assurance shall be an integral part of hazardous drug preparation. In order to assure containment, especially in operations preparing large volumes of hazardous drugs, environmental sampling to detect uncontained hazardous drugs needs to be performed routinely: e.g., initially as a benchmark and at least every 6 months. This sampling shall include surface wipe sampling of the working area of BSC and CAI, counter tops where finished preparations are placed, areas adjacent to BSC and CAI, including the floor directly under the working area, and patient administration areas. Common marker hazardous drugs that can be assayed include cyclophosphamide, ifosfamide, methotrexate, and fluorouracil. If any measurable contamination (cyclophosphamide levels greater than 1.00 ng/cm2 has been found to cause human uptake) is found by any of these quality assurance procedures, practitioners shall make the decision to identify, document, and contain the cause of contamination. Such action may include retraining, thorough cleaning, and improving engineering controls.

- Disposal of all hazardous drug wastes shall comply with all applicable federal and state regulations. All personnel who perform routine custodial waste removal and cleaning activities in storage and preparation areas for hazardous drugs shall be trained in appropriate procedures to protect themselves and prevent contamination. The NIOSH Publication No. 2004-165 at www.cdc.gov/niosh/docs/2004-165/ and the references under the heading Sterile Hazardous Preparations at www.ashp.org/SterileCpd/ are recommended sources for education and training in principles and practices of safety with hazardous drugs.

- The BSC and Compounding Aseptic Isolator (CAI) (barrier isolators) optimally shall be 100% vented to the outside air through HEPA filtration (see the Ventilated cabinet section at www.cdc.gov/niosh/docs/2004-165/).

- Other related sections—Radiopharmaceuticals—Refer to USP Chapter 797, Radiopharmaceuticals for specific information.

This summary is not intended to take the place of reading and understanding USP Chapter 797 and other related standards (NIOSH, OSHA, and JCAHO).

Principal Engineering Controls

Closed Systems

There are two official definitions related to what is considered a closed system. A closed system is defined as a device that does not exchange unfiltered air or contaminants with the adjacent environment. Another definition is a closed-system drug-transfer device, which is a drug-transfer device that mechanically prohibits the transfer of environmental contaminants into toxicity, reproductive toxicity in humans, organ toxicity at low doses in humans or animals, genotoxicity, or new drugs that mimic existing hazardous drugs in structure or toxicity.

Consider using devices such as closed-system transfer devices, glove bags, and needleless systems when transferring hazardous drugs from primary packaging (such as vials) to dosing equipment (such as infusion bags, bottles, or pumps). Closed systems limit the potential for generating aerosols and exposing workers to sharps. Remember that a closed-system transfer device is not an acceptable substitute for a ventilated cabinet and should be used *only* within a ventilated cabinet. Furthermore, use appropriate PPE and work practices even when you are using a closed-system.

Administer drugs safely by using protective medical devices (such as needleless and closed systems) and techniques (such as priming of IV tubing by pharmacy personnel inside a ventilated cabinet or priming inline with no drug solutions).

Do not use supplemental engineering or process controls (such as needleless systems, glove bags, and closed-system drug-transfer devices) as a substitution for ventilated cabinets (BSCs), even though such controls may reduce the potential for exposure when preparing and administering hazardous drugs.

A closed system for delivery of cytotoxic drugs can reduce or eliminate human exposure to cancer chemotherapy drugs in the workplace. A closed system consists of a set of disposable containment devices that connect the original drug vial, syringe and IV injection or infusion set together into a completely sealed pathway. The system's double membrane prevents drug leakage and keeps the connections dry. A built-in expansion chamber equalizes system pressure to prevent the release of toxic aerosols and vapors. A protector with a flexible bulb fits onto the drug vial and equalizes air pressure in the vial during drug preparation when air or diluents are injected or withdrawn. The system's double membrane is designed to prevent leaks during drug transfers and disconnections. The injector element uses a needle that is never exposed, preventing needle-stick injuries and avoiding leakage during injection. The connector allows for a dry-spike connection. Because it is a closed system, hazardous drugs are contained throughout the entire process of drug transfer, preparation, transport, administration, and disposal. An example of a closed system sold in the United States is the PhaSeal's®Baxa Corp., manufactured by the Baxa Corporation (www.baxa.com/) and/or www.isips.org/presentations/PhaSeal/player.html.

Locking Systems

Luer-lock® fittings is preferred over using push connections on syringes, tubing, and IV sets. Luer-Lok® at various manufacturers fittings or other brands should always be used during drug transfers from vials to syringes or from syringes to intravenous sets.

Clearlink® Baxter combines standard set technology with unique design characteristics including a nonlatex, clear polycarbonate housing, a large easy-to-swab injection surface and a silicone-based double design. This cost-effective access system virtually eliminates needle-stick injuries during IV set access procedures. Safety focused health-care workers: Clearlink® Baxter's double seal design helps prevent back pressure and leakage since the seal tightens in relation to increased back pressure. This unique design also helps prevent valve leakage, a potential safety issue for blood-borne pathogens. Patient safety: the clear housing enables visualization of the fluid path. Clinicians can monitor what is happening inside the valve, helping them detect precipitates from incompatible drugs or blood clots resulting from inadequate flushing. Other features: needleless, reduces needle-stick injuries, and helps facilities meet OSHA safety standards; robust double seal design—helps prevent back pressure leakage; fewer system components—streamlines inventory/purchasing process.

Cytotoxic Sharps Containers

Exposures to hazardous drugs may occur through inhalation, skin contact, skin absorption, ingestion, or injection. Inhalation and skin contact/absorption are the most likely routes of exposure, but unintentional ingestion from hand to mouth contact and unintentional injection through a needle-stick or sharps injury are also possible. Place empty vials and sharps such as needles and syringes in chemotherapy waste containers designed to protect workers from injuries and dispose of them by incineration at a regulated medical waste facility. *Do not* place hazardous drug–contaminated sharps in red sharps containers that are used for infectious wastes, since these are often autoclaved or microwaved. Cytotoxic sharps containers mist be appropriately identified and disposed of in accordance with local policy and SOPs.

Emergency Eyewash and Showers

If all protective measures fail and an employee receives a chemical splash, then emergency eyewash and shower should be installed near the preparation and administration areas to comply with American National Standards Institute (ANSI) Z358.1-2004. ANSI Z358.1-2004 establishes minimum performance requirements for eyewash and shower equipment for the emergency treatment of the eyes or body of a person who has been exposed to injurious materials. Eyewash fountains should be tested weekly and documented by allowing the water to run for at least 3 minutes to ensure proper operation and to flush stagnant water from the water supply lines.

Employees should familiarize themselves with the location and operation of the nearest emergency eyewash and shower. Always flood the eyes for at least 15 to 30 minutes to be sure there is no residue of the corrosive liquid. Flush from the eye outward. After thorough washing, seek medical care. This is because serious damage may have already occurred before the eye was thoroughly rinsed and/or the damage may not be immediately apparent.

Isolator Barrier Used for Hazardous Drugs (Cytotoxic Drugs)

Compounding isolator is generally defined as a class of isolator designed for use during pharmacy drug compounding. Compounding isolators utilize an airtight glove/glove port design that allows the user to perform hands-on tasks inside the isolator without compromising the intended performance of the isolator.

There are two types of compounding isolators, each named according to their design objective: Compounding Aseptic Isolator and Compounding Aseptic Containment Isolator. Among other features, the compounding isolator achieves its design objective through the following:

- The intentional use of air pressure relationships that define the direction of airflow in/out of the cabinet.
- The use of airflow capture velocities to capture and remove aerosolized drug product near its point of generation.
- The use of high-efficiency filtration systems (HEPA minimum) to capture aerosolized drug preparations and particulate contamination.
- The use of external venting to remove vaporized hazardous drugs from work chamber and from the pharmacy.
- The use of material transfer processes that allow material transfer in/out of the compounding isolator without compromising worker exposure to undesirable levels of airborne drug or unwittingly compromising the sterility of the compounding environment.

Name of Isolator	Type of Isolator	Purpose	Building Exhaust Requirements	Placement of Barrier Isolator
Compounding Aseptic Containment Isolator— nonrecirculating	Negative pressure with total exhaust	Compounding hazardous drugs including those that volatilize (cytotoxic drugs)	Must be properly connected from building in accordance with air solution regulators	Must be located in an area devoted to hazardous drug naming. Preferred to be located in a clean room. If located in an uncontrolled room, it should be proven that the isolator prevents transfer of unfiltered room air into the isolator during material transfer or compounding operations

The isolator design should facilitate physical disinfection of all work surfaces. Interior seams should be shaped and sized to facilitate easy cleaning. All interior surfaces should be easily reached through the gloves to accommodate cleaning. If the interior is designed in a manner that does not permit easy physical disinfection of all surfaces, an alternative gaseous decontamination process must be developed and validated.

Manipulations within a barrier isolator are conducted through a glove/sleeve (gauntlet) assembly. Two types of glove/sleeve assemblies are available:

1. One-Part: The one-part assembly is where the glove and sleeve are of a single, unbroken unit.
2. Two-Part: The two-part assembly is where the glove and sleeve are separate and are connected at the sleeve (gauntlet) by some type of seal system. The two-part system allows for the relatively simple change-out of gloves.

The type of work conducted in the isolator and the disinfectants that will be used should be taken into consideration in determining the glove material. Commonly used materials include Neoprene®DuPont, Hypalon®DuPont, nitrile, and latex. The gloves must have sufficient chemical resistance to stand up to decontaminating chemicals, cleaning agents, and process materials. Special gloves developed for use with chemotherapy agents is appropriate for cytotoxic drugs applications. It is common practice to use a double glove system to minimize the possibility of a tear or leak to compromise the environment within the isolator. An ordinary latex glove or chemo gloves can be worn underneath the isolator glove and changed as needed. Glove life will be affected by the cleaning agents, solvents, and process materials (cytotoxic drugs, etc.). A faulty glove will represent a potential route of exposure to the product and may expose the operator to hazardous drugs. Gloves should be inspected daily for pinholes as well as breaches at seams, gaskets, and seals. A regular replacement program should be established so gloves are replaced before a breach of integrity occurs or chemical breakthrough occurs.

The transfer of materials into and out of the isolator is one of the greatest potential sources of contamination. There are three basic types of pass-through that are employed in the design of an open compounding-isolator system—static air, dilution airflow, and unidirectional airflow. In all cases, the pass-through must be designed to effectively isolate the interior of the isolator from the room when materials are transported in and out, and where containment is required, isolate the operator and room from the hazardous drugs.

Static Pass-Through: In its most basic form, a static pass-through is a box with doors on two sides that is sealed to the isolator. Materials are placed into the pass-through from the outside door. After the materials are placed inside, the outside door is closed. The inside door can then be opened and materials passed through to the isolator. The process is reversed for material removal from the isolator.

Dilution and Unidirectional Airflow Pass-Through: Improvements over the static air pass-through are dilution control and unidirectional pass-through because the particulate level in the pass-through can be reduced before opening the door to the main body of the isolator. Airborne particulate levels can be reduced with a dilution-controlled pass-through or virtually eliminated with a unidirectional pass-through.

To prevent direct exposure between the compounding isolator main chamber and the room, both pass-through doors should not be open at the same time. The installation of door interlocks may be used to prevent simultaneous opening, and timers may be used to aid operators. The interior pressure of the compounding aseptic isolator should be sufficient to prevent air movement from the pass-through to the main work chamber and in the case of compounding aseptic containment isolators; both prevent air movement from the pass-through to the main work chamber and contain the hazardous preparation for operator protection. Manufacturer validation of the appropriate time required and procedures before opening either the exterior or the interior door should be provided.

A benefit of unidirectional airflow pass-through is that the materials can be removed from the outer packaging in the pass-through prior to entry into the compounding chamber. This will reduce the potential of contamination build up in the compounding area when the packaging is opened. The goal of compounding isolators is to "isolate" the work area from the surrounding room and any potential source of contamination.

Regardless of the isolator type, opening and closing the pass-through to the room may allow some room air into the pass-through. Additionally, there will be some surface contamination on the material that is brought into the unit via the pass-through. A dilution-controlled isolator dilutes out the airborne contamination over time. A unidirectional isolator will flush out the contamination almost immediately with a continuous bath of HEPA filtered air. Any airborne contamination that is brought in through the pass-through with the product is swept away, carried to the return, and removed from the work zone. Note that for both unidirectional and turbulent flow isolators, provisions should be made to address the issue of surface contamination on inbound materials.

Care should be taken to avoid the ingress of any airborne particles from the external environment by induction at product ingress locations such as the pass-through door. This induction can occur from local turbulent flow causing air swirls or backflows into the isolator from the room in both positive and negative pressure isolators. Additionally, negative pressure isolators are more susceptible to drawing room air in to the work chamber, so the operation of the pass-through must incorporate this condition into the overall design of the isolator.

Ergonomic Considerations in Isolators: Working in an isolator can often involve long periods with arms in a relatively still position. Comfortable working conditions are obviously very important. Consideration to worker comfort is recommended as part of any isolator purchase. Some manufacturers have height adjustors available as part of their units. This should allow a relatively easy transition from short to tall operators or from sitting to standing working positions. In addition, the design should have front view screen and glove ports sized and positioned to allow comfortable and efficient work. It should be noted that height adjustors might not work with units connected to an external exhaust system. Flexible duct connections may help but may limit the length of travel.

Placement and Clean Zone Classification: USP Chapter 797 requires a minimum cleanliness classification of ISO class 5 for the compounding zone within the isolator. ISO (International Organization for Standardization) class 5 should be stated as follows; class 5 at 0.5 μm particles under dynamic operating conditions. What is less clear is what classification the surrounding room needs to meet. USP 797 states, "The contamination reduction conditions and procedures in this section include LAFWs (laminar airflow workbenches) being located within buffer or room areas that maintain at least an ISO Class 8." "It is preferred, but not necessary, to locate barrier isolators within such a buffer air quality area."

Compounding isolators should be placed in an ISO class 7 (Note: The USP Sterile Compounding Expert Panel required ISO Class 8 in chapter 797, but is on record as recommending ISO in the next revision) cleanroom unless they can prove the following:

1. The compounding isolator truly isolates the work area from the room. Isolator zone particulate levels should not increase from static conditions at any time by either material transfer or product manipulation.
2. Aseptic technique is aided by a flow of HEPA filtered air across the entire work area and process-generated contamination is immediately pulled from the isolator return grilles.
3. Compounding aseptic containment isolators must be located in an area that is devoted to that purpose alone and is restricted to authorized personnel.

Isolator barriers must be certified in accordance with manufacturer's specifications every six months or sooner if repairs are made or the unit is relocated by an NSF International or equivalent certified technician, and documentation must be maintained in accordance with local regulations.

Introduction to Applied Toxicology

General

"All substances are poisons—the difference is in the dose." This aphorism is attributed to Paracelsus. It illustrates that the potential for harm is widespread and all chemicals could be toxic but the degree of harm that a chemical can inflict on a human or any other living being depends on the dose or the degree of exposure as well as on other factors.

Toxicity is a physiological property of matter that defines the capacity of a chemical to harm or injure a living organism by other than mechanical means. The toxicity of a chemical depends upon the degree of exposure. In other words, the risk (i.e., that product of the likelihood and the severity of harm) from a toxic hazard depends on the exposure.

Hazard is regarded as the probability that this toxic concentration in the body will occur. Many factors contribute to determining the degree of hazard; that is, the physical state of the substance, route of entry, dosage, physiological state, environmental variable, engineering controls, personal protective equipment used, and many others.

A toxic substance cannot produce systemic injury unless it gains entry into the bloodstream (body). Common route of entries are ingestion, injection, skin absorption, and inhalation. The material and its specific properties will determine which routes will be potential paths for exposure. For example, a cytotoxic drug provided in a tablet or capsule form would have less potential for exposing the person administrating the medicine body than if provided in a liquid form that must be diluted, that is if the tablets or capsules were not crushed or opened or handled with bare hands prior to administrating it to the patient.

Many of the MSDSs are written based on the *worst case* for pharmaceutical manufacturing not in a clinical setting. A reasonable person would expect a worker in a drug manufacturing process to have a greater opportunity for exposure than a pharmacist working with cytotoxic drugs in a biological safety cabinet or barrier isolator.

All toxicological considerations are based on the dose-response relationship. The dose-response relationship is the correlation between the amount of exposure to a toxic substance and the resulting effect on the body. A toxic substance cannot produce systemic injury unless it gains entry into the bloodstream (body). Common route of entries are ingestion, injection, skin absorption and inhalation. The material and its specific properties will determine which routes will be potential paths for exposure.

In a typical healthcare facility, cytotoxic (antineoplastic) drugs are anticancer agents used to treat patients, but the drugs also have toxic effects on healthy cells, and thus pose a health risk to those employees who are involved in their transportation, preparation, storage, administration, and disposal. Workers risking occupational exposure include pharmacists, pharmacy technicians, nurses, physicians, respiratory therapists, housekeeping staff, hazardous waste collection staff, and safety and health staff.

Health Effects

Many of the cytotoxic drugs are investigational drugs. Investigational drugs by definition are drugs whereby toxicological properties have not been fully investigated, *particularly* as it pertains to occupational exposure of workers. In some cases, toxicological information for certain CDs is solely based on animal studies, while in other cases it is extrapolated from clinical (therapeutic) exposure data. Several of the drug manufacturers provided exposure data based on manufacturing operations, where possibilities for occupational exposure is higher than in a clinical environmental. It is prudent to limit exposure by using appropriate engineering, personal protective equipment, and best practices/administrative procedures, since in most cases there are no established safe occupational exposure limits (OEL) to investigational (cytotoxic) drugs.

Drugs come in several different forms and can have different effects on your body. Some chemicals cause "acute" problems that you feel right away such as breathing difficulties, nausea, headache, allergic reactions, skin injury, hearing disorders, eye problems, and rashes. Other drugs cause "chronic" problems where the effects of exposure may not be evident for months or even years. An example of chronic affects are carcinogens, *teratogen*, reproductive effects (male and female), and miscarriages, as well as chromosomal damage (mutagens).

How CDs Enter the Body

There are four basic ways a chemical can enter the body: inhalation, ingestion, absorption, and injection. Working with cytotoxic drugs, exposure is mainly through inhaling droplets or dusts. Some CDs can also be absorbed through the skin, from eye contact, accidental injection, or by swallowing food/beverages, or smoking, which are contaminated with CDs.

What You Can Do to Prevent Exposure to Cytotoxic Drugs

Ensure that you have completed all required training to perform your job duties and that you have obtaining medical clearance to work with CDs. Prior to handling CDs, review the Manufacturer's Material Safety Data Sheet and other secondary sources of technical information (such as this handbook). Select the appropriate personal protective equipment (PPE) based on this information and wear the selected PPE properly. Ensure that PPE are properly worn and that engineering controls are working properly prior to commencing handling CDs or contaminated materials. Review emergency procedures and ensure appropriate spill kits are available within the immediate work area. Locate the emergency shower/eye wash located in your area in case contact with CDs occurs. Follow local SOPs, this handbook, and guidance found in the references section listed in section 3.23.

How to Read and Understand a
Material Safety Data Sheet (MSDS)

Section I: Basic Product Information/Material Identification

1. Trade Name or Synonym—Self-Explanatory
2. Manufacturer's Name and Address—Self-Explanatory
3. Emergency Telephone Number—Self-Explanatory
4. Chemical Name of Product—Self-Explanatory
5. Date Prepared—Signifies the date the original MSDS information was complied or last updated. This information should be used to verify whether a new MSDS has been updated or is a duplicate of current MSDS on file.
6. Optional information—Name of person who prepared the MSDS.

Section II: Hazardous Ingredients/Identity Information

1. Which chemicals are covered—The percentage concentration of each substance in a mixture may also be listed, but not required.
2. What are the names of the chemicals—A trade name is the brand name; a generic name describes a family or group of chemicals, i.e., chlorinated hydrocarbons. The law says that chemical names must also be listed.
3. The chemical or specific name is the one that describes the specific chemical. The chemical name is the easiest name to use when doing research on the health effects of chemicals they represent.
4. The CAS number is a number given by the Chemical Abstract Service to each chemical. While different, may have the same name, but they will all have their own CAS number, which can be used to look up information.
5. The MSDS must list the chemical names of all hazardous ingredients, which make up more than 1% of the mixture (or 0.1% for cancer-causing substances). Listing only the trade name, only the CAS number, or only the generic name is not acceptable.

Section III: Physical/Chemical Data

1. Boiling Point: The temperature in degrees F at which a liquid boils (becomes a vapor) under normal atmospheric conditions. The lower the boiling point, the quicker it evaporates, and the easier it is to inhale. Chemicals with boiling points below 100°C (212°F) require special caution.
2. Vapor Pressure of saturated vapor above the liquid in mercury at 68° F. A high vapor pressure indicates that a liquid will evaporate easily. Liquids with high vapor pressure may be especially hazardous if you are working with them in a confined space or an enclosed area.
3. Vapor Density: If the vapor density is less than one, it will tend to rise in air. If the vapor density is greater than one, it will fall in air and concentrate in the bottom of tanks or confined spaces.
4. Specific Gravity: If the specific gravity is greater than one, the substance will sink in water; if less than one, it will float on top of water.

5. Evaporation Rate: This is the rate at which a substance evaporates compared to either ether, which evaporates quickly, or butyl acetate, which evaporates slowly. If the substance has an evaporation rate greater than one, it evaporates faster than the comparison substance.

Section IV: Fire and Explosion Hazard Data

This section should provide information on the fire hazards of a product and special precautions necessary to extinguish a fire.

1. Flash Point: This is the lowest temperature at which a liquid gives off enough vapor to form a mixture with air that can be ignited by a spark. Liquid with a flash point below 100° F is considered flammable. Liquid with a flash point between 100° and 200° F is combustible.
2. Extinguishing Media: This section should specify what kind of fire extinguisher to use.
3. Special fire fighting procedures and unusual fire and explosion hazards.

Section V: Reactivity Data

When stored improperly, some chemicals can react with other chemicals and release dangerous materials. This section describes the reaction of chemicals when they are mixed together with other chemicals, or when stored or handled improperly.

Section VI: Health Hazard Data

This section describes the health effects of the products, including signs and symptoms of exposure, and medical conditions made worse by exposure. Acute (short-term) and chronic (long-term) effects of exposure must always be included. Furthermore, this section must contain information on target organs (liver, kidneys, or central nervous system), signs or symptoms of exposure, medical conditions generally aggravated by exposure, and emergency first aid.

Section VII: Precautions for Safe Handling and Use (Spill or Leak Procedures)

This section contains information on proper equipment to use and what precautions to follow if a spill or leak occur. It should also describe safe waste disposal methods and precautions to be taken in handling and storing.

Section VIII: Control Measures

This section must contain list of control measures that can reduce or eliminate the hazard, including ventilation and other engineering controls, safe work practices, and personal protective equipment.

The Hazardous Material Information System (HMIS) is a computerized information management system containing information concerning characteristics of hazardous materials, which exist throughout the Department of Defense (DoD). One aspect of this system is the DOD hazardous chemical warning system, which establishes a method of communicating standardized warning information to DoD personnel when manufacturer's labels cannot be used or to supplement existing labels. The HMIS label, Like the NFPA 704 diamond, provides hazardous information. HMIS uses color for type of hazard and numbers for the degree of the hazard, 4 being the most hazardous. Furthermore, the HMIS system can provide information on the type of personal protective equipment (PPE) that should be used when handling this material. In this category, a letter is used to indicate what combination of PPE should be used to provide adequate protection. When available, HMIS information is furnished in the Safety and Health Handbook for Cytotoxic Drugs for specific cytotoxic drugs and will assist in filling out Hazardous Material Information System Labels as depicted below and will assist in manually filling out a DoD Hazardous Material Warning Label (DOD Form 2521 and DOD Form 2522).

HMIS	
HEALTH [blue]	
FIRE HAZARD [red]	
REACTIVITY [yellow]	
PERSONAL PROTECTION [white]	

PPE Categories

A = Safety glasses
B = Safety glasses, chemical gloves
C = Safety glasses, chemical gloves, chemical apron
D = Face shield, chemical gloves, chemical apron
E = Safety glasses, chemical gloves, dust respirator
F = safety glasses, chemical gloves, chemical apron, dust respirator
G = Safety glasses, gloves, vapor respirator
H = Splash goggles, chemical gloves, chemical apron, vapor respirator
I = Safety glasses, gloves, dust and vapor respirator
J = Splash goggles, gloves, chemical apron, dust and vapor respirator

K = Air line hood or mask, gloves, full chemical suit, boots
N = Splash goggles
O = Face shield
P = Chemical (Chemo) gloves
X = Ask Supervisor or Standard Operating Procedure
— = None specified by manufacturer but PPE may be required for your task—ask your supervisor

Note: Before using any respirator/mask, check with your supervisor, safety representative, and/or industrial hygiene staff for assistance.

When HMIS information is available, it is furnished in the Safety and Health Handbook for Cytotoxic Drugs, section 2.2, under the Health and Safety Hazards heading, and will assist in filling out Hazardous Material Information System Labels as depicted below, and in manually filling out a DoD Hazardous Material Warning Label (DOD Form 2521 and DOD Form 2522).

Hazardous Material Information System (HMIS) Example

HEALTH	2*
FIRE HAZARD	0
REACTIVITY	0
PERSONAL PROTECTION	-

National Fire Protection Association (NFPA) 704 Hazard Diamond

The NFPA Hazard Diamond is similar to the HMIS system described in the preceding Section 3.14. Both have four sections colored blue, red, yellow, and white. The higher the number, the more hazardous. Numbers range from 0 to 4. HMIS uses colored bars, while NFPA uses colored diamonds. HMIS attempts to convey full health warning information to all employees, while NFPA is meant primarily for fire fighters and other emergency responders. The following example will demonstrate how the NFPA 704 system works:

6-Thioguanine (154-42-7)
NFPA 704 Hazard Diamond

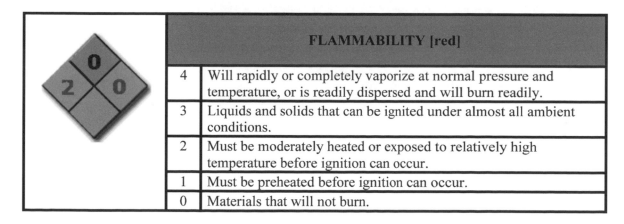

	HEALTH [blue]	
4	Very short exposure could cause death or serious residual injury even though prompt medical attention is given.
3	Short exposure could cause serious temporary or residual injury even though prompt medical attention is given.
2	Intense or continued exposure could cause temporary incapacitation or possible residual injury unless prompt medical attention is given.
1	Exposure under fire conditions would offer no hazard beyond that of ordinary combustion materials.
0	Exposure under fire conditions would offer no hazard beyond that of ordinary combustible materials.

	FLAMMABILITY [red]	
4	Will rapidly or completely vaporize at normal pressure and temperature, or is readily dispersed and will burn readily.
3	Liquids and solids that can be ignited under almost all ambient conditions.
2	Must be moderately heated or exposed to relatively high temperature before ignition can occur.
1	Must be preheated before ignition can occur.
0	Materials that will not burn.

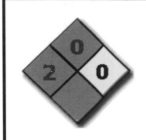	INSTABILITY [yellow]	
	4	Readily capable of detonation or of explosive decomposition or reaction at normal temperatures and pressures.
	3	Capable of detonation or explosive reaction, but requires a strong initiating source or must be heated under confinement before initiation, or reacts explosively with water.
	2	Normally unstable and readily undergo violent decomposition but do not detonate. Also may react violently with water or may form potentially explosive mixtures with water.
	1	Normally stable, but become unstable at elevated temperatures and pressures or may react with water with some release of energy, but not violently.
	0	Normally stable, even under fire exposure conditions, and are not reactive with water.

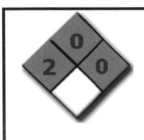	SPECIAL HAZARDS [white]	
	This section is used to denote special hazards. There are only two NFPA 704 approved symbols:	
	OX	This denotes an oxidizer, a chemical, which can greatly increase the rate of combustion/fire.
	W	Unusual reactivity with water. This indicates a potential hazard using water to fight a fire involving this material.
		Other symbols may be unofficially used. They are **ACID, ALK** (Alkaline/Base) & **COR** (corrosive).

United States Consensus Occupational Exposure Level(s)/Limits for Cytotoxic Drugs

Drug Nomenclature/ Chemical Abstracts System Registry Number (CAS)	Agency	Standard	Method(s)
ARSENIC TRIOXIDE (CAS: 1327-53-3)★ ★As Inorganic Compounds Arsenic (AS) (CAS: 7440-38-2)	OSHA	OSHA PEL: 0.01 MG/M3 (AS) ACTION LEVEL 5 µG/M3 TWA 8-HRS (AS) (REFER TO 29 CFR 1910.1018)	OSHA 1D-105 ALTERNATE OSHA 1006 NIOSH 7901
ARSENIC TRIOXIDE (CAS: 1327-53-3)★ ★As Inorganic Compounds Arsenic (AS) (CAS: 7440-38-2)	NIOSH	NIOSH REL: C 0.002 MG/M3 (AS)/15 MIN; CA NIOSH IDLH: 5 mg(AS).m3	OSHA 1D105 NIOSH 7901
ARSENIC TRIOXIDE (CAS: 1327-53-3)★ ★As (AS)	ACGIH	ACGIH TLV: 0.01 MG/M3 TWA; CA (A1—CONFIRMED HUMAN CARCINOGEN)	OSHA 1D105 NIOSH 7901
CARBOPLATIN (PARAPLATIN) (DIAMMINE)★ (C6H12N2O4Pt) (CAS: 41575-94-5) (CAS: 7440-06-4) ★As Pt	NIOSH	NIOSH REL: 2 µG/M3 TWA	NIOSH 7303; ICP-AES
CARBOPLATIN (PARAPLATIN) (DIAMMINE)★ (C6H12N2O4Pt) (CAS: 41575-94-5) (CAS: 7440-06-4) ★As (Pt)	OSHA	OSHA PLATINUM PEL : 2 µG/M3 TWA	OSHA ID130SG— AAS/GF OSHA ID-121

Drug Nomenclature/ Chemical Abstracts System Registry Number (CAS)	Agency	Standard	Method(s)
CARBOPLATIN (PARAPLATIN) (DIAMMINE) (C6H12N2O4Pt) (CAS: 41575-94-5) (CAS: 7440-06-4)	ACGIH	ACGIH TLV: 2 μG/ M3 TWA	N.O.S.
CISPLATIN (CIS-PLATIN) (PLATINOL AQ) (CAS: 15663-27-1)	OSHA	OSHA PEL: 0.002 MG/ M3 TWA (AS Pt)	OSHA ID 121 OSHA CSI SLCI; AAS/GF
CISPLATIN (CIS-PLATIN) (PLATINOL AQ) (CAS: 15663-27-1)	NIOSH	NIOSH REL 0.002 MG/ M3 TWA (Pt)	OSHA ID 121 OSHA CSI
CISPLATIN (CIS-PLATIN) (PLATINOL AQ) (CAS: 15663-27-1)	ACGIH	ACGIH TLV 0.002 MG/ M3 TWA	OSHA ID 121 OSHA CSI
NITROGEN MUSTARD-2, CHLORMETHINE (MECHLORETHANMINE) (CAS: 51-75-2) (CAS: 55-86-7)	TSG	TSG WORKING GROUP: 0.02 MG/M3 TWA HN-1: AIRBORNE EXPOSURE LIMIT (AS RECOMMENDED BY THE SURGEON GENERAL'S WORKING GROUP, U.S. DEPARTMENT OF HEALTH AND HUMAN SERVICES) = 0.003 MG/M^3 AS A TIME-WEIGHTED AVERAGE (TWA) FOR THE WORKPLACE. NO STANDARDS EXIST FOR HN-2 OR HN-3.	N.O.S.
NITROGEN MUSTARD-2, CHLORMETHINE (MECHLORETHANMINE) (CAS: 51-75-2) (CAS: 55-86-7)	DOE	TEEL-0: 1.25 MG/M3; TEEL-1: 4 MG/M3 TEEL-2 29 MG/M3; TEEL-3 29 MG/M3 (PEAK 15 MIN TWA PERIOD)	N.O.S.
NITROGEN MUSTARD-2, CHLORMETHINE (MECHLORETHANMINE) (CAS: 51-75-2) (CAS: 55-86-7)	EPA	ACUTE★ EXPOSURE GUIDELINE LEVELS (AEGLs) (MG/M3)	N.O.S.

Drug Nomenclature/ Chemical Abstracts System Registry Number (CAS)	Agency	Standard	Method(s)
		AEGL 1 10 MIN NR 30 MIN NR 60 MIN NR 4 HR NR 8 HR NR	
		AEGL 2 10 MIN 0.013 30 MIN 0.044 60 MIN 0.022 4 HR 0.0056 8 HR 0.0028	
		AEGL 3 10 MIN 2.2 30 MIN 0.74 60 MIN 0.37 4 HR 0.093 8 HR 0.047 (★Humans Resulting rrom Once-in-a-Lifetime, or Rare, Exposure to Airborne Chemicals)	
VINORELBINE TARTRATE (NAVELBINE) (CAS: C44H52N408) (CAS: 71486-72-2) (CAS: 125317-39-7)	ACGIH	ACGIH TLV STEL 0.5 MG/M3	N.O.S.
ANY CYTOTOXIC DRUGS THAT HAS AN ANALYTICAL METHOD WHICH CAN BE A SENTINEL FOR OTHER DRUGS THAT HAS NO ACCEPTABLE ANALYTICAL METHOD	VOLUNTARY (PRUDENT INDUSTRIAL HYGIENE PRACTICE)	ESCAL—ESTABLISHED BY THE FACILITY HAZARDOUS DRUGS COMMITTEE (CHEMICAL ALARA) (REFER TO SECTION 3.9, RATIONALE FOR THE ENVIRONMENTAL SENTINEL CONTAMINATION ACTION LEVEL (ESCAL) CONCEPT).	REFER TO CYTOTOXIC DRUG TABLES WITHIN THIS HANDBOOK

Note: Refer to Section 3.1 for acronyms, abbreviations, and definitions.

Cytotoxic Drugs

International Consensus Occupational Exposure Limits/
Occupational Exposure Standards Excluding the United States
(Sorted by Country)

Drug Nomenclature Chemical Abstracts Service Registry Number (CAS)	Country/Agency	Occupational Exposure Limit/Standard	Sampling Method(s)
ARSENIC TRIOXIDE (CAS: 1327-53-3)★ ★As (AS)	ARAB REPUBLIC OF EGYPT/NOT OTHERWISE SPECIFIED (N.O.S.)	OEL-TWA 0.2 MG(AS)/M3	N.O.S.
ARSENIC TRIOXIDE (CAS: 1327-53-3)★ ★As (AS)	AUSTRALIA/N.O.S	OCCUPATIONAL EXPOSURE LIMIT— AUSTRALIA CARCINOGEN, JUL 2008 OEL-TWA 0.05 MG(AS)/ M3; CARCINOGEN OEL-TWA 0.2 MG(SE)/M3	N.O.S.
CISPLATIN, PLATINOL AQ (CAS: 15663-27-1)	AUSTRALIA/N.O.S.	OEL-TWA 1 MG/M3	N.O.S.
ARSENIC TRIOXIDE (CAS: 1327-53-3)	AUSTRIA/N.O.S.	OCCUPATIONAL EXPOSURE LIMIT— TRK 0.1 MG/M3 (INHALABLE), JAN 2006	N.O.S.
ARSENIC TRIOXIDE (CAS: 1327-53-3)★ ★As Inorganic Compounds Arsenic (AS) (CAS: 7440-38-0)	BELGIUM/N.O.S.	OCCUPATIONAL EXPOSURE LIMIT— TIME-WEIGHTED AVERAGE 0.1 MG(AS)/M3, CARCINOGEN, MAR 2002 (INORGANIC ARSENIC)	N.O.S.

Drug Nomenclature Chemical Abstracts Service Registry Number (CAS)	Country/Agency	Occupational Exposure Limit/Standard	Sampling Method(s)
CISPLATIN, PLATINOL AQ (CAS: 15663-27-1)	BELGIUM/N.O.S.	OCCUPATIONAL EXPOSURE LIMIT— TIME-WEIGHTED AVERAGE 0.002 MG(PT)/M3, MAR 2002	N.O.S.
ARSENIC TRIOXIDE (CAS: 1327-53-3)★ ★As (AS)	CANADA/N.O.S.	TWA 0.05 (MG(AS)/M3)	N.O.S.
ARSENIC TRIOXIDE (CAS: 1327-53-3)★ ★As (AS)	DENMARK/N.O.S.	OCCUPATIONAL EXPOSURE LIMIT— TIME-WEIGHTED AVERAGE 0.01 MG(AS)/M3, OCT 2002 OEL- TWA 0.05 MG(AS)/M3	N.O.S.
ARSENIC TRIOXIDE (CAS: 1327-53-3)	FINLAND/N.O.S.	OCCUPATIONAL EXPOSURE LIMIT— CARCINOGEN, JAN 1993	N.O.S.
ARSENIC TRIOXIDE (CAS: 1327-53-3)★ ★As (AS)	FRANCE/N.O.S.	OEL-STEL 0.2 PPM; CARCINOGEN OEL- TWA 0.2 MG(AS)/M3	N.O.S.
ARSENIC TRIOXIDE (CAS: 1327-53-3)	FRANCE/N.O.S.	OCCUPATIONAL EXPOSURE LIMIT— VME 0.2 MG/M3, CONTINUOUS CARCINOGEN, FEB 2006	N.O.S.
ARSENIC TRIOXIDE (CAS: 1327-53-3)	GERMANY/N.O.S.	CARCINOGEN OEL	N.O.S.
ARSENIC TRIOXIDE (CAS: 1327-53-3)	GERMANY/N.O.S.	SPITZENBEGRENZUNG: 0.4 MG/M3 MAK: 0.1 MG/M3 (TRGS900), 1999	N.O.S.
ARSENIC TRIOXIDE (CAS: 1327-53-3)★ ★As (AS)	HONG KONG/N.O.S.	OCCUPATIONAL EXPOSURE LIMIT— TIME-WEIGHTED AVERAGE 0.01 MG (AG)/M3	N.O.S.

Drug Nomenclature Chemical Abstracts Service Registry Number (CAS)	Country/Agency	Occupational Exposure Limit/Standard	Sampling Method(s)
CISPLATIN, PLATINOL AQ (CAS: 15663-27-1)	HONG KONG/N.O.S.	OCCUPATIONAL EXPOSURE LIMIT—0.0002 MG(Pt)/M3	N.O.S.
ARSENIC TRIOXIDE (CAS: 1327-53-3)	HUNGARY/N.O.S.	OCCUPATIONAL EXPOSURE LIMIT—CEILING CONCENTRATION 0.1 MG/M3, CARCINOGEN, SEP 2000	N.O.S.
CISPLATIN, PLATINOL AQ (CAS: 15663-27-1)	HUNGARY/N.O.S.	OCCUPATIONAL EXPOSURE LIMIT—TIME-WEIGHTED AVERAGE 0.002 MG(PT)/M3, SEP 2000	N.O.S.
ARSENIC TRIOXIDE (CAS: 1327-53-3)	JAPAN/N.O.S.	CARCINOGEN OEL-STEL 0.5 PPM;	N.O.S.
CISPLATIN, PLATINOL AQ (CAS: 15663-27-1)	JAPAN/N.O.S.	OCCUPATIONAL EXPOSURE LIMIT—0.001 MG(PT)/M3, SEN, APR 2007	N.O.S.
ARSENIC TRIOXIDE (CAS: 1327-53-3)★ ★As (AS)	KOREA/N.O.S.	OCCUPATIONAL EXPOSURE LIMIT—TIME-WEIGHTED AVERAGE 0.2 MG(AS)/M3, 2006	N.O.S.
ARSENIC TRIOXIDE (CAS: 1327-53-3)	MEXICO/N.O.S.	OCCUPATIONAL EXPOSURE LIMIT—TIME-WEIGHTED AVERAGE 0.5 MG/M3 (PRODUCTION), 2004	N.O.S.
CARBOPLATIN (PARAPLATIN) (DIAMMINE) (C6H12N2O4PT) (CAS: 41575-94-5) (CAS: 7440-06-4)	N.O.S.	N.O.S.	N.O.S.

Drug Nomenclature Chemical Abstracts Service Registry Number (CAS)	Country/Agency	Occupational Exposure Limit/Standard	Sampling Method(s)
CARBOPLATIN (PARAPLATIN) (DIAMMINE) (C6H12N2O4PT) (CAS: 41575-94-5) (CAS: 7440-06-4)	N.O.S.	N.O.S.	N.O.S.
CARBOPLATIN (PARAPLATIN) (DIAMMINE) (C6H12N2O4PT) (CAS: 41575-94-5) (CAS: 7440-06-4)	N.O.S.	N.O.S.	N.O.S.
NITROGEN MUSTARD-2, CHLORMETHINE (MECHLORETHANMINE) (CAS: 51-75-2) (CAS: 55-86-7)	N.O.S.	N.O.S.	N.O.S.
VINORELBINE TARTRATE (NAVELBINE) (C44H52N4O8) (CAS: 71486-72-2) (CAS: 125317-39-7)	N.O.S.	N.O.S.	N.O.S.
ARSENIC TRIOXIDE (CAS: 1327-53-3)	NETHERLAND/N.O.S.	TGG 15 MIN: 0.05 MG/M3 (OK) TGG 8 HRS: 0.025 MG/M3 (OK) (NATIONALE MAC-LIJST), 2000	N.O.S.
AZATHIOPRINE, AZANIN, IMUREL, TABTHIOPRINE, IMURAN (CAS: 446-86-6)	NETHERLANDS/DUTCH HEALTH COUNCIL (GEZONDHEIDSRAAD)	0.005 MG/M3 TGG-8U	N.O.S.
CISPLATIN, PLATINOL AQ (CAS: 15663-27-1)	NETHERLANDS/DUTCH HEALTH COUNCIL (GEZONDHEIDSRAAD)	0.00005 MG/M3 TGG-8U	N.O.S.
ARSENIC TRIOXIDE (CAS: 1327-53-3)★ ★As (AS)	NEW ZEALAND/N.O.S.	OCCUPATIONAL EXPOSURE LIMIT— TIME-WEIGHTED AVERAGE 0.05 MG(AS)/M3, CARCINOGEN, JAN 2002	N.O.S.

Drug Nomenclature Chemical Abstracts Service Registry Number (CAS)	Country/Agency	Occupational Exposure Limit/Standard	Sampling Method(s)
CISPLATIN, PLATINOL AQ (CAS: 15663-27-1)	NEW ZEALAND/N.O.S.	OCCUPATIONAL EXPOSURE LIMIT—TIME-WEIGHTED AVERAGE 0.002 MG(PT)/M3, SEN, JAN 2002	N.O.S.
ARSENIC TRIOXIDE (CAS: 1327-53-3)★ ★As (AS)	NORWAY/N.O.S.	OCCUPATIONAL EXPOSURE LIMIT—TIME-WEIGHTED AVERAGE 0.01 MG(AS)/M3, JAN 1999	N.O.S.
ARSENIC TRIOXIDE (CAS: 1327-53-3)	PHILIPPINES/N.O.S.	OCCUPATIONAL EXPOSURE LIMIT—TIME-WEIGHTED AVERAGE 0.1 MG/M3, CARCINOGEN, JAN 1993	N.O.S.
ARSENIC TRIOXIDE (CAS: 1327-53-3)★ ★As (AS)	PHILIPPINES/N.O.S.	OEL-TWA 0.5 MG(AS)/M3	N.O.S.
ARSENIC TRIOXIDE (CAS: 1327-53-3)★ ★As (AS)	POLAND/N.O.S.	OCCUPATIONAL EXPOSURE LIMIT—TIME-WEIGHTED AVERAGE 0.01 MG(AS)/M3, JAN 1999 OEL-TWA 0.3 MG(AS)/M3	N.O.S.
ARSENIC TRIOXIDE (CAS: 1327-53-3)★ ★As (AS)	SLOVAKIA/N.O.S.	OEL-TWA 0.2 MG(AS)/M3; STEL 0.6 MG(AS)/M3	N.O.S.
ARSENIC TRIOXIDE (CAS: 1327-53-3)★ ★As (AS)	SWEDEN/N.O.S.	OCCUPATIONAL EXPOSURE LIMIT—TIME-WEIGHTED AVERAGE 0.01 MG(AS)/M3, CARCINOGEN, JUN 2005 OEL-SWEDEN: TWA 0.03 MG(AS)/M	N.O.S.

Drug Nomenclature Chemical Abstracts Service Registry Number (CAS)	Country/Agency	Occupational Exposure Limit/Standard	Sampling Method(s)
CISPLATIN, PLATINOL AQ (CAS: 15663-27-1)	SWEDEN/N.O.S.	OCCUPATIONAL EXPOSURE LIMIT—TIME-WEIGHTED AVERAGE 1 MG (PT)/M3 (TOTAL DUST), JUN 2005	N.O.S.
ARSENIC TRIOXIDE (CAS: 1327-53-3)* *As (AS)	SWITZERLAND/N.O.S.	OCCUPATIONAL EXPOSURE LIMIT—MAK- WEEK 0.1 MG(AS)/M3, CARCINOGEN, DEC 2006 CARCINOGEN JAN 2009 OEL-TWA 0.15 MG/M3	N.O.S.
CISPLATIN, PLATINOL AQ (CAS: 15663-27-1)	SWITZERLAND/N.O.S.	OCCUPATIONAL EXPOSURE LIMIT—MAK- WEEK 0.002 MG(PT)/M3, DEC 2006	N.O.S.
ARSENIC TRIOXIDE (CAS: 1327-53-3)	SWITZERLAND/SUVA	MAK: 0.1 MG/M3, 1997	N.O.S.
AZATHIOPRINE, AZANIN, IMUREL, TABTHIOPRINE, IMURAN (CAS: 446-86-6)	UK/HSE	OEL-MAXIMUM EXPOSURE LIMIT (MEL): 5 μ/M3 (CEILING LIMIT; NOT TIME-WEIGHTED)	N.O.S.
CISPLATIN, PLATINOL AQ (15663-27-1)	UK/HSE	OEL—0.002 MG/M3 TWA	N.O.S.

Note: Refer to Section 3.1 for acronyms, abbreviations, and definitions.

International Consensus Occupational Exposure Limits/
Occupational Exposure Standards Excluding the United States
(Sorted by Drug Nomenclature)

Drug Nomenclature Chemical Abstracts Service Registry Number (CAS)	Country/Agency	Occupational Exposure Limit/Standard	Sampling Method(s)
ARSENIC TRIOXIDE (CAS: 1327-53-3)★ ★As (AS)	ARAB REPUBLIC OF EGYPT/NOT OTHERWISE SPECIFIED (N.O.S.)	OEL-TWA 0.2 MG(AS)/M3	N.O.S.
ARSENIC TRIOXIDE (CAS: 1327-53-3)★ ★As (AS)	AUSTRALIA/N.O.S	OCCUPATIONAL EXPOSURE LIMIT— AUSTRALIA CARCINOGEN, JUL 2008 OEL-TWA 0.05 MG(AS)/ M3; CARCINOGEN OEL-TWA 0.2 MG(SE)/M3	N.O.S.
ARSENIC TRIOXIDE (CAS: 1327-53-3)	AUSTRIA/N.O.S.	OCCUPATIONAL EXPOSURE LIMIT— TRK 0.1 MG/M3 (INHALABLE), JAN 2006	N.O.S.
ARSENIC TRIOXIDE (CAS: 1327-53-3)★ ★As Inorganic Compounds Arsenic (AS) (CAS: 7440- 38-0)	BELGIUM/N.O.S.	OCCUPATIONAL EXPOSURE LIMIT— TIME-WEIGHTED AVERAGE 0.1 MG(AS)/M3, CARCINOGEN, MAR 2002 (INORGANIC ARSENIC)	N.O.S.
ARSENIC TRIOXIDE (CAS: 1327-53-3)★ ★As (AS)	CANADA/N.O.S.	TWA 0.05 (MG(AS)/M3)	N.O.S.

Drug Nomenclature Chemical Abstracts Service Registry Number (CAS)	Country/Agency	Occupational Exposure Limit/Standard	Sampling Method(s)
ARSENIC TRIOXIDE (CAS: 1327–53–3)★ ★As (AS)	SLOVAKIA/N.O.S.	OEL-TWA 0.2 MG(AS)/M3; STEL 0.6 MG(AS)/M3	N.O.S.
ARSENIC TRIOXIDE (CAS: 1327–53–3)★ ★As (AS)	DENMARK/N.O.S.	OCCUPATIONAL EXPOSURE LIMIT—TIME-WEIGHTED AVERAGE 0.01 MG(AS)/M3, OCT 2002 OEL-TWA 0.05 MG(AS)/M3	N.O.S.
ARSENIC TRIOXIDE (CAS: 1327–53–3)★ ★As (AS)	FRANCE/N.O.S.	OEL-STEL 0.2 PPM; CARCINOGEN OEL-TWA 0.2 MG(AS)/M3	N.O.S.
ARSENIC TRIOXIDE (CAS: 1327–53–3)	FINLAND/N.O.S.	OCCUPATIONAL EXPOSURE LIMIT—CARCINOGEN, JAN 1993	N.O.S.
ARSENIC TRIOXIDE (CAS: 1327–53–3)	FRANCE/N.O.S.	OCCUPATIONAL EXPOSURE LIMIT—VME 0.2 MG/M3, CONTINUOUS CARCINOGEN, FEB 2006	N.O.S.
ARSENIC TRIOXIDE (CAS: 1327–53–3)	GERMANY/ N.O.S.	CARCINOGEN OEL	N.O.S.
ARSENIC TRIOXIDE (CAS: 1327–53–3)	GERMANY/N.O.S.	SPITZENBEGRENZUNG: 0.4 MG/M3 MAK: 0.1 MG/M3 (TRGS900), 1999	N.O.S.
ARSENIC TRIOXIDE (CAS: 1327–53–3)	HUNGARY/N.O.S.	OCCUPATIONAL EXPOSURE LIMIT—CEILING CONCENTRATION 0.1 MG/M3, CARCINOGEN, SEP 2000	N.O.S.
ARSENIC TRIOXIDE (CAS: 1327–53–3)	JAPAN/N.O.S.	CARCINOGEN OEL-STEL 0.5 PPM;	N.O.S.
ARSENIC TRIOXIDE (CAS: 1327–53–3)★ ★As (AS)	KOREA/N.O.S.	OCCUPATIONAL EXPOSURE LIMIT—TIME-WEIGHTED AVERAGE 0.2 MG(AS)/M3, 2006	N.O.S.

Drug Nomenclature Chemical Abstracts Service Registry Number (CAS)	Country/Agency	Occupational Exposure Limit/Standard	Sampling Method(s)
ARSENIC TRIOXIDE (CAS: 1327-53-3)	MEXICO/N.O.S.	OCCUPATIONAL EXPOSURE LIMIT— TIME-WEIGHTED AVERAGE 0.5 MG/M3 (PRODUCTION), 2004	N.O.S.
ARSENIC TRIOXIDE (CAS: 1327-53-3)	NETHERLANDS/N.O.S.	TGG 15 MIN: 0.05 MG/ M3 (OK) TGG 8 HRS: 0.025 MG/M3 (OK) (NATIONALE MAC-LIJST), 2000	N.O.S.
ARSENIC TRIOXIDE (CAS: 1327-53-3)★ ★As (AS)	NEW ZEALAND/N.O.S.	OCCUPATIONAL EXPOSURE LIMIT— TIME-WEIGHTED AVERAGE 0.05 MG(AS)/M3, CARCINOGEN, JAN 2002	N.O.S.
ARSENIC TRIOXIDE (CAS: 1327-53-3)★ ★As (AS)	NORWAY/N.O.S.	OCCUPATIONAL EXPOSURE LIMIT— TIME-WEIGHTED AVERAGE 0.01 MG(AS)/M3, JAN 1999	N.O.S.
ARSENIC TRIOXIDE (CAS: 1327-53-3)★ ★As (AS)	HONG KONG/N.O.S.	OCCUPATIONAL EXPOSURE LIMIT— TIME WEIGHTED AVERAGE 0.01 MG (AG)/M3	N.O.S.
ARSENIC TRIOXIDE (CAS: 1327-53-3)	PHILIPPINES/N.O.S.	OCCUPATIONAL EXPOSURE LIMIT— TIME-WEIGHTED AVERAGE 0.1 MG/M3, CARCINOGEN, JAN 1993	N.O.S.
ARSENIC TRIOXIDE (CAS: 1327-53-3)★ ★As (AS)	PHILIPPINES/N.O.S.	OEL-TWA 0.5 MG(AS)/M3	N.O.S.
ARSENIC TRIOXIDE (CAS: 1327-53-3)★ ★As (AS)	POLAND/N.O.S.	OCCUPATIONAL EXPOSURE LIMIT— TIME-WEIGHTED AVERAGE 0.01 MG(AS)/M3, JAN 1999 OEL-TWA 0.3 MG(AS)/M3	N.O.S.

Drug Nomenclature Chemical Abstracts Service Registry Number (CAS)	Country/Agency	Occupational Exposure Limit/Standard	Sampling Method(s)
ARSENIC TRIOXIDE (CAS: 1327-53-3)★ ★As (AS)	SWEDEN/N.O.S.	OCCUPATIONAL EXPOSURE LIMIT— TIME-WEIGHTED AVERAGE 0.01 MG(AS)/M3, CARCINOGEN, JUN 2005 OEL-SWEDEN: TWA 0.03 MG(AS)/M	N.O.S.
ARSENIC TRIOXIDE (CAS: 1327-53-3)★ ★As (AS)	SWITZERLAND/N.O.S.	OCCUPATIONAL EXPOSURE LIMIT— MAK- WEEK 0.1 MG(AS)/M3, CARCINOGEN, DEC 2006 CARCINOGEN JAN 2009 OEL-TWA 0.15 MG/M3	N.O.S.
ARSENIC TRIOXIDE (CAS: 1327-53-3)	SWITZERLAND/SUVA	MAK: 0.1 MG/M3, 1997	N.O.S.
AZATHIOPRINE, AZANIN, IMUREL, TABTHIOPRINE, IMURAN (CAS: 446-86-6)	UK/HSE	OEL-MAXIMUM EXPOSURE LIMIT (MEL): 5 µ/M3 (CEILING LIMIT; NOT TIME-WEIGHTED)	N.O.S.
AZATHIOPRINE, AZANIN, IMUREL, TABTHIOPRINE, IMURAN (CAS: 446-86-6)	NETHERLANDS/ DUTCH HEALTH COUNCIL (GEZONDHEIDSRAAD)	0.005 MG/M3 TGG-8U	N.O.S.
CARBOPLATIN (PARAPLATIN) (DIAMMINE) (C6H12N2O4PT) (CAS: 41575-94-5) (CAS: 7440-06-4)	N.O.S.	N.O.S.	N.O.S.
CARBOPLATIN (PARAPLATIN) (DIAMMINE) (C6H12N2O4PT) (CAS: 41575-94-5) (CAS: 7440-06-4)	N.O.S.	N.O.S.	N.O.S.

Drug Nomenclature Chemical Abstracts Service Registry Number (CAS)	Country/Agency	Occupational Exposure Limit/Standard	Sampling Method(s)
CARBOPLATIN (PARAPLATIN) (DIAMMINE) (C6H12N2O4PT) (CAS: 41575-94-5) (CAS: 7440-06-4)	N.O.S.	N.O.S.	N.O.S.
CISPLATIN, PLATINOL AQ (CAS: 15663-27-1)	AUSTRALIA/N.O.S.	OEL-TWA 1 MG/M3	N.O.S.
CISPLATIN, PLATINOL AQ (15663-27-1)	UK/HSE	OEL—0.002 MG/M3 TWA	N.O.S.
CISPLATIN, PLATINOL AQ (CAS: 15663-27-1)	NETHERLANDS/DUTCH HEALTH COUNCIL (GEZONDHEIDSRAAD)	0.00005 MG/M3 TGG-8U	N.O.S.
CISPLATIN, PLATINOL AQ (CAS: 15663-27-1)	BELGIUM/N.O.S.	OCCUPATIONAL EXPOSURE LIMIT— TIME-WEIGHTED AVERAGE 0.002 MG(PT)/M3, MAR 2002	N.O.S.
CISPLATIN, PLATINOL AQ (CAS: 15663-27-1)	HONG KONG/N.O.S.	OCCUPATIONAL EXPOSURE LIMIT 0.0002 MG(Pt)/M3	N.O.S.
CISPLATIN, PLATINOL AQ (CAS: 15663-27-1)	HUNGARY/N.O.S.	OCCUPATIONAL EXPOSURE LIMIT— TIME-WEIGHTED AVERAGE 0.002 MG(PT)/M3, SEP 2000	N.O.S.
CISPLATIN, PLATINOL AQ (CAS: 15663-27-1)	JAPAN/ N.O.S.	OCCUPATIONAL EXPOSURE LIMIT— 0.001 MG(PT)/M3, SEN, APR 2007	N.O.S.
CISPLATIN, PLATINOL AQ (CAS: 15663-27-1)	NEW ZEALAND/N.O.S.	OCCUPATIONAL EXPOSURE LIMIT— TIME-WEIGHTED AVERAGE 0.002 MG(PT)/M3, SEN, JAN 2002	N.O.S.
CISPLATIN, PLATINOL AQ (CAS: 15663-27-1)	SWEDEN/N.O.S.	OCCUPATIONAL EXPOSURE LIMIT— TIME-WEIGHTED AVERAGE 1 MG (PT)/ M3 (TOTAL DUST), JUN 2005	N.O.S.

Drug Nomenclature Chemical Abstracts Service Registry Number (CAS)	Country/Agency	Occupational Exposure Limit/Standard	Sampling Method(s)
CISPLATIN, PLATINOL AQ (CAS: 15663-27-1)	SWITZERLAND/N.O.S.	OCCUPATIONAL EXPOSURE LIMIT— MAK- WEEK 0.002 MG(PT)/M3, DEC 2006	N.O.S.
NITROGEN MUSTARD-2, CHLORMETHINE (MECHLORETHANMINE) (CAS: 51-75-2) (CAS: 55-86-7)	N.O.S.	N.O.S.	N.O.S.
VINORELBINE TARTRATE (NAVELBINE) (C44H52N408) (CAS: 71486-72-2) (CAS: 125317-39-7)	N.O.S.	N.O.S.	N.O.S.

Note: Refer to Section 3.1 for acronyms, abbreviations, and definitions.

Summary of Internal Occupational Exposure Levels for Cytotoxic Drugs as Listed in Section 2.1 (Sorted by Drug Name)

Drug Name OELS (Internal—Occupational Exposure Levels)

Chemical Abstracts Service Registry Number (CAS)

Drug Name OELS / Chemical Abstracts Service Registry Number (CAS)	Manufacturer Company	Standard(s)	Method(s)
ARSENIC TRIOXIDE, TRISENOX (CAS: 91327-53-3)	ASG	0.1 MG/M3 AGS TRK (Inhalable Dust Fraction)	Not Otherwise Specified
ASASTROZOLE (CAS: 120511-73-1)	Astrazeneca	TWA 0.0001 mg/m3	Not Otherwise Specified
ASPARAGINASE (CAS: 9015-68-3)	Merck	OEL: Merck 10 μ/m3 8-hr TWA	Not Otherwise Specified
BICALUTAMIDE, CASODEX (CAS: 90357-06-5)	Astrazeneca	BICALUTAMIDE (CASODEX) BICALUTAMIDE(CASODEX) OEL: Astrazeneca 0.01 mg/m3 COM	Not Otherwise Specified
BLEOMYCIN (CAS: 67763-87-5)	Bedford Labs	BLEOMYCIN OEL: Bedford Labs 50 mg/m3	Not Otherwise Specified
BUSULFA (MYLERAN) (CAS: 55-98-1)	GW and GSK	BUSULFA (MYLERAN) OEL GW OEL GSK (same) 1.0 μ/m3 (OEL GW/GSK 2005)	Not Otherwise Specified
CHLORAMBUCIL, LEUKERAN (CAS: 305-03-3)	GSK	CHLORAMBUCIL OEL–GSK 0.5 μ/m3 (8 hr TWA)	Not Otherwise Specified
CHLORMETHINE HYDROCHLORIDE (CAS: 55-86-7)	Not Otherwise Specified		Not Otherwise Specified

Acute Exposure Guideline Levels (Proposed)—(mg/m3)

	10 MIN	30 MIN	60 MIN	4 HR	8 HR
AEGL 1	NR	NR	NR	NR	NR
AEGL 2	3.7	3.7	3.0	1.9	1.2
AEGL 3	11.0	11.0	9.1	5.7	3.7

NR = Not recommended due to insufficient data per company.

Acute Exposure Guideline Levels (mg/m3)

	10 MIN	30 MIN	60 MIN	4 HR	8 HR
AEGL 1	NR	NR	NR	NR	NR
AEGL 2	0.13	0.044	0.022	0.0056	0.0028
AEGL 3	2.2	0.74	0.37	0.093	0.047

NR = Not recommended due to insufficient data.

Substance (CAS)	Company	OEL / Exposure Limit	Monitoring methods and references
CISPLATIN (CAS: mixture)	Bristol-Myers Squibb	CISPLATIN OEL OEL–Bristol-Myers Squibb PLATINOL–AQ(CISPLATIN) (2005) 0.00002 mg/m3 TWA (8 hr)	Monitoring methods and references: NIOSH Method S191 OR 7300; Measurement Method: Particulate Filter; Acid/ Reagen; Graphite Furnace Atomic Absorption Spectrometry; NIOSH II(7) # S191
CLADRIENINE, LEUSTATIN (CAS: 4291-63-8)	Bedford Lab Ben Venue Labs Pharmaceutical Research Insti. J&J	OEL: Bedford Lab and Ben Benue Laboratories, Inc. 2.5 µ/m3 TWA Pharmaceutical Research Institute and J&J 1996 OEL 0.0025 mg/m3 TWA	Not Otherwise Specified
CYTARABINE, CYTOSAR-U (CAS: 147-94-4)	Pharmacia UP John	OEL: Pharmacia & UP John 2 µG/M3 TWA	Not Otherwise Specified
DACTINOMYCIN (CAS: 50-76-0)	Merck Sharp & Dohme	DACTINOMYCIN OEL—Merck, Sharp & Dohme DACTINOMYCIN Zero Exposure★ Merck Exposure Control Limit (ECL); ★Zero exposure is an internally derived exposure control limit based on the carcinogenic potential of the compound.	Not Otherwise Specified
ELOXATIN LYOPHILIZED, OXALIPLATIN (CAS: 61825-94-3)	Sanofi Winthrop IND	OEL Sanofi Winthrop IND ELOXATIN LYOPHILIZED Exposure Band: 0.1–5 µG/m3 Exposure Limit: 10 mg/m3	Not Otherwise Specified
ERBITUX (CAS: 205923-56-4)	Bristol-Myers Squibb	OEL: Bristol-Myers Squibb Company 0.01 MG/M3	Not Otherwise Specified

Drug Name OELS (Internal—Occupational Exposure Levels) Chemical Abstracts Service Registry Number (CAS)	Manufacturer Company	Standard(s)	Method(s)
ETOPOSIDE, VEPESID (CAS: 33419-42-0) (CAS: 33419-42-9)	Pharmacia ★ UP John Bristol Myers Squibb	Pharmacia & UP John exposure limit for ETOPOSIDE Occupational Exposure–TWA: The exposure limit will be at the no detection (ND) limit. OEL–Bristol Myers Squibb VEPESID 0.000014 mg/m3 TWA 8-hr (dust control)★ ★Adherence to this target level should protect most employees who handle this drug from experiencing adverse effects from this substance; however, exposure to this substance should be maintained as low as reasonably possible. Pharmacia and UP John Exposure Limit for ETOPOSIDE Occupational Exposure—TWA: The exposure limit will be at the no detection (ND) limit.	Not Otherwise Specified
FLOXURIDINE, 5-FUDR (CAS: 0-91-9)	Bedford Lab	OEL: Bedford Lab 10 μ/m3	Not Otherwise Specified
GANCICLOVIR (CAS: 84245-13-6)	Roche and Hoffman-LA Syntex	OEL: Roche and Hoffman-LA IOELV: 5 μg/m3 sampling on glass fiber and chemical determination of the active compound (EG HPLC). OEL:Syntex (GANCICLOVIR) 5 μg/m3 (8 hr TWA) OEL–Roche: 0.005 mg/m3	Not Otherwise Specified
GEMCITABINE (CAS: 95058-81-4)	Lilly	OEL: Lilly Exposure Guidance/Method GEMCITABINE (95058-81-4) LEG 0.3 μg/m3 TWA for 8 hours, LEG 0.2 μg/m3 for 12 hours; Excursion Limit 2.4 μg/m3 for no more than a total of 30 min.	Not Otherwise Specified

GEMTUZUMAB OZOGAMYCIN (CAS: 220578-59-6)	American Home Products	OEL MYLOTARGGEMTUZUMAB OZOGAMICIN (American Home Products) 0.1 µg/m3	Not Otherwise Specified
GOSERELIN ACETATE, ZOLADEX (CAS: 65807-02-5) (CAS: 145781-92-6)	Astrazenca	OEL: Astrasenca ZOLADEX (GOSERELIN ACETATE) 0.0025 mg/m3 STEL/Ceiling	Not Otherwise Specified
HYDROXYUREA (CAS: 127-07-1)	Bristol-Myers Squibb	OEL–Bristcl-Myers Squibb OEL/Exposure Guidelines 0.1 mg/m3 8-hour TWA Adherence to the exposure guideline will ensure that a worker is not exposed to more than 0.1% of the lowest recommended oral therapeutic dose of HYDROXYUREA and should protect employees who handle HYDROXYUREA from experiencing pharmacological effects of this drug. This substance is a weak mutagen. Adherence to the exposure guideline should minimize the potential for mutagenic changes to occur ir the cells of persons who handle this material.	Not Otherwise Specified
IFOSFAMIDE (CAS: 3778-73-2) (CAS: 66849-33-0) (CAS: 66849-34-1) (CAS: 84711-20-6) (CAS: 19767-45-4)	Bristol-Myers Squibb	OEL—Bristol-Myers Squibb IFOSFAMIDE 0.1 µ/m3 ★ TWA ★Bristol-Myers Squibb dust control target Exposure Guideline Summary: IFOSFAMIDE is a cytotoxic drug used alone or in combination with other chemotherapeutic drugs to treat various types of cancer. A dust control target of 0.1 µ/m3 in air (8-hour time-weighted average concentration) has been established for workplace exposure to IFOSFAMIDE. Adherence to this target level should protect most employees who handle this drug from experiencing adverse effects from this substance; however, exposure to this substance should be maintained as low as reasonably possible.	Not Otherwise Specified

Drug Name OELS (Internal—Occupational Exposure Levels) Chemical Abstracts Service Registry Number (CAS)

Drug Name OELS (Internal—Occupational Exposure Levels) Chemical Abstracts Service Registry Number (CAS)	Manufacturer Company	Standard(s)	Method(s)
IMURAN, AZATHIOPRINE (CAS: 446–86–6)	Glaxco Wellcome	IMURAN (AZATHIOPRINE) 3 µ/m3 (15 min TWA) OEL–GSK 3 mg/m3 (8–hr TWA)★ carcinogen, reproductive hazard, skin sensitizer ★Occupational Hygiene Air Monitoring Methods: An occupational/industrial hygiene monitoring method has been developed for this material. For advice on suitable monitoring methods, consult your local occupational or industrial hygiene specialist, health and safety department, or the health and safety group identified. OEL–UK maximum exposure limit (MEL): 5 µ/m3 (ceiling limit; not time–weighted)	Not Otherwise Specified
LEUPRORELIN. LEUPRORELIN ACETATE SALT (CAS: 53714–56–0) (CAS: 74381–53–6)	Abbott Labs Innovators	OEL Abbott Laboratories LEUPROLIDE ACETATE 0.05 µ/m3 TWA (8 hrs) OEL Innovators 20 mg/m3 TWA	Not Otherwise Specified
LEVAMISOLE (CAS: 14769–73–4)	Janssen Pharmaceutica	LEVAMISOLE OEL—Janssen Pharmaceutica 0.15 mg/m3	Not Otherwise Specified
MECHLORETHANMINE OEL (CAS: 51–75–2) (CAS: 55–56–7)	Company N.O.S.	MECHLORETHANMINE OEL Acute exposure guideline levels (AEGLS) (mg/m3) <table><tr><td></td><td>10 MIN</td><td>30 MIN</td><td>60 MIN</td><td>4 HR</td><td>8 HR</td></tr><tr><td>AEGL 1</td><td>NR</td><td>NR</td><td>NR</td><td>NR</td><td>NR</td></tr><tr><td>AEGL 2</td><td>0.13</td><td>0.044</td><td>0.022</td><td>0.0056</td><td>0.0028</td></tr><tr><td>AEGL 3</td><td>2.2</td><td>0.74</td><td>0.37</td><td>0.093</td><td>0.047</td></tr></table> NR = Not recommended due to insufficient data	Not Otherwise Specified
MEGESTROL (CAS: 595–33–5) (CAS: 3562–63–8)	Pharmacia & UPJohn	OEL: Pharmacia & UPJohn /Pharmacia & UPJohn 40 µg/m3 TWA	Not Otherwise Specified

Substance	Source	OEL	
MELPHALAN, ALKERAN (CAS: 148-82-3) (CAS: 8057-25-8)	GW GSK	OEL–GW 1.0 μ/M3 8-hr TWA (one MSDS) 1.0 μ/M3 8-hr TWA (one MSDS) 0.0025 mg/m3 (maximum exposure limit) (MSDS)(1996) OEL–GW OEL–GSK (same) 4.0 μ/m3 8-hr TWA	Not Otherwise Specified
MERCAPTOPURINE MONHYDRATE, PURINETHOL tablets (CAS: 6112-76-1) (CAS: 50-44-2)	GSK	OEL-GSK MERCAPTOPURINE MONHYDRATE (PURINETHOL tablets) 10 μ/m3 (8-hr TWA) (reproductive hazard; carcinogen)	Not Otherwise Specified
METHOTREXATE (CAS: 59-05-2)	American Pharm Partners, Inc. American Cyanamid	OEL: American Pharmaceutical Partners, Inc. OEL–METHOTREXATE: 0.5 μ/m³ OEL—American Cyanamid OEL—METHOTREXATE: 0.0007 mg/m3 OEL—American Cyanamid METHOTREXATE Adult non–child bearing potential 5 consecutive days: 0.02 mg/m3 5 consecutive days: 0.01 mg/m3 Repeated at 7- to 9-day intervals Daily exposure for 5 days or more: 0.001 mg/m3 Interrupted by not more than 2 days (e.g., continuous repetition of a 5 day/week shift)	Not Otherwise Specified
MITOXANTRONE (CAS: 70476-82-3) (CAS: 65271-80-9)	AHPC Lederle Lab	OEL–AHPC–OEG NOVANTRONE MITOXANTRONE HCL 0.2 μg/m3 OEL—Lederle Laboratories NOVANTRONE MITOXANTRONE HCL ACCO PEL: 0.016 mg/m3 once/month; 0.003 mg/m3 5 consecutive exposures per month	Not Otherwise Specified

Drug Name OELS (Internal— Occupational Exposure Levels) Chemical Abstracts Service Registry Number (CAS)	Manufacturer Company	Standard(s)	Method(s)
OXYLATODIAMMINEPL, PLATINUM (CAS: mixture)	Bristol-Myers Squibb	OEL Bristol-Myers Squibb 2 µg/m3 (sensitizer) Bristol-Myers Squibb Exposure Guidelines Summary: Adherence to this guideline should protect employees from experience the therapeutic and/or adverse effects of this drug. Recommended Industrial Hygiene Monitoring Methods: Contact the Bristol-Myers Squibb AIHA accredited industrial hygiene laboratory at 732–227–7368.	Not Otherwise Specified
PEMETREXED, ALIMTA (CAS: 150399–23–8)	Lilly	PEMETREXED (ALIMTA) Lilly Exposure Guide 0.3 micrograms/m3 TWA for 8 or 12 hours. 3.6 micrograms/m3 for no more than a total of 30 minutes (excursion limit)	Not Otherwise Specified
PENTAMIDINE (CAS: 140–64–7)	Abbott Lab	OEL: Abbott Lab 0.1 mg/m3	Not Otherwise Specified
PENTOSTATIN, NIPENT (CAS: 53910–25–1)	Warner-Lambert	OEL: Warner-Lambert 0.014 mg/m3 TWA	Not Otherwise Specified
RITUXAN, RITUXIMAB (CAS: 174722–31–7)	Hoffman–La Roche	OEL—Hoffmann–La Roche Threshold value (Roche) air—Category 1 (Roche group directive K1, annex 3): IOELV >500 µg/m3	Not Otherwise Specified
TAMOXIFEN, NOLVADEX (CAS: 10540–29–1) (CAS: 54965–24–1)	Zeneca	OEL—Zeneca OEL TAMOXIFEN (NOLVADEX) TWA mg/m3 0.01	Not Otherwise Specified

Substance	Manufacturer	OEL	
TAXOL, PACLITAXEL (CAS: 33069-62-4)	Bristol-Myers Squibb	OEL Bristol-Myers Squibb PACLITAXEL: 0,0000 mg/m3 TWA 8 hrs BMS dust control★ target ★PACLITAXEL is a potent stabilizer of microtubules in vitro and in vivo. It is quite toxic when administered systemically and has potential to cause chromosome damage in human cells. It is being evaluated in clinical trails as a therapy for various types of cancer, especially ovarian and breast cancer. A dust control target of 0.0008 mg/m3 in air (8-hr time-weighted average concentration in air) has been established for workplace exposure to PACLITAXEL. Adherence to this target level should protect most employees who handle this drug from experience adverse effects from this substance. However, exposure to this substance should be maintained as low as reasonably possible.	Not Otherwise Specified
TEMODAR, TEMOZOMIDE (CAS: 85622-93-1)	Schering	OEL-Schering TEMODAR Schering OEG: 2 µg/m3	Not Otherwise Specified
THIOGUANINE (CAS: 154-42-7)	GSK	OEL-GSK THIOGUANINE 10 µ/m3 (8-hr TWA) GSK Exposure Controls: An exposure control approach (ECA) is established for operations involving this material based upon the OEL/occupational hazard category and the outcome of a site- or operation-specific risk assessment. Refer to the exposure control matrix for more information about how ECAs are assigned and how to interpret them.	Not Otherwise Specified
THIOTEPA (CAS: 52-24-4)	American Cyanamd	OEL: American Cyanamid 0.0014 mg/m3 THIOTEPA OEL: American Cyanamid and Ben Venue Laboratories 0.0014 mg/m3 0.01 mg/m3 TWA	Not Otherwise Specified
TOPOTECAN (CAS: 123948-87-8) (CAS: 119413-54-6)	GSK	OEL-GSK OEL-TOPOTECAN 0.03 µ/m3 (8-hr TW/A)	Not Otherwise Specified

Drug Name OELS (Internal—Occupational Exposure Levels) Chemical Abstracts Service Registry Number (CAS)	Manufacturer Company	Standard(s)	Method(s)
VINBLASTINE (CAS: 143–67–9) (CAS: 865–21–4) ?	N.O.S.	OEL: LEG 0.47 µg/m3 TWA For 12 hours Excursion Limit: 5.64 mg/m3 for no more than a total of 30 minutes. "Worse case" computer aided prediction of spray/mist or fume/dust components and concentration: Composite exposure standard for mixture (TWA): 3.0000 mg/m3. Operations, which produce a spray/mist or fume/dust, introduce particulates to the breathing zone. If the breathing zone concentration of any of the components listed below is exceeded, "worst case" considerations deem the individual to be overexposed. Breathing Zone Mixture Component Conc. mg/m3 Conc. (%) VINBLASTINE SULFATE: 3.0000 0.7	Not Otherwise Specified
VINCRISTINE. LEUROCRISTINE (CAS: 2067–78–2) (CAS: 57–22–7)	Lilly	OEL: Lilly 0.14 G/M3 PER 12 HOURS EXCURSION LIMIT 1.68 µG/M3 (30 MINS)	Not Otherwise Specified
VINORELBINE TARTRATE, VINORELBINE (CAS: 125317–39–7) (CAS: 71486–22–1)	GSK Bedford Lab (Ben Venue Lab, Inc.)	GSK OEL 0.5 µ/m3 (8-hr TWA) OEL: Bedford (Ben Venue Lab, Inc.) Laboratories 0.5 mcg/m3 8-hr TWA	Not Otherwise Specified Not Otherwise Specified
XELODA, CAPECITABINE (CAS: 154361–50–9) (CAS: 158798–73–3)	Hoffman–La Roche, Inc. PHARMACIA & UPJohn Camtosar	OEL: Hoffman–La Roche, Inc. mg/m3 TWA OEL: Pharmacia & UPJohn OEL: Camtosar 0.4 µg/m3 TWA	Not Otherwise Specified

Note: Internal established OELs as listed in the cytotoxic drug tables within this guide; refer to the acronyms, abbreviations, and definitions table, appendix 3.1.

Summary of Internal Occupational Exposure Levels for Cytotoxic Drugs as Listed in Section 2.1 (Sorted by Manufacturer Name)

OELS (Internal–Occupational Exposure Levels) Chemical Abstracts Service Registry Number (CAS)	Manufacturer Company	Standard(s)	Method(s)
PENTAMIDINE (CAS: 140-64-7)	Abbott Lab	OEL: Abbott Lab 0.1 mg/m3	Not Otherwise Specified
LEUPRORELIN. LEUPRORELIN ACETATE SALT (CAS: 53714-56-0) (CAS: 74381-53-6)	Abbot Labs Innovators	OEL Abbott Laboratories LEUPROLIDE ACETATE 0.05 µ/m3 TWA (8 hrs) OEL Innovators 20 ng/m3 TWA	Not Otherwise Specified
MITOXANTRONE (CAS: 65271-80-9) (CAS: 70476-82-3)	AHPC Lederle Lab	OEL-AHPC-OEG NOVANTRONE MITOXANTRONE HCL 0.2 µg/m3 OEL–Lederle Laboratories NOVANTRONE MITOXANTRONE HCL ACCO PEL: 0.016 mg/m3 once/month 0.003 mg/m3 5 consecutive exposures per month	Not Otherwise Specified
THIOTEPA (CAS: 52-24-4)	American Cyanamid	OEL: American Cyanamid 0.0014 mg/m3 THIOTEPA OEL: American Cyanamid and Ben Venue Laboratories 0.0014 mg/m3 0.01 mg/m3 TWA	Not Otherwise Specified

GEMTUZUMAB OZOGAMYCIN (CAS: 220578-59-6)

American Home Products

OEL MYLOTARGEMTUZUMAB OZOGAMICIN (American Home Products)
0.1 µg/m3

Not Otherwise Specified

METHOTREXATE (CAS: 59-05-2)

American Pharm Partners, Inc.

OEL: American Pharmaceutical Partners, Inc.
OEL-METHOTREXATE: 0.5 µ/m³

Not Otherwise Specified

American Cyanamid

OEL–American Cyanamid
OEL-METHOTREXATE: 0.0007 mg/m3

OEL–American Cyanamid
METHOTREXATE

Adult non–child bearing potential

5 consecutive days: 0.02 mg/m3

5 consecutive days: 0.01 mg/m3 repeated at 7– to 9–day intervals

Daily exposure for 5 days or more: 0.001 mg/m3
Interrupted by not more than 2 days (e.g., continuous repetition of a 5 day/week shift)

ARSENIC TRIOXIDE, TRISENOX (CAS: 91327-53-3)

ASG

0.1 mg/m3 AGS TRK (Inhalable Dust Fraction)

Not Otherwise Specified

Acute Exposure Guideline Levels (AEGLS) (proposed) (mg/m3)

	10 MIN	30 MIN	60 MIN	4 HR	8 HR
AEGL 1	NR	NR	NR	NR	NR
AEGL 2	3.7	3.7	3.0	1.9	1.2
AEGL 3	11.0	11.0	9.1	5.7	3.7

NR = Not recommended due to insufficient data per company.

GOSERELIN ACETATE, ZOLADEX (CAS: 65807-02-5) (CAS: 145781-92-6)

Astrazenca

OEL: ASTRAZENCA
ZOLADEX (GOSERELIN ACETATE)
0.0025 mg/m3 STEL/Ceiling

Not Otherwise Specified

OELS
(Internal—Occupational Exposure Levels)

Chemical Abstracts Service Registry Number (CAS)	Manufacturer Company	Standard(s)	Method(s)
ASASTROZOLE (CAS: 120511-73-1)	Astrazenca	TWA 0.0001 mg/m3	Not Otherwise Specified
BICALUTAMIDE, CASODEX (CAS: 90357-06-5)	Astrazenca	BICALUTAMIDE (CASODEX) BICALUTAMIDE(CASODEX) OEL: Astrazenca 0.01 mg/m3 COM	Not Otherwise Specified
FLOXURIDINE, 5-FUDR (CAS: 0-91-9)	Bedford Labs	OEL: Bedford Lab 10 μ/m3	Not Otherwise Specified
BLEOMYCIN (CAS: 67763-87-5)	Bedford Labs	BLEOMYCIN OEL: Bedford Labs 50 ng/m3	Not Otherwise Specified
CLADRIENINE, LEUSTATIN (CAS: 4291-63-8)	Bedford Lab Ben Venue Labs Pharmaceutical Research Instit. J&J	OEL: Bedford Lab and Ben Venue Laboratories, Inc. 2.5 μ/m3 TWA Pharmaceutical Research Institute and J&J 1996 OEL 0.0025 mg/m3 TWA	Not Otherwise Specified
CISPLATIN (CAS: MIXTURE)	Bristol-Myers Squibb	CISPLATIN OEL OEL–Bristol-Myers Squibb PLATINOL-AQ (CISPLATIN) (2005): 0.00002 mg/m3 TWA (8-hr)	Monitoring Methods and References: NIOSH Method S191 or 7300; measurement method: particulate filter; acid/ reagent; graphite furnace atomic absorption spectrometry; NIOSH II(7) # S191

ERBITUX (CAS: 205923-56-4)	Bristol-Myers Squibb	OEL: Bristol-Myers Squibb Company 0.01 mg/m3	Not Otherwise Specified

HYDROXYUREA (CAS: 127-07-1) — Bristol-Myers Squibb

OEL–Bristol-Myers Squibb

OEL/Exposure Guidelines
0.1 mg/m3 8-hrTWA

Adherence to the exposure guideline will ensure that a worker is not more than 0.1% of the lowest recommended oral therapeutic dose of HYDROXYUREA and should protect employees who handle HYDROXYUREA from experiencing pharmacological effects of this drug. This substance is a weak mutagen. Adherence to the exposure guideline should minimize the potential for mutagenic changes to occur in cells of persons who handle this material.

Not Otherwise Specified

TAXOL. PACLITAXEL (CAS: 33069-62-4) — Bristol-Myers Squibb

OEL Bristol-Myers Squibb
PACLITAXEL 0,0000 mg/m3 TWA 8 hrs
BMS Dust Control★ Target

★PACLITAXEL is a potent stabilizer of microtubules in vitro and in vivo. It is quite toxic when administered systemically and has potential to cause chromosome damage in human cells. It is being evaluated in clinical trials as a therapy for various types of cancer, especially ovarian and breast cancer. A dust control target of 0.0008 mg/m3 in air (8-hr time-weighted average concentration in air) has been established for workplace exposure to PACLITAXEL. Adherence to this target level should protect most employees who handle this drug from experiencing adverse effects from this substance. However, exposure to this substance should be maintained as low as reasonably possible.

Not Otherwise Specified

OELS

(Internal–Occupational Exposure Levels)

Chemical Abstracts Service Registry Number (CAS)	Manufacturer Company	Standard(s)	Method(s)
IFOSFAMIDE (CAS: 3778-73-2) (CAS: 66849-33-0) (CAS: 66849-34-1) (CAS: 84711-20-6) (CAS: 19767-45-4)	Bristol-Myers Squibb	OEL–Bristol-Myers Squibb IFOSFAMIDE 0.1 μ/m3 ★ TWA ★Bristol-Myers Squibb Dust Control Target Exposure Guidelines Summary: IFOSFAMIDE is a cytotoxic drug used alone or in combination with other chemotherapeutic drugs to treat various types of cancer. A dust control target of 0.1 μ/m3 in air (8–hr time–weighted average concentration) has been established for workplace exposure to IFOSFAMIDE. Adherence to this target level should protect most employees who handle this drug from experiencing adverse effects from this substance. However, exposure to this substance should be maintained as low as reasonable possible.	Not Otherwise Specified
OXYLATODIAMMINEPL, PLATINUM (CAS: mixture)	Bristol-Myers Squibb	OEL Bristol-Myers Squibb: 2 μg/m3 (sensitizer) Bristol-Myers Squibb Exposure Guidelines Summary: Adherence to this guideline should protect employees from experiencing the therapeutic and/or adverse effects of this drug. Recommended Industrial Hygiene Monitoring Methods: Contact the Bristol-Myers Squibb AIHA accredited industrial hygiene laboratory at 732–227–7368.	Not Otherwise Specified
MECHLORETHANMINE OEL (CAS: 51-75-2) (CAS: 55-56-7)	Company N.O.S.	MECHLORETHANMINE OEL Acute Exposure Guideline Levels (AEGLS) (mg/m3)	Not Otherwise Specified

	10 MIN	30 MIN	60 MIN	4 HR	8 HR
AEGL 1	NR	NR	NR	NR	NR
AEGL 2	0.13	0.044	0.022	0.0056	0.0028
AEGL 3	2.2	0.74	0.37	0.093	0.047

NR = Not recommended due to insufficient data.

Substance	Manufacturer	Exposure Limits	Not Otherwise Specified
IMURAN, AZATHIOPRINE (CAS: 446-86-6)	Glaxo Wellcome	IMURAN (AZATHIOPRINE) 3 µ/m3 (15 min TWA) OEL-GSK 3 mg/m3 (8-hr TWA)* carcinogen, reproductive hazard, skin sensitizer *Occupational Hygiene Air Monitoring Methods: An occupational/industrial hygiene monitoring method has been developed for this material. For advice on suitable monitoring methods, consult your local occupational or industrial hygiene specialist, health and safety department, or the health and safety group identified. CEL-UK maximum exposure limit (MEL): 5 µ/m3 (ceiling limit; not time-weighted)	Not Otherwise Specified
CHLORAMBUCIL, LEUKERAN (CAS: 305-03-3)	GSK	CHLORAMBUCIL OEL-GSK 0.5 µ/m3 (8-hr TWA)	Not Otherwise Specified
MERCAPTOPURINE MONHYDRATE, PURINETHOL tablets (CAS: 6112-76-1) (CAS: 50-44-2)	GSK	CEL-GSK MERCAPTOPURINE MONHYDRATE (PURINETHOL tablets) 10 µ/m3 (8-hr TWA) (reproductive hazard, carcinogen)	Not Otherwise Specified
THIOGUANINE (CAS: 154-42-7)	GSK	CEL-GSK THIOGUANINE: 10 µ/m3 (8-hr TWA) GSK Exposure Controls: An exposure control approach (ECA) is established for operations involving this material based upon the OEL/occupational hazard category and the outcome of a site- or operation-specific risk assessment. Refer to the exposure control matrix for more information about how ECAs are assigned and how to interpret them.	Not Otherwise Specified
TOPOTECAN (CAS: 123948-87-8) (CAS: 119413-54-6)	GSK	CEL-GSK CEL-TOPOTECAN 0.03 µ/m3 (8-hr TWA)	Not Otherwise Specified
VINORELBINE TARTRATE, VINORELBINE (CAS: 125317-39-7) (CAS: 71486-22-1)	GSK, Bedford Lab (Ben Venue Lab, Inc.)	GSK OEL 0.5 µ/m3 (8-hr TWA) CEL: Bedford (Ben Venue Lab, Inc.) Laboratories 0.5 mcg/m3 (8-hr TWA)	Not Otherwise Specified

OELS (Internal–Occupational Exposure Levels) Chemical Abstracts Service Registry Number (CAS)	Manufacturer Company	Standard(s)	Method(s)
MELPHALAN, ALKERAN (CAS: 148-82-3) (CAS: 8057-25-8)	GW	OEL-GW 1.0 µg/m3 (8-hr TWA) (one MSDS) 1.0 µg/m3 (8-hr TWA) (one MSDS) 0.0025 mg/m3 (maximum exposure limit) (MSDS)(1996)	Not Otherwise Specified
	GSK	OEL-GW OEL-GSK (same) 4.0 µg/m3 (8-hr TWA)	
BUSULFA (MYLERAN) (CAS: 55-98-1)	GW and GSK	BUSULFA (MYLERAN) OEL GW OEL GSK (same) 1.0 µg/m3 (OEL GW/GSK 2005)	Not Otherwise Specified
RITUXAN, RITUXIMAB (CAS: 174722-31-7)	Hoffman–La Roche	OEL–Hoffman–La Roche Threshold value (Roche) air—category 1 (Roche group directive K1, annex 3): IOELV >500 µg/m3	Not Otherwise Specified
XELODA, CAPECITABINE (CAS: 154361-50-9) (CAS: 158798-73-3)	Hoffmann–La Roche, Inc. Pharmacia & UPJohn Camtosar	OEL: Hoffmann–La Roche, Inc. 0.01 mg/m3 TWA OEL: Pharmacia & UPJohn OEL Camtosar 0.4 µg/m3 TWA	Not Otherwise Specified
LEVAMISOLE (CAS: 14769-73-4)	Janssen Pharmaceutica	LEVAMISOLE OEL–Janssen Pharmaceutica 0.15 mg/m3	Not Otherwise Specified
GEMCITABINE (CAS: 95058-81-4)	Lilly	OEL: Lilly Exposure Guidance Method: GEMCITABINE (95058-81-4) LEG 0.3 µg/m3 TWA for 8 hrs, LEG 0.2 µg/m3 for 12 hrs; excursion limit 2.4 µg/m3 for no more than a total of 30 minutes	Not Otherwise Specified
PEMETREXED, ALIMTA (CAS: 150399-23-8)	Lilly	PEMETREXED (ALIMTA) Lilly Exposure Guide 0.3 micrograms/m3 TWA for 8 or 12 hours 3.6 micrograms/m3 for no more than a total of 30 minutes (excursion limit)	Not Otherwise Specified

VINCRISTINE, LEUROCRISTINE (CAS: 2067–78-2) (CAS: 57–22-7)	Lilly	OEL: Lilly 0.14 g/m3 per 12 hours Excursion Limit 1.68 µg/m3 (30 mins)	Not Otherwise Specified
ASPARAGINASE (CAS: 9015–68-3)	Merck	OEL: Merck 10 µ/m3 8-hr TWA	Not Otherwise Specified
DACTINOMYCIN (CAS: 50–76-0)	Merck Sharp & Dohme	DACTINOMYCIN OEL–Merck, Sharp & Dohme DACTINOMYCIN Zero Exposure★ Merck Exposure Control Limit (ECL): ★Zero exposure is an internally derived exposure control limit based on the carcinogenic potential of the compound.	Not Otherwise Specified
VINBLASTINE (CAS: 143–67-9) (CAS: 865-21-4)	N.O.S.	OEL: LEG 0.47 µg/m3 TWA for 12 hrs Excursion Limit: 5.64 mg/m3 for no more than a total of 30 minutes.	Not Otherwise Specified

"Worse case" computer-aided prediction of spray/mist or fume/dust components and concentration:

Composite Exposure Standard for Mixture (TWA): 3.0000 mg/m3. Operations, which produce a spray/mist or fume/dust, introduce particulates to the breathing zone. If the breathing zone concentration of any of the components listed below is exceeded, "worst case" considerations deem the individual to be overexposed.

Breathing Zone Mixture
Component
conc. mg/m3
conc. (%)

VINBLASTINE SULFATE
3.0000
0.7

OELS (Internal–Occupational Exposure Levels)

Chemical Abstracts Service Registry Number (CAS)	Manufacturer Company	Standard(s)	Method(s)
CHLORMETHINE HYDROCHLORIDE (CAS: 55-86-7)	Not Otherwise Specified	Acute Exposure Guideline Levels (AEGLS) (mg/m3) (see table below)	Not Otherwise Specified
CYTARABINE, CYTOSAR-U (CAS: 147-94-4)	Pharmacia UPJohn	OEL: Pharmacia & UPJohn 2 µg/m3 TWA	Not Otherwise Specified
ETOPOSIDE, VEPESID (CAS: 33419-42-0) (CAS: 33419-42-9)	Pharmacia & UPJohn / Bristol-Myers Squibb	Pharmacia & UPJohn Exposure Limit for ETOPOSIDE Occupational Exposure–TWA: The exposure limit will be at the no detection (ND) limit. OEL–Bristol-Myers Squibb VEPESID: 0.000014 mg/m3 TWA 8-hr (dust control)★ ★Adherence to this target level should protect most employees who handle this drug from experiencing adverse effects from this substance; however, exposure to this substance should be maintained as low as reasonably possible. Pharmacia and UPJohn Exposure Limite for ETOPOSIDE Occupational Exposure–TWA: The exposure limit will be at the no detection (ND) limit.	Not Otherwise Specified
MEGESTROL (CAS: 595-33-5) (CAS: 3562-63-8)	Pharmacia & UPJohn	OEL: Pharmacia & UPJohn/Pharmacia & UPJohn 40 µg/m3 TWA	Not Otherwise Specified

	10 MIN	30 MIN	60 MIN	4 HR	8 HR
AEGL 1	NR	NR	NR	NR	NR
AEGL 2	0.13	0.044	0.022	0.0056	0.0028
AEGL 3	2.2	0.74	0.37	0.093	0.047

NR = Not recommended due to insufficient data.

Compound	Manufacturer	OEL	
GANCICLOVIR (CAS: 84245–13–6)	Roche and Hoffmann-LA	OEL: Roche and Hoffmann-LA IOELV: 5 μg/m3 sampling on glass fiber and chemical determination of the active compound (e.g., HPLC).	Not Otherwise Specified
	Synex	OEL: Syntex (GANCICLOVIR) 5 μg/m3 (8-hr TWA) OEL-Roche: 0.005 mg/m3	
ELOXATIN LYOPHILIZED, OXALIPLATIN (CAS: 61825–94–3)	Sanofi Winthrop IND	OEL Sanofi Wintrhop IND ELOXATIN LYOPHILIZED Exposure Band: 0.1–5 μg/m3 Exposure Limit: 10 mg/m3	Not Otherwise Specified
TEMODAR, TEMOZOMIDE (CAS: 85622–93–1)	Schering	OEL-Schering TEMODAR Schering OEG: 2 μg/m3	Not Otherwise Specified
PENTOSTATIN, NIPENT (CAS: 53910–25–1)	Warner-Lambert	OEL: Warner–Lambert 0.014 mg/m3 TWA	Not Otherwise Specified
TAMOXIFEN, NOLVADEX (CAS: 10540–29–1) (CAS: 54965–24–1)	Zeneca	OEL-Zeneca OEL TAMOXIFEN (NOLVADEX) TWA mg/m3 0.01	Not Otherwise Specified

DRUG NAME	CARCINOGEN*	MUTAGEN*	TERATOGEN*	REPRODUCTIVE* (FEMALE AND/OR MALE)	OTOTOXIC	TOXIC
5-FLUOROURACIL (51-21-8)	YES (IARC-G3)	YES (MSDS)	YES (NIH MSDS) (P65)	YES (MSDS)	?	MOD (NIH MSDS)
6-MERCAPTOPURINE (50-44-2) (6112-76-1)	YES—WEAK (NIH MSDS) (BERK)	YES (UMCP) (MSDS)	YES (UMCP) (MSDS)	YES (MSDS)	?	ACUTELY (NIH)
6-THIOGUANINE (154-42-7)	YES (BC-CAN)	YES (BC CAN) (UMCP)	YES (NIH/P65) (UMCP)	?	?	ACUTELY (NIH MSDS)
ADRIAMYCIN HCL (23214-92-8) (25316-40-9)	YES (IARC-G2A) (NTP-C2) (UMCP)	YES (UMCP) (MSDS)	YES (UMCP/P65)	YES (MALE P65) (MSDS)	?	HIGHLY TOXIC (MSDS)
ALTRETAMINE (645-05-6)	YES (MSDS)	YES (MSDS)	YES (P65)	YES (P65/MSDS)	?	TOXIC (MSDS)
ARSENIC TRIOXIDE (1327-53-3)	YES (IARC-G1) (NTP-C1) (OSHA) (NIOSH) (BERK) (ACGIH) (P65)	YES (MSDS)	YES (UMCP/MSDS)	?	?	ACUTELY (UMCP) HIGHLY TOXIC (MSDS)
AVASTIN (216974-75-3)	?	?	YES (MSDS)	YES (MSDS)	?	?
BICALUTAMIDE (CASODEX) (90357-06-5)	YES (CA ANIMAL-MSDS)	?	YES (ANIMAL-MSDS)	YES (REP ANIMAL-MSDS)	?	?
CARBOPLATIN (41575-94-4) (7440-06-4)	YES (MSDS)	YES (UMCP) (MSDS)	YES (MSDS)	YES (MSDS)	YES (HAIN)	HIGHLY (MSDS)

Drug (CAS No.)						
CYCLOPHOSPHAMIDE (50-18-0) (6055-19-2) (60007-96-7) (60030-72-0) (6007-95-6)	YES (NTP-C1) (IARC-G1) (BERK) (UMPC)	YES (MSDS)	YES (UMCP/P65) (MSDS)	YES (P65) (CENTRE COL)	YES (HAIN)	ACUTELY (MSDS)
ETOPOSIDE (33419-42-0)	YES (IARC-G2A) (NTP) (MSDS)	YES (UMCP) (MSDS)	YES (UMCP) (MSDS)	?	?	TOXIC (MSDS)
GEMZAR (95058-81-4) (12211-03-9)	?	YES (MSDS)	?	YES (MSDS) (NFPA)	?	SKIN PERM (MSDS)
GOSERELIN ACETATE (65807-02-5)	?	?	YES (P65)	YES (P65 MALE/ FEMALE)	?	?
HYDROXYUREA (HU) (127-07-1)	YES (IARC-G3)	YES (UMCP)	YES (UMCP/P65)	YES (P65)	?	TOXIC (MSDS)
LEUPROLIDE AC DEPOT (53714-56-0)	?	YES (RTECS)	YES (P65)	YES (P65)(MSDS)	?	TOXIC (MSDS)
MEGESTROL (MEGACE) (595-33-5) (3562-63-8)	YES (IARC-G1/ MSDS)	?	YES (P65/MSDS)	YES (MSDS)	?	?
METHOTREXATE (59-05-2)	YES (IARC-G3) (BERK)	YES (MSDS)	YES (UMCP/P65)	YES (MSDS)	YES (SEARCH)	ACUTELY (NIH)
OXALIPLATIN (61825-94-3)	LIMITED (MSDS)	?	?	?	?	?
RITUXAN (174722-31-7)	?	?	?	?	?	?

DRUG NAME	CARCINOGEN*	MUTAGEN*	TERATOGEN*	REPRODUCTIVE* (FEMALE AND/OR MALE)	OTOTOXIC	TOXIC
STREPTOZOCIN (18883-66-4) (66395-18-4) (66395-17-3)	YES (IARC-G2B) (NTP-C2)	YES (NIH MSDS) (MSDS)	YES (NIH MSDS) (P65)	YES (P65) (MSDS)	?	?
TAMOXIFEN CITRATE (10540-29-1) (54965-24-1)	YES (IARC-G1/P65) (NTP-C1)	YES (MSDS)	YES (P65)	YES (MSDS)	?	TOXIC (MSDS)
TAXOTERE (114977-28-5)	?	?	?	?	?	MOD (MSDS)
VELCADE (179324-69-7)	?	?	?	YES (MSDS)	?	YES (MSDS)
VINBLASTINE (SULFATE) (143-67-9) (865-21-4)	YES (IARC-G3) (BERK)	YES (UMCP) (MSDS)	YES (UMCP) (P65) (NIH MSDS)	YES (MSDS)	YES (SEARCH)	YES (NIH MSDS)
VINCRISTINE (2068-78-2) (57-22-7)	YES (IARC-G3) (MSDS)	YES (UMCP)	YES (UMCP/P65)	YES (MSDS)	YES (HAIN)	YES (MSDS)

*Used most conservative definitions from various organization, such as IARC, NTP, NIEHS–NIH, and others.

Hazardous Drugs (Cytotoxic) Program Self-Assessment   3.20

Facility Name: _____   Project # _____
Start Date _____/_____/_____   End Date _____/_____/_____

Program Elements	Regulatory	Y	N	NA	Remarks
Hazardous Drugs Safety and Health Program					
Has a hazardous drugs officer (HD officer) been appointed by the commander? Contact Information: NAME: PHONE: LOCATION: Ideal candidates: Safety and health representative, nurses, and industrial hygienists.	USACHPPM TG 149, Part 1, Chapter 2, 2-2, a. Prudent Safety Practice				
Has a hazardous drugs committee been established? Representatives from: Medical & nursing staffs; pharmacy; occupational health; preventative medicine, hospital education and training; safety; logistics, including housekeeping, and maintenance.	USACHPPM TG 149, Part 1, Chapter 2, 2-2, b. OSHA Tech Manual, Sec VI: Chapter 2, V, A, 2.				

Program Elements	Regulatory	Y	N	NA	Remarks
Is a written hazardous drugs safety and health plan (HDSHP) published and implemented?	OSHA Tech Manual, Sec VI: Chapter 2, V, A, 2.				
Are HD references available (i.e., USACHPPM TG 149, OSHA Tech Manual, 29 CFR 1910, etc.) with a minimum content of:	USACHPPM TG 149, Part 1, Chapter 2, 2-3				
Described methods used to systematically identify, evaluate, and prevent or control work place hazards;					
Identification and evaluation methods, that is, job hazard analyses, general safety inspections, reviews of employee reports of unsafe/unhealthy working conditions, accident and incident reports, OSHA Log;	Prudent Safety Practice				
Prevention and control methods to include engineering and administrative controls, safe work practices, and PPE used to prevent or minimize occupational exposures;					
Ventilation Systems—BSCs, Barrier Isolators, etc., and certification and maintenance;	Prudent Safety Practice				
The technical basis for selection of engineering controls IAW ALARA program.					
SOPs related to Cytotoxic Drugs, HAZCOM, emergency preparedness, HAZMAT, etc.;					
Investigational Drugs—statement related to compliance with AR 40-7.					

Program Elements	Regulatory	Y	N	NA	Remarks
Healthcare workers having potential occupational exposure to hazardous drugs received training prior to working with HD. Healthcare workers must understand the safety and health hazards of HDs and safe work practices;					
Supervisors must be trained to evaluate work area and how to detect safety and health hazards, to insure control measures are functional and properly used, reinforce worker training and safe work practices;	OSHA Tech Manual, Sec VI: Chapter 2, V, A, 1. Prudent Safety Practice USACHPPM TG 149, Part 1, Chapter 2, 2-3, h.				
Medical surveillance and examination must be provided to HD workers (refer to Medical Surveillance section of this checklist);	Prudent Safety Practice				
Recordkeeping—required to keep records to show that the HDSHP is carried out as it was designed (refer to Recordkeeping section of this checklist);					
A written ALARA program has been implemented and used to perform effectiveness evaluations?					
Are effectiveness evaluations performed IAW guidelines?					
HD officer will perform a HDSHP evaluation at least annually; and update the HDSHP as necessary;					
The HD committee and the MTF safety committee should review the annual effectiveness evaluations, incidents reports, injuries and equipment failures. Provide program improvement suggestions; and					

Program Elements	Regulatory	Y	N	NA	Remarks
Work area supervisors should update SOPs as needed, but at least once every three years.					
Are orientation and refresher training requirements being met?	OSHA Tech Manual, Sec VI: Chapter 2, VIII, A, B & C				
Are shipping/receiving personnel, physicians, nurses, pharmacists, respiratory therapists, housekeepers, maintenance workers, hazardous waste handlers and emergency response trained in hazards of the HDs in their work areas(s) and the safe work practices?	USACHPPM TG 149, Part 1, Chapter 3, 3-1 Prudent Safety Practice **29 CFR 1910.1200** USACHPPM TG 149, Part 1, Chapter 3, 3-2				
Meet or exceed HAZCOM program requirements?	OSHA Tech Manual, Sec VI: Chapter 2, IX;				
Written program and inventories;	USACHPPM TG 149, Part 1, Chapter 3, 3-3, a.				
Warning labels present;					
MSDSs and other safety and health information concerning HDs are maintained and available 7/24;					
Training consists of health hazards, primary exposure routes, carcinogenic evaluations, acute exposure treatment, chemical inactivators, solubility, stability, and volatility; engineering controls, PPE, spill procedures, first aid, and waste disposal methods.					
Are training recordkeeping maintained for at least three years?	Manual, Sec VI: Chapter 2, IX; USACHPPM TG 149, Part 1, Chapter 3, 3-3, a.				
Receipt, Storage, and Handling					
Are receipt, storage, and handling requirements being met?	OSHA Tech Manual, Sec VI, Chapter 2, V, C, 6				

Program Elements	Regulatory	Y	N	NA	Remarks
Is access to all areas where hazardous drugs are stored limited to specified authorized staff? Posted?	USACHPPM TG 149, Part 2, Chapter 7 (7–1 through 7–5)				
Are storage areas secured from unauthorized personnel?					
Are warning labels used to identify cytotoxic drugs containers, shelves, and bins?					
Are stored in a separate storage area away from other drugs?					
Are storage facilities designed to provide a secured storage area with barriers at the front to prevent falling to the floor?					
Are hazardous drugs requiring refrigeration stored separately from nonhazardous drugs in individual bins designed to prevent breakage and contain leakage?					
Is an explosive-proof refrigerator available for flammable items?					
Are written policies and standard procedures for preparing hazardous drugs maintained and followed?					
All personnel who handle cytotoxic and other hazardous agents should have access to the procedures pertaining to their responsibilities. Deviations from the standard procedures must not be permitted except under defined circumstances.					
Are written procedures for handling damaged packages of hazardous drugs followed?					

Program Elements	Regulatory	Y	N	NA	Remarks
Are staffs trained in handling damaged/leaking packages?					
Are secondary containers used during transportation of cytotoxic drugs in case of breakage and leaking containers?					
Is a SOP in place for handling broken, leaking, contaminated drug containers, packages, etc.?					
Has a hazard analysis been conducted for each task and appropriate PPE are being used?					
Has personnel transporting cytotoxic drugs been placed on cytotoxic occupational health medical exam track?					
General engineering controls (refer to Engineering Control section)					
General PPE (refer to PPE section)					
Are staffs included on the medical surveillance program for cytotoxic drugs?					
Medical surveillance (refer to the Medical Surveillance section)					
Is a method for orienting all involved personnel to the special nature of the hazardous drugs in question and the policies and procedures that govern their handling present?	29 CFR 910.1200 OSHA Tech Manual, Sec VI: Chapter 2, VI				
Are employees trained to clean up spills using appropriate information?					

Program Elements	Regulatory	Y	N	NA	Remarks
Is sufficient information maintained and made available to employees concerning safe use of the hazardous drugs in the work area, that is, HAZCOM policy, MSDSs, and other technical sources of information?					
Are MSDS information and related information available to employee 24/7?					
Are staffs trained in responding to cytotoxic spills?					
Are (approved) spill kits available?					
Are hand washing facilities available in area nearby?					
Is an established first aid protocol in placed?					
Are receiving cytotoxic drugs cartons/packages verified as being noncontaminated?					
Are eyewash and emergency showers readily accessible? Tested and documented? Weekly?					
Pharmacy Preparation Areas					
Are pharmacy preparation areas requirements being met?	OSHA Tech Manual, Sec VI: Chapter 2, IV, A				
Are chemotherapy drugs wastes placed in properly labeled sharp container for disposal IAW local SOP, state and federal regulations?	USACHPPM TG 149, Part 2, Chapter 8, 8-1 through 8-6				

Program Elements	Regulatory	Y	N	NA	Remarks
Is pharmacy staff that receives cytotoxic drugs been identified to receive medical surveillance with emphasis on cytotoxic drugs?					
Are access to all areas where hazardous drugs are stored limited to specified authorized staff? Posted?					
Are warning labels used to identify cytotoxic drugs containers, shelves, and bins?					
Are written procedures for handling damaged packages of hazardous drugs followed?					
Are employees trained in handling damaged packages?					
Are cytotoxic drugs packages upon receipt handled with chemotherapy-approved gloves or with double-gloved hands and stored in a separate storage area away from other drugs?	Prudent Safety Practices				
Are storage facilities designed to provide a secured storage area with barriers at the front to prevent falling to the floor?					
Are hazardous drugs requiring refrigeration stored separately from nonhazardous drugs in individual bins designed to prevent breakage and contain leakage? Flammable CD is stored in an explosive-proof refrigerator?					
Are written policies and standard procedures for preparing hazardous drugs maintained and followed?					

Program Elements	Regulatory	Y	N	NA	Remarks
All personnel who handle cytotoxic and other hazardous agents should have access to the procedures pertaining to their responsibilities. Deviations from the standard procedures must not be permitted except under defined circumstances.					
Is a method for orienting all involved personnel to the special nature of the hazardous drugs in question and the policies and procedures that govern their handling present?					
Is a system established for verifying and documenting acceptable staff performance of and conformance with established procedures maintained?					
Is sufficient information maintained and made available to employees on safe use of the hazardous drugs in the work area, that is, HAZCOM policy, MSDSs, and other technical sources of information?					
Engineering controls (refer to the Engineering Control section)					
General PPE (refer to the PPE section)					
Medical surveillance (refer to the Medical Surveillance section)					
Are cytotoxic drugs spills properly cleaned up according to SOP and only by trained staff?					
Is sufficient information maintained and made available to employees on safe use of the hazardous drugs in the work area, that is, HAZCOM policy, MSDSs, and other technical sources of information?					

Program Elements	Regulatory	Y	N	NA	Remarks
Are staffs trained in responding correctly to cytotoxic spills?					
Are (approved) spill kits available?					
Are appropriate SOPs developed and implemented?					
Cytotoxic drugs administration controls; certification and decontamination of engineering devices; spill cleanup; waste disposal; housekeeping; proper use of PPE and engineering controls					
Is an established first aid protocol in placed?					
Are hands washing facilities available in area nearby?					
Are hazardous drugs labeled with a warning label stating the need for special handling?					
Are procedures for administering hazardous drugs preventing the accidental exposure of patients and staff and contamination of the work environment?					
Hazardous (cytotoxic) drug waste is disposed of in accordance with all applicable state, federal, and local regulations for the handling of hazardous and toxic waste?					
Are work surfaces decontaminated at least once per day and always after a spill of potentially cytotoxic drugs?					

Program Elements	Regulatory	Y	N	NA	Remarks
Are eyewash and emergency showers readily accessible? Tested and documented? Weekly?					
Clinical Administration Areas					
Are clinical administration areas requirements being met?	OSHA Tech Manual, Sec VI: Chapter 2, IV, B				
Are access to all areas where hazardous (cytotoxic) drugs are administered limited to specified authorized staff and authorized patients? Posted?	USACHPPM TG 149, Part 2, Chapter 9, 9-1 through 9-5				
Are staffs on medical surveillance for cytotoxic drugs?					
Are storage areas secured from unauthorized personnel?					
Are warning labels used to identify cytotoxic drugs containers, shelves, and bins?					
Are stored in a separate storage area away from other drugs?					
Are written policies and standard procedures for preparing hazardous drugs maintained and followed?					
All personnel who handle cytotoxic and other hazardous agents should have access to the procedures pertaining to their responsibilities. Deviations from the standard procedures must not be permitted except under defined circumstances.					
Are written procedures for handling hazardous drugs followed?					

Program Elements	Regulatory	Y	N	NA	Remarks
Are chemotherapy gloves or doubled gloves being used when handling cytotoxic drugs?					
Are workers exposed to potential eye contact with hazardous drugs provided appropriate PPE? (refer to PPE section)					
Are appropriate engineering controls (eyewash and emergency shower) available?					
Engineering controls (refer to the Engineering Controls section)					
General PPE (refer to the PPE section)					
Are staffs on medical surveillance program for cytotoxic drugs?					
Medical surveillance (refer to the Medical Surveillance section)					
Are eyewash and emergency showers readily accessible? Tested and documented?					
Are closed systems and/or Leur-Lock devices being used routinely?					
Is an established first-aid protocol in placed?					
Are hand washing facilities available in area?					
Are hazardous drugs labeled with a warning label stating the need for special handling?					

Program Elements	Regulatory	Y	N	NA	Remarks
Are hazardous (cytotoxic) drug wastes disposed of in accordance with all applicable state, federal, and local regulations for the handling of hazardous and toxic waste?					
Is MSDS information and related information available 24/7?					
Are staffs trained in responding to cytotoxic spills?					
Are (approved) spill kits available?					

Housekeeping and Waste Management

Housekeeping and waste management requirements being met:	OSHA Tech Manual, Sec VI: Chapter 2, IV, C.				
Are hazardous (cytotoxic) drug wastes disposed of in accordance with all applicable state, federal, and local regulations for the handling of hazardous and toxic waste?	USACHPPM TG 149, Part 2, Chapter 10, 10-1 through 10-6				
Are staffs on the medical surveillance program for cytotoxic drugs?					
Are chemotherapy gloves used when urine and other excreta from patients receiving hazardous drugs are being handled? Skin contact and splattering should be avoided during disposal. While it may be useful to post a list of drugs that are excreted in urine and feces and the length of time after drug administration during which precautions are necessary, an alternative is to select a standard duration (e.g., 48 hours) that covers most of the drugs and is more easily remembered.					

Program Elements	Regulatory	Y	N	NA	Remarks
Are gloves discarded after each use and immediately if contaminated?					
Are gowns discarded on leaving the patient-care area and immediately if contaminated?					
Are hands washed thoroughly after hazardous drugs are handled?					
Are disposable linen or protective pads used for incontinent or vomiting patients?					
Nondisposable linen contaminated with a hazardous drug should be handled with gloves and treated similarly to that for linen contaminated with infectious material. One procedure is to place the linen in specially marked water-soluble laundry bags. These bags (with the contents) should be prewashed; then the linens should be added to other laundry for an additional wash. Items contaminated with hazardous drugs should not be autoclaved unless they are also contaminated with infectious material.					
Is sufficient information maintained and made available to employees on safe use of the hazardous drugs in the work area, that is, HAZCOM policy, MSDSs, and other technical sources of information?					
Engineering controls (refer to the Engineering Controls section)					
General PPE (refer to the PPE section)					

Program Elements	Regulatory	Y	N	NA	Remarks
Are staffs on medical surveillance program for cytotoxic drugs?					
Medical surveillance (refer to the Medical Surveillance section)					
Are eyewash and emergency showers readily accessible? Tested and documented?					
Is an established first-aid protocol in placed?					
Emergency Response (Spills)					
Emergency response (spills) requirements:	OSHA Tech Manual, Sec VI: Chapter 2, V, C, 5.				
Are staffs trained to response to spills? Small Spills Large Spills	USACHPPM TG 149, Part 2, Chapter 11, 11-1 through 11-5				
Are appropriate PPEs available for every potential response scenario?	29 CFR 1910.120 USACHPPM TG 275				
Selection based on hazards and specifications from the manufacturer?					
Are spill kits and other supplies available when needed?					
Are spilled cytotoxic drugs MSDSs and other technical information referring to spill clean-up information (deactivators, incompatible substances, first aid, etc.) available?					
Is the local spill procedure (SOP) incorporated into the facility emergency response plan?					

Program Elements	Regulatory	Y	N	NA	Remarks
Has coordination occurred with external emergency response organizations (post, city, county)?					
Engineering controls (refer to the Engineering Controls section)					
General PPE (refer to the PPE section)					
Are staffs on medical surveillance program for cytotoxic drugs?					
Medical surveillance (refer to the Medical Surveillance section)					
Personal Protective Equipment (PPE)					
Are PPE program requirements being met? OSHA's new final standard on personal protective equipment, 29CFR 1910 132, Subpart I, imposes several new and important requirements relating to basic safety and health programs. The standard adds new general requirements for the selection and use of personal protective equipment (PPE). Included in these requirements are the following: • Employers must conduct a hazard assessment to determine if hazards presented necessitate the use of PPE. • Employers must certify in writing that the hazard assessment was conducted. • PPE selection must be made on the basis of a hazard assessment and affected workers properly trained. • Defective or damaged PPE must not be used.	OSHA Tech Manual, Sec VI: Chapter 2, I–X USACHPPM TG 149, Part 2, Chapter 6, 6-1 through 6-4 29CFR 1910.132 "General Requirements" 29 CFR 1910.133, "Eye and Face Protection" 29 CFR 1910.134, "Respiratory Protection" 29 CFR 1910.135, "Head Protection" 29 CFR 1910.136, "Occupational Foot Protection" 29 CFR 1910.138, "Hand Protection"				

Program Elements	Regulatory	Y	N	NA	Remarks
• Established training requirements for employees using PPE must be established. This should include requirements for employees to demonstrate an understanding of the training. • Employer must certify in writing that training programs were provided and understood.	ANSI, Z87.1-1989, "Eye and Face Protection" ANSI Z41.1-1991, Protective Footwear" ANSI Z89.1-1986, "Industrial Head Protection" USACHPPM TG 275				
Are hazard assessments completed for each task or area and documented?					
Are PPE selection based upon hazard assessments?					
Respiratory protection program in place?					
Vision protection program in place?					
Hand and foot protection program in place?					
Is documentation of exposure maintained and shared with appropriate departments?					
Are air samples conducted?					
Is contamination monitoring conducted?					
Are bioassays performed as part of a medical surveillance program?					
Defective or damaged PPE not being used?					
Are PPE furnished to staff at no cost?					
PPE training complete and documented?					

Program Elements	Regulatory	Y	N	NA	Remarks
Description of eye and face protection used (Brand/Model/Stock #) and location:					
Respirators (Brand/Type/Model: _____) mists and dusts vapors					
Eye and face shields (Brand/Type/Model: _____) (Complies with standards?)					
Gloves (Brand/Type/Model: _____)					
Gowns/shoe covers: (Brand/Type/Model: _____)					
Are gloves discarded after each use and immediately if contaminated?					
Are gowns discarded on leaving the patient-care area and immediately if contaminated?					
Are hands washed thoroughly before and after donning/doffing appropriate gloves?					
Are appropriate gloves used to handle HDs? Never without gloves?					
Are hands washed thoroughly before and after donning/doffing appropriate gloves?					

Program Elements	Regulatory	Y	N	NA	Remarks
Maintenance Activities					
Maintenance (biomedical) requirements:	OSHA Tech Manual, Sect VI, Chapter2, VII, A, 4.				
Are staffs on the medical surveillance program for cytotoxic drugs?	USA CHPPM TG 149, Part 1, Chapter 3, 2-2, a.				
Is sufficient information maintained and made available to employees on safe use of the hazardous drugs in the work area, that is, HAZCOM policy, MSDSs, and other technical sources of information?	OSHA Tech Manual, Sect VI, Chapter2, VII, A, 4. USACHPPM TG 149, Part 1, Chapter 2, 2-2, b. USACHPPM TG 149, Part 1, Chapter 2, 2-3, b.				
All maintenance workers received orientation and refresher training?	USACHPPM TG 149, Part 2, Chapter 5, 5-1, d.				
Is contaminated equipment deactivated using appropriate deactivators and verification sampling is conducted to verify the equipment is contamination free?	USACHPPM TG 149, Part 2, Chapter 5 USACHPPM TG 149, Part 2, Chapter 8, 8-5 Prudent Safety Practices				
Are appropriate PPE used when potential of exposure to cytotoxic drugs exists?					
Selected based on hazards and manufacturers' specifications?					
Is there a decommissioning SOP and has it been implemented?					
Engineering controls (refer to the Engineering Controls section)					
General PPE (refer to the PPE section)					
Medical Surveillance (refer to the Medical Surveillance section)					
How is cytotoxic drugs contamination detected?					

Program Elements	Regulatory	Y	N	NA	Remarks
Is there a maintenance representation on the hazardous drug committee?					
Are procedures in place to verify that ventilation systems are operational?					
Are certifications performed every six months and whenever the BSC is moved or repaired? Contractor Qualified. HAZCOM information provided? Records Maintained IAW HDSHP or JCAHO?					
Procedure implemented to verify decontamination of equipment and spill areas?					
Who has the responsibility for the oversight for release of equipment and declaring spill areas safe for routine work?					
Are (approved) spill kits available?					
When renovations are performed, does all equipment meet new standards (i.e., OSHA, NFPA, JCOHA, Army, ASHP, etc.)?					
Are hand washing facilities available in area nearby?					
Are eyewash and emergency showers readily accessible? Tested and documented?					
Is an established first-aid protocol in place?					

Program Elements	Regulatory	Y	N	NA	Remarks
Engineering Controls					
Are engineering controls appropriately used?	USACHPPM TG 149, Part 2, Chapter 5, 5-1 through 5-3				
Are BSCs and/or BARRIER ISOLATORS used for cytotoxic drugs preparation and vented 30%, 70%, or 100% outside? 100% preferred.	OSHA Tech Manual, Sect VI, Chapter 2, I through X.				
Are certifications of BSCs and Barrier Isolator units performed every six months or when serviced? Documentation available?					
Is decontaminated equipment and spill areas verified and certified before release?					
When repaired or removed from service or replaced, are equipment decontamination and verification samples taken to validate the decontamination? Is appropriate technical information used in determining decontamination/ deactivation?					
Are barrier isolators' gloves replaced prior to cytotoxic drugs breakthrough?					
What method is used to verify breakthrough?					
Are workers who are not protected by the containment environment of a BSC provided respiratory protection when handling hazardous drugs or potential for exposure?					
Are closed systems and/or Leur-Lock devices being used routinely? With BSCs?					

Program Elements	Regulatory	Y	N	NA	Remarks
General Safety					
Are general safety requirements being met?	OSHA Tech Manual, Sect VI, Chapter 1, IV, C.				
Eating, drinking, handling contact lenses, applying cosmetics, and mouth pipetting are prohibited in areas where cytotoxic drugs are handled, prepared, administered, and stored.					
Standard operating practices and procedures are written and followed.					
These SOPs should include experimental protocols, daily housekeeping, waste disposal, and emergency plans covering accidental spills, personal contamination, and security procedures. Inhalation is one of the four modes of entry for chemical exposure. "Sniff-testing" should not be done.					
Never pipette by mouth. Always use a bulb to pipette.					
Do not drink, eat, smoke, or apply cosmetics in the laboratory or chemical storage areas.					
No food, beverage, tobacco, or cosmetics products are allowed in the laboratory or chemical storage areas at any time. Cross contamination between these items and chemicals or samples is an obvious hazard and should be avoided.					
Exiting or Egress					
• Are all exits marked with an exit sign and illuminated by a reliable light source?					
• Are the directions to exits, when not immediately apparent, marked with visible signs?					

Program Elements	Regulatory	Y	N	NA	Remarks
• Are doors, passageways or stairways, that are neither exits nor access to exits and which could be mistaken for exits, appropriately marked "NOT AN EXIT," "TO BASEMENT," "STOREROOM," and the like?					
• Are exit signs provided with the word "EXIT" in lettering at least 5 inches high and the stroke of the lettering at least 1/2 inch wide?					
• Are exit doors side-hinged?					
• Are all exits kept free of obstructions?					
• Are at least two means of egress provided from elevated platforms, pits, or rooms where the absence of a second exit would increase the risk of injury from hot, poisonous, corrosive, suffocating, flammable, or explosive substances?					
• Are there sufficient exits to permit prompt escape in case of emergency?					
Exit Doors					
• Are doors that are required to serve as exits designed and constructed so that the way of exit travel is obvious and direct?					
• Are windows that could be mistaken for exit doors made inaccessible by means of barriers or railings?					
• Are exit doors openable from the direction of exit travel without the use of a key or any special knowledge or effort when the building is occupied?					
• Where panic hardware is installed on a required exit door, will it allow the door to open by applying a force of 15 pounds or less in the direction of the exit traffic?					

Program Elements	Regulatory	Y	N	NA	Remarks
• Are doors on cold storage rooms provided with an inside release mechanism that will release the latch and open the door even if it is padlocked or otherwise locked on the outside? • Where exit doors open directly onto any street, alley, or other area where vehicles may be operated, are adequate barriers and warnings provided to prevent employees stepping into the path of traffic? • Are doors that swing in both directions and are located between rooms where there is frequent traffic provided with viewing panels in each door?					

Medical Surveillance—Occupational Health Program

Program Elements	Regulatory	Y	N	NA	Remarks
Are medical surveillance requirements being met? Does HD personnel receive medical surveillance to include: Replacement, transfer, or termination medical examinations; and Examinations tailor-based on potential exposure and specific toxic profiles of drugs. Are periodic examinations performed IAW army and manufacturer's guidance (yearly, every 2- to 3-year basis, and after an acute exposure)? Are incident examinations initiated post acute exposure? Are local pregnancy policies and SOPs explained through education and counseling to HD (cytotoxic) workers during training and during medical surveillance?	OSHA Tech Manual, Sec VI: Chapter 2, VI, A–F. USACHPPM TG 149, Part 2, Chapter 4, 4-1 through 4-6 29 CFR 1910.1020 AR 40-5 (f) USACHPPM TG 275				

Program Elements	Regulatory	Y	N	NA	Remarks
Is an employee cytotoxic drugs registry established and maintained to include the following information:					
Records of drugs and quantities handled (include what form the drug is in, that is, capsule, injection, implant, aerosol, and so on					
Hours spent handling these drugs per week					
Number of preparations/ administrations per week					
Engineering controls and PPE used					
Description of the worker duties					
Are medical records reviewed to determine if trends are detected?					
Are records maintained for duration of employment plus 30 years?					
Have workers been informed of their rights to access their medical records?					
Records and Recordkeeping					
Are employee exposure and medical records maintained and stored properly?					
The medical record for each employee is to be preserved and maintained for at least the duration of employment plus 30 years.					
Each employee exposure record shall be preserved and maintained for at least 30 years.					
Each analysis using employee exposure or medical records shall be preserved and maintained for at least 30 years.					

Program Elements	Regulatory	Y	N	NA	Remarks
If an employee, or their designated representative, requests a copy of the employee's health record, the facility is to provide a copy within 15 days of the request, or provide facilities to make copies at no cost, or loan the records to employee or designated representative so that copies can be made.					
References Occupational Safety and Health Administration (OSHA) Technical Manual, Sec VI: Chapter 1 and Chapter 2. USACHPPM Technical Guide 149, Guidelines for Controlling Occupational Exposure to Hazardous Drugs, June 2001 American National Standards Institute, American National Standard ANSI Z41-1991, "Personnel Protection—Protective Footwear." American National Standards Institute, American National Standard ANSI Z87.1-1989, "Practice for Occupational and Educational Eye and Face Protection." American National Standards Institute, American National Standard ANSI Z89.1-1986, "Safety Requirements for Industrial Head Protection." OSHA Standard 29 CFR 1910.120, "Hazardous Waste Operations and Emergency Response." OSHA Standard 29 CFR 1910.132, "General Requirements"					

Program Elements	Regulatory	Y	N	NA	Remarks
OSHA Standard 29 CFR 1910.133, "Eye and Face Protection"					
OSHA Standard 29 CFR 1910.134, "Respiratory Protection"					
OSHA Standard 29 CFR 1910.135, "Head Protection"					
OSHA Standard 29 CFR 1910.136, "Occupational Foot Protection"					
OSHA Standard 29 CFR 1910.138, "Hand Protection"					
OSHA Standard 29 CFR 1910.1020, "Access to Employee and Medical Records"					
OSHA Standard 29 CFR 1910.1200, "Hazard Communication"					
USACHPPM TG 275, Personal Protective Equipment Guide for Military Medical Treatment Facility Personnel Handling Casualties from Weapons of Mass Destruction and Terrorism Events, August 2003					
AR 40–5, Preventive Medicine					

Facility Name: _____   Project # _____

Auditor's Name: _____   Manager: _____

Dept./Clinic: _____   Ph # _____

Building: _____   Room(s) _____

Start Date _____/_____/_____   End Date _____/_____/_____

Auditor's Signature   Date:

Clinic/Department/Pharmacy Representative Signature   Date:

CC:
HD Officer, HDSH Committee, Facility Safety Officer, Facility Industrial Hygienist/Preventive Medicine, Occupational Health Clinic

Cytotoxic Drugs Listed as Characteristic Hazardous Waste by EPA (United States) 3.21

GENERIC NAME	BRAND NAME	CHEMICAL ABSTRACT SYSTEM REGISTRY NUMBER	RTECS
ARSENIC TRIOXIDE	TRISENOX	1327-53-3	CG3325000
CHLORAMBUCIL	LEUKERAN, AMBOCHLORIN	305-03-3	ES7525000
CYCLOPHOSPAMIDE	CYTOZAN, NEOSAR	50-18-0 6055-19-2 60007-96-7 60030-72-0 6007-95-6 MIXTURE	RP6157750 RP5950000
DAUNOMYCIN	DAUNORUBICIN, CERUBIDIN, DAUNOXOME, RUBIDOMYCIN	23541-50-6 20830-81-3	HB7878000
DIETHYSTIBESTROL	DES, STILPHOSTROL	18883-66-4 522-40-7 66395-18-4 66395-17-3	LZ5775000
MELPHALAN	ALKERAN, L-PAM, MYLERAN, PHENYLALANIME MUSTARD	148-82-3 8057-25-8	AY3675000
MITOMYCIN C STREPTOZOTOCIN	MITOMYCIN, MUTAMYCIN	50-07-7	CN0700000
URACIL MUSTARD	URAMUSTINE, (5-[(BIS(2-CHLOROETHYL) AMINO)] URACIL)	66-75-1	YQ8925000

Note: Chemotherapy waste contaminated with listed hazardous waste chemotherapy drugs is listed hazardous waste and must be managed as hazardous waste. Chemotherapy waste contaminated with characteristic hazardous waste chemotherapy drugs should be tested to determine if the mixture is a characteristic hazardous waste; if you do not test the chemotherapy waste, you should manage it as characteristic hazardous waste. Containers that held hazardous waste chemotherapy drugs, and do not meet the definition of "empty," are hazardous waste when discarded. Hazardous waste regulations may change at any time; it behooves you to contact your local hazardous waste expert.

NATIONAL OEL(S)	INTERNATIONAL OEL(S)	NFPA HMIS	MIDI	UN GUIDE #	EPA WASTE CODE
OSHA: 0.01 MG/M3 (AS) ACTION LEVEL 5 μG/M3 TWA 8-HRS (AS) (REFER TO 29 CFR 1910.1018) NIOSH REL: C 0.002 MG/M3 (AS)/15 MIN; CA DOE: TEEL-3: 9.1 MG/M3 ACGIH TLV: 0.01 MG/M3 TWA; CA	CANADA: TWA 0.05 (MG(AS)/M) UK MEL: 0.1 MG/M3 TWA	NFPA 3,0,0 NFPA 3,0,2 HMIS 3*,0,0,- HMIS 3,0,0,E	HW01	UN 1561 GUIDE 151	P012 D004
N.O.S	N.O.S	NFPA 2,0,0 HMIS N.O.S.	HW01	UN 2811 GUIDE 154	U035
N.O.S	N.O.S	NFPA 2,0,0 NFPA 3,1,1 NFPA 2,1,0 HMIS 2,1,0,E HMIS 2*,0,0,-	HW01	UN 2811 GUIDE 154	U058
N.O.S	N.O.S	NFPA 1,0,0 NFPA 2,1,0 NFPA 2,0,0 NFPA 3,0,0 HMIS 2*,1,0,A HMIS 3*,0,0,- HMIS 3,0,9,X	HW01	UN 2811 GUIDE 154 UN 2810 GUIDE 153	U059
N.O.S	N.O.S	NFPA 2,1,0 HMIS 2,1,0,E HMIS 0*,0,0,- NFPA 2,0,0	N.O.S.	N.O.S. N.O.S.	U089 U206
DOE: TEEL-3 23.0 MG/M3	N.O.S.	NFPA 3,0,0	HW01	UN 2811 GUIDE 154 UN 3249 GUIDE 151	U150
N.O.S.	N.O.S.	NFPA 4,1,0 HMIS 4*,1,0,A	HW01	UN2811 GUIDE 154	U010 U206
N.O.S.	N.O.S.	N.O.S.	HW01	UN2811 GUIDE 154	U237

Summary of Cytotoxic Drugs Solubility and Insolubility in Water and/or Alcohol

The solubility and insolubility of a cytotoxic drug* is useful in determining if alcohol or water-based cleaning solutions will be effective in cleaning up spills. If not soluble, the spilled materials are spread around the surface contaminating a larger area and will be tracked into other areas. Specific cytotoxic drug solubility and insolubility information is available in sections 2.1 and 2.2.

Approximate Number of Table Entries	Various Soluble (Miscible) and Insoluble Categories
88	Alcohol** Insoluble (Includes Unknowns and Conflicts)
19	Alcohol** Soluble
71	Water Soluble
36	Water Insoluble (Includes Unknowns and Conflicts)
8	Both Water and Alcohol** Soluble
28	Both Water and Alcohol** Insoluble (Includes Unknowns and Conflicts)

Notes: *Refer to section 2.2 "Comprehensive Cytotoxic Drugs Tables," which contains specific solubility data.
**Alcohol includes isopropyl, ethyl (ethanol), or dehydrated alcohol.

References

40 CFR 261.5. *Identification and Listing of Hazardous Waste.*

40 CFR 264. *Standards for Owners and Operators of Hazardous Waste Treatment, Storage, and Disposal Facilities.*

40 CFR 265. *Interim Status Standards for Owners and Operators of Hazardous Waste Treatment, Storage, and Disposal Facilities.*

42 CFR 84. *Approval of Respiratory Protective Devices.*

Acampora, A., L. Castiglia, N. Miraglia, M. Pieri, C. Soave, F. Liotti, and N. Sannolo. A Case Study: Surface Contamination of Cyclophosphamide Due to Working Practices and Cleaning Procedures in Two Italian Hospitals. *Ann. Occup. Hyg.* 49 (2005): 611–18.

Allwood, M., Wright, A., and Stanley, P., eds. *Cytotoxic Handbook.* 4th ed. Abingdon, UK: Radcliffe Medical Press, 2003.

Amato, D., and J. S. Niblett. Neutropenia from Cyclophosphamide in Breast Milk. *Med. J. Aust.* 1 (1977): 383–84.

American Academy of Pediatrics, Committee on Drugs. Transfer of Drugs and Other Chemicals into Human Milk. *Pediatrics* 93 (1994): 137–50.

American Conference of Government Industrial Hygienists. *Threshold Limit Values for Chemical Substances and Physical Agents and Biological Exposure Indices.* Cincinnati: American Conference of Government Industrial Hygienists, 1993.

American Conference of Governmental Industrial Hygienists (ACGIH). *Industrial Ventilation: Manual of Recommended Practice.* 23rd ed. Cincinnati: American Conference of Government Industrial Hygienists, 1998.

American Hospital Formulary Service Drug Information. Bethesda, MD: American Society of Hospital Pharmacists, Inc., 1992.

American Medical Association Council for Scientific Affairs. Guidelines for Handling Parenteral Antineoplastics. *JAMA* 253 (1985): 1590–592.

ANSI Z88.2 American National Standards Institute. *American National Standard Practices for Respiratory Protection.* New York: American National Standards Institute, 1989.

ANSI Z88.6 American National Standards Institute. American National *Standard for Respiratory Protection—Respirator Use— Physical Qualifications for Personnel.* New York: American National Standards Institute, 1984.

ANSI Z88.10-2001 American National Standards Institute. American National *Standard for Respirator Fit Testing Methods.*

ANSI Z87.1-1989 (R 1998). *Practice for Occupational/Educational Eye and Face Protection.*

ANSI Z9.5-1992. American National *Standard for Laboratory Ventilation.*

ANSI Z87.1-1989. American National *Standard Practice for Occupational and Educational Eye and Face Protection.*

ANSI Z358.1-2004. American National *Standard for Emergency Eyewash and Shower Equipment.*

American Society of Heating, Refrigeration and Air Conditioning Engineers, Inc. (ASHRAE). Laboratories (chap. 14). *ASHRAE Handbook.* Atlanta, GA: ASHRAE, 1982.

American Society of Hospital Pharmacists (ASHP). ASHP Technical Assistance Bulletin on Handling Cytotoxic and Hazardous Drugs. *Am. J. of Hosp. Pharm.* 47 (1990): 1033–49.

ASHP Guidelines on Handling Hazardous Drugs. ASHP Council on Professional Affairs and ASHP Board of Directors, November 28, 2005.

American Society of Health-System Pharmacists. ASHP Technical Assistance Bulletin on Handling Cytotoxic Drugs in Hospitals. *Am. J. Hosp. Pharm.* 42 (1985): 131–37.

Anderson, R. W., W. H. Puckett, W. J. Dana, et al. Risk of Handling Injectable Antineoplastic Agents. *Am. J. Hosp. Pharm.* 39 (1982): 1881–887.

Barek, J., J. Cvaccka, J. Zima, M. De Meo, M. Laget, J. Michelon, and M. Castegnaro. Chemical Degradation of Wastes of Antineoplastic Agents Amsacrine, Azathioprine, Asparaginase and Thiotepa. *Ann. Occup. Hyg.* 42 (1998): 259–66.

Barek, J., S. Hansel, M. H. Sportouch, J. Cvaccka, J. Zima, M. De Meo, M. Laget, J. Michelon, and M. Castegnaro. Chemical Degradation of Wastes of Antineoplastic Agents. *Cancer Detection and Prevention* 22 (1998), supp. 1.

Barry, L. K., and R. B. Booher. Promoting the Responsible Handling of Antineoplastic Agents in the Community. *Oncol. Nurs. Forum.* 12 (1985): 40–46.

Barstow, J. Safe Handling of Cytotoxic Agents in the Home. *Home Healthcare Nurse* 3 (1986): 46–47.

Bennett, P. N., I. Matheson, L. J. Notarianni, A. Rane, and D. Reinhardt. Monographs on Individual Drugs. In *Drugs and Human Lactation*, edited by P. N. Bennett, 269–70. 2nd ed. Amsterdam: Elsevier, 1996.

Bos, R. P., and P. J. M. Sessink. Biomonitoring of Occupational Exposure to Cytostatic Anticancer Drugs. *Rev. Environ. Health* 12 (1997): 43–58.

Bristol-Myers Squibb Pharmaceutical Group. *Reverse-Phase HPLC for Determination of Taxol in Dust Samples Collected on Teflon Filters.* New Brunswick, NJ: Bristol-Myers Squibb Pharmaceutical Group, 1993.

Burton, L. C., and C. A. James. Rapid Method for the Determination of Ifosfamide and Cyclophosphamide in Plasma by High-Performance Liquid Chromatography with Solid-Phase Extraction. *J. Chromatog.* 431 (1988): 450–54.

Castegnaro, M., J. Adams, M. A. Armour, et al., eds. *Laboratory Decontamination and Destruction of Carcinogens in Laboratory Wastes: Some Antineoplastic Agents.* International Agency for Research on Cancer Scientific Publication 73. Fair Lawn, NJ: Oxford University Press, 1985.

Castegnaro, M., M. De Meo, M. Laget, J. Michelon, L. Garren, M. H. Sportouch, and S. Hansel. Chemical Degradation of Wastes of Antineoplastic Agents 2: Six Anthracyclines: Idarubicin, Doxorubicin, Epirubicin, Pirarubicin, Aclarubicin, and Daunorubicin. *Int. Arch. Occup. Environ. Health* 70 (1997): 378–84.

Chrysostomou, A., A. A. Morley, and R. Sehadri. Mutation Frequency in Nurses and Pharmacists Working with Cytotoxic Drugs. *Aust. N. Z. J. Med.* 14 (1984): 831–34.

Clark, C. Occupational Exposure to Cytotoxic Drugs. *Pharm. J.* 263 (1999): 65–68.

Clinical Oncological Society of Australia. Guidelines and Recommendations for Safe Handling of Antineoplastic Agents. *Med. J. Aust.* 1 (1983): 426–28.

Cloak, M. M., T. H. Connor, K. R. Stevens, et al. Occupational Exposure of Nursing Personnel to Antineoplastic Agents. *Oncol. Nurs. Forum* 12 (1985): 33–39.

Connor, T. H. External Contamination of Antineoplastic Drug Vials. *Hosp. Pharm. Eur.* Nov/Dec 2005, 52–54.

Connor, T. H., R. W. Anderson, P. J. Sessink, et al. Surface Contamination with Antineoplastic Agents in Six Cancer Treatment Centers in Canada and the United States. *Am. J. Health-Syst. Pharm.* 56 (1999): 1427–432.

Connor, T. H., R. W. Anderson, P. J. Sessink, and S. M. Spivey. Effectiveness of a Closed-System Device in Containing Surface Contamination with Cyclophosphamide and Ifosfamide in an I.V. Admixture Area. *Am. J. Health-Syst. Pharm.* 59 (2002): 68–72.

Connor, T. H., P. J. M. Sessink, B. R. Harrison, J. R. Pretty, B. G. Peters, R. M. Alfaro, A. Bilos, G. Beckmann, M. R. Bing, L. M. Anderson, and R. DeChristoforo. Surface Contamination of Chemotherapy Drug Vials and Evaluation of New Vial-Cleaning Techniques: Results of Three Studies. *Am. J. Health-Syst. Pharm.* 62 (2005): 475–84.

Connor, T. H., J. C. Theiss, R. W. Anderson, et al. Re-evaluation of Urine Mutagenicity of Pharmacy Personnel Exposed to Antineoplastic Agents. *Am. J. Hosp. Pharm.* 43 (1986): 1236–39.

Connor, T. H., P. Van Balen, and P. J. Sessink. Monitoring for Hazardous Drugs in the Operating Room. *Ann. Surg. Oncol.* 10 (2002): 821–22.

Coulam, C. B., T. P. Moyer, N. S. Jiang, and H. Zincke. Breast-Feeding after Renal Transplantation. *Transplant Proc.* 14 (1984): 605–9.

Crauste-Manciet, S., P. J. M. Sessink, S. Ferrari, J.-Y. Jomier, and D. Brossard. Environmental Contamination with Cytotoxic Drugs in Healthcare Using Positive Air Pressure Isolators. *Ann. Occup. Hyg.* 49 (2005): 619–28.

Delporte, J. P., P. Chenoix, and P. Hubert. Chemical Contamination of the Primary Packaging of 5-Fluorouracil RTU Solutions Commercially Available on the Belgian Market. *Eur. Hosp. Pharm.* 5 (1999): 119–21.

De Vries, E. G. E., A. G. J. Van Der Zee, D. R. A. Uges, and D. Th. Sleijfer. Excretion of Platinum into Breast Milk. *Lancet* 1 (1989): 497.

deWerk Neal, A., R. A. Wadden, and W. L. Chiou. Exposure of Hospital Workers to Airborne Antineoplastic Agents. *Am. J. Hosp. Pharm.* 40 (1983): 597–601.

DHHS Publication No. 93-8395. *Biosafety in Microbiological and Biomedical Laboratories.*

DoD 6055.5-M. *Occupational Health Surveillance Manual.*

Durodola, J. I. Administration of Cyclophosphamide during Late Pregnancy and Early Lactation: A Case Report. *J. Natl. Med. Assoc.* 71 (1979): 165–66.

Egan, P. C., M. E. Costanza, P. Dodion, M. J. Egorin, and N. R. Bachur. Doxorubicin and Cisplatin Excretion into Human Milk. *Cancer Treat. Rep.* 69 (1985): 1387–89.

Emergency Response Guidebook. U.S. Department of Transportation, 1990.

Falck, K., P. Grohn, M. Sorsa, et al. Mutagenicity in Urine of Nurses Handling Cytostatic Drugs. *Lancet.* 1 (1979): 1250–51.

Favier, B., L. Gilles, C. Ardiet, and J. F. Latour. External Contamination of Vials Containing Cytotoxic Agents Supplied by Pharmaceutical Manufacturers. *J. Oncol. Pharm. Practice* 9 (2003): 15–20.

Favier, B., L. Gilles, J. F. Latour, M. Desage, F. Giammarile. Contamination of Syringe Plungers during the Sampling of Cyclophosphamide Solutions. *J. Oncol. Pharm. Practice* 11 (2005): 1–5.

Favier, B., F. M. Rull, H. Bertucat, C. Pivot, G. LeBoucher, D. Charlety, V. Dubois, M. C. Veyre, C. Ardiet, and J. F. Latour. Surface and Human Contamination with 5-Fluorouracil in Six Hospital Pharmacies. *J. Pharmacie Clinique* 20 (2001): 157–62.

Greenberger, P. A., Y. K. Odeh, M. C. Frederiksen, and A. J. Atkinson Jr. Pharmacokinetics of Prednisolone Transfer to Breast Milk. *Clin. Pharmacol. Ther.* 53 (1993): 324–28.

Gregoire, R. E., R. Segal, and K. M. Hale. Handling Antineoplastic-Drug Admixtures at Cancer Centers: Practices and Pharmacist Attitudes. *Am. J. Hosp. Pharm.* 44 (1987): 1090–95.

Grekas, D. M., S. S. Vasiliou, and A. N. Lazarides. Immunosuppressive Therapy and Breast-Feeding after Renal Transplantation. *Nephron* 37 (1984): 68.

Hedmer, M., A. Georgiadi, E. Rämme Bremberg, B. A. G. Jönsson, and S. Eksborg. *Ann. Occup. Hyg.* 49 (2005): 629–37.

Hemminki, K., P. Kyyronen, and M. L. Lindbohm. Spontaneous Abortions and Malformations in the Offspring of Nurses Exposed to Anesthetic Gases, Cytostatic Drugs and Other Potential Hazards in Hospitals, Based on Registered Information of Outcome. *J. Epidemiol. Community Health* 39 (1985): 141–47.

Hewitt, J. B. *Health Effects of Occupational Exposure to Antineoplastic Drugs: An Integrative Research Review, Prepared for the Occupational Disease Panel.* Industrial Diseases Standards Panel, Ministry of Labour Ontario, Canada, 1997.

Hirst, M., S. Tse, D. G. Mills, et al. Occupational Exposure to Cyclophosphamide. *Lancet.* 1 (1984): 186–88.

Hoy, R. H., and L. M. Stump. Effect of an Air-Venting Filter Device on Aerosol Production from Vials. *Am. J. Hosp. Pharm.* 41 (1984): 324–26.

IARC Monographs on the Evaluation of the Carcinogenic Risk of Chemicals to Humans: International Agency for Research on Cancer. International Agency for Research on Cancer.

Jagun, O., M. Ryan, and H. A. Waldrom. Urinary Thioether Excretion in Nurses Handling Cytotoxic Drugs. *Lancet.* 2 (1982): 443–44.

Johns, D. G., L. D. Rutherford, P. C. Keighton, and C. L. Vogel. Secretion of Methotrexate into Human Milk. *Am. J. Obstet. Gynecol.* 112 (1972): 978–80.

Joint Commission on Accreditation of Healthcare Organizations. *Comprehensive Accreditation Manual for Hospitals: The Official Handbook.* Chicago: Joint Commission on Accreditation of Healthcare Organizations, 2001.

Jones, R. B., R. Frank, and T. Mass. Safe Handling of Chemotherapeutic Agents: A Report from the Mount Sinai Medical Center. *Ca. Cancer J. Clin.* 33 (1983): 258–63.

Kamilli, I., and U. Gresser. Allopurinol and Oxypurinol in Human Breast Milk. *Clin. Invest.* 71 (1993): 161–64.

Kiffmeyer, T. K., H.-J. Götze, M. Jursch, and U. Lüders. Trace Enrichment, Chromatographic Separtation and Biodegradation of Cytostatic Compounds in Surface Water. *Fresenius J. Anal. Chem.* 361 (1998): 185–91.

Kiffmeyer, T. K., K. G. Ing, and G. Schoppe. External Contamination of Cytotoxic Drug Packing: Safe Handling and Cleaning Procedures. *J. Onc. Pharm. Practice* 6 (2000): 13.

Kiffmeyer, T. K., C. Kube, S. Opiolka, P. Sessin, et al. Vapour Pressures, Evaporation Behaviour and Airborne Concentrations of Hazardous Drugs: Implications for Occupational Safety. *Pharmaceutical Journal* 268, no. 7188 (2002): 331–37.

Kleinberg, M. L., and M. J. Quinn. Airborne Drug Levels in a Laminar Flow Hood. *Am. J. Hosp. Pharm.* 38 (1981): 1301–333.

Kromhout, H., F. Hoek, R. Uitterhoeve, R. Huijbers, R. F. Overmars, R. Anzion, and R. Vermeulen. Postulating a Dermal Pathway for Exposure to Antineoplastic Drugs among Hospital Workers: Applying a Conceptual Model to the Results of Three Workplace Surveys. *Ann. Occup. Hyg.* 44 (2000): 551–60.

Labuhn, K., B. Valanis, R. Schoeny, K. Loveday, and W. M. Vollmer. Nurses' and Pharmacists Exposure to Antineoplastic Drugs: Findings from Industrial Hygiene Scans and Urine Mutagenicity Tests. *Cancer Nursing* 21 (1998): 79–89.

Larson, R. R., M. B. Khazaeli, and H. K. Dillon. Monitoring Method for Surface Contamination Caused by Selected Antineoplastic Agents. *Am. J. Health-Syst. Pharm.* 59 (2002): 270–77.

Lassila, O., A. Toivanen, and E. Nordman. Immune Function In Nurses Handling Cytostatic Drugs. *Lancet.* 1980 Aug; 2: 482.

Leboucher, G., F. Serratrice, V. Bertholle, L. Thore, and M. Bost. Evaluation of Platinum Contamination of a Hazardous Drug Preparation Area in a Hospital Pharmacy. *Bull Cancer* 89 (200): 949–55.

List of Known or Suspect Carcinogens. Colgate University Chemical Management.

List of Known or Suspect Carcinogens. University of Maryland, College Park.

Lunn, G., E. B. Sansone, A. W. Andrews, and L. C. Hellwig. Degradation and Disposal of Some Antineoplastic Drugs. *J. Pharm. Sci.* 78 (1989): 652–59.

Mader, R. M., B. Rizovski, and G. G. Steger. On-Line Solid-Phase Extraction and Determination of Paclitaxel in Human Plasma. *J. Chromatog. B.* 769 (2002): 357–61.

Mason, H. J., S. Blair, C. Sams, K. Jones, et al. Exposure to Antineoplastic Drugs in Two UK Pharmacy Units. *Ann. Occup. Hyg.* 49, no. 7 (2005): 603–10.

Mason, H. J., J. Morton, S. J. Garfitt, S. Iqbal, and K. Jones. Cytotoxic Drug Contamination on the Outside of Vails Delivered to a Hospital Pharmacy. *Ann. Occup. Hyg.* 47 (2003): 681–85.

McAbee, R. R., B. J. Gallucci, and H. Checkoway. Adverse Reproductive Outcomes and Occupational Exposure among Nurses. *AAOHN J.* 41 (1993): 110–19.

McDevitt, J. J., P. S. J. Lees, and M. A. McDiarmid. Exposure of Hospital Pharmacists and Nurses to Antineoplastic Agents. *J. Occup. Med.* 35 (1993): 57–60.

McDiarmid, M. A. Medical Surveillance for Antineoplastic-Drug Handlers. *Am. J. Hosp. Pharm.* 47, no. 5: 1061–66

McDiarmid, M. A., T. Egan, M. Furio, et al. Sampling for Airborne Fluorouracil in a Hospital Drug Preparation Area. *Am. J. Hosp. Pharm.* 43 (1986): 1942–45.

McKenna, R., E. R. Cole, and U. Vasan. Is Warfarin Contraindicated in the Lactating Mother? *J. Pediatr.* 103 (1983): 325–27.

Micoli, G., R. Turci, M. Arpellini, and C. Minoia. Determination of 5-Fluorouracil in Environmental Samples by Solid-Phase Extraction and High-Performance Liquid Chromatography with Ultraviolet Detection. *J. Chromatog. B.* 750 (2001): 25–32.

Minoia, C., R. Turci, C. Sottani, A. Schiavi, L. Perbellini, S. Angeleri, F. Draicchio, and P. Apostoli. Application of High Performance Liquid Chromatography/Tandem Mass Spectrometry in the Environmental and Biological Monitoring of Health Care Personnel Occupationally Exposed to Cyclophosphamide and Ifosfamide. *Rapid Commun. Mass Spectrom.* 12 (1998): 1485–493.

Minoia, C., R. Turci, C. Sottani, A. Schiavi, L. Perbellini, S. Angeleri, F. Frigerio, F. Draicchio, and P. Apostoli. Risk Assessment Concerning Hospital Personnel Participating in the Preparation and Administration of Antineoplastic Drugs [Italian]. *Giornale Italiano di Medicina del Lavoro ed Ergonomia* 21 (1999): 93–107.

National Institute for Occupational Safety and Health. *Preventing Occupational Exposures to Antineoplastic and Other Hazardous Drugs in Healthcare Settings.* Retrieved March 25, 2004.

National Sanitation Foundation. *Class II (Laminar Flow) Biohazard Cabinetry.* National Sanitation Foundation Standard no. 49. Ann Arbor, MI: National Sanitation Foundation, 1976.

National Study Commission on Cytotoxic Exposure. *Consensus Responses to Unresolved Questions Concerning Cytotoxic Agents.* March 1984. Available from Louis P. Jeffrey, Sc.D., Director of Pharmacy Services, Rhode Island Hospital, Provincetown, RI 02902.

National Study Commission on Cytotoxic Exposure. *Recommendations for Handling Cytotoxic Agents.* September 1984. Available from Louis P. Jeffrey, Sc.D., Director of Pharmacy Services, Rhode Island Hospital, Provincetown, RI 02902.

National Study Commission on Cytotoxic Exposure. *Consensus Responses to Unresolved Questions Concerning Cytotoxic Agents.* February 1986. Available from Louis P. Jeffrey, Sc.D., Director of Pharmacy Services, Rhode Island Hospital, Provincetown, RI 02902.

National Study Commission on Cytotoxic Exposure. *Position Statement: The Handling of Cytotoxic Agents by Women Who Are Pregnant, Attempting to Conceive, or Breast Feeding.* January 1987. Available from Louis P. Jeffrey, Sc.D., Director of Pharmacy Services, Rhode Island Hospital, Provincetown, RI 02902.

National Study Commission on Cytotoxic Exposure: Recommendations for Handling Cytotoxic Agents. Available at http://ctep.cancer .gov/handbook/append_13.html. Accessed October 9, 2003.

Navy Reference (Ref). *Reproductive and Developmental Hazards: A Guide for Occupational Health Professionals.* Navy Environmental Health Center, Technical Manual NEHC-TM-OEM 6260.01A. Portsmouth, VA: Navy Environmental Health Center.

Nikula, E., K. Kiviniitty, J. Leisti, et al. Chromosome Aberrations in Lymphocytes of Nurses Handling Cytostatic Agents. *Scand. J. Work Environ. Health* 10 (1984): 71–74.

NIOSH Publication No. 88-119. *Guidelines for Protecting the Safety and Health of Health Care Workers.*

NIOSH Publication No. 83-2621. *Recommendations for the Safe Handling of Parenteral Antineoplastic Drugs.*

NIOSH Publication No. 97-135. NIOSH Alert - *Preventing Allergic Reactions to Natural Rubber Latex in the Workplace.*

NIOSH Publication No. 2004-65. NIOSH ALERT - *Preventing Occupational Exposure to Antineoplastic and Other Hazardous Drugs in Healthcare Setting.*

Norppa, H., M. Sorsa, H. Vainio, et al. Increased Sister Chromatid Exchange Frequencies In Lymphocytes Of Nurses Handling Cytostatic Drugs. *Scand. J. Work Environ. Health* 6 (1980): 299–301.

Nygren, O., B. Gustavsson, L. Strom, and A. Friberg. Cisplatin Contamination on the Outside of Drug Vials. *Ann. Occup. Hyg.* 46 (2002): 555–57.

Nygren, O., and C. Lundgren. Determination of Platinum in Workroom Air and in Blood and Urine from Nursing Staff Attending Patients Receiving Cisplatin Chemotherapy. *Int. Arch. Occ. Environ. Health* 70 (1997): 209–14.

Peelen, S., N. Roeleveld, D. Heederick, H. Krombout, and W. deKort. *Toxic Effects on Reproduction in Hospital Personnel*. The Netherlands: Dutch Ministry of Society Affairs and Employment, 1999.

Penn, I. Occurrence of Cancer in Immune Deficiencies. *Cancer* 34 (1974): 858–66.

Pethran, A., K. Hauff, and H. Hessel. Biological, Cytogenetic and Ambient Monitoring of Exposure to Antineoplastic Drugs. *J. Oncol. Pharm. Practice* 4 (1998): 57.

Polovich, M., C. S. Blecher, E. M. Glynn-Tucker, et al. *Handling of Hazardous Drugs*. Oncology Nursing Society (ONS), 2003.

Power, L. A., R. W. Anderson, R. Cortopassi, J. R. Gera, and R. M. Lewis Jr. Update on Safe Handling of Hazardous Drugs: The Advice of Experts. *Am. J. Hosp. Pharm.* 47, no. 5: 1050–60.

Preventing Occupational Exposure to Antineoplastic and Other Hazardous Drugs in Healthcare Settings. NIOSH ALERT, September 2004.

Primary Containment for Biohazards: Selection, Installation and Use of Biological Safety Cabinets. 2nd ed. U.S. Department of Health and Human Services Public Health Service Centers for Disease Control and Prevention and National Institutes of Health, September 2000.

Prudent Practices for Handling Hazardous Chemicals in Laboratories. Washington, DC: National Academy Press, 1995.

Pyy, L., M. Sorsa, and E. Hakala. Ambient Monitoring of Cyclophosphamide in Manufacture and Hospitals. *Am. Ind. Hyg. Assoc. J.* 49 (1988): 314–17.

Quality Standard for the Oncology Pharmacy Service with Commentary. Published by the Institute for Applied Healthcare Sciences (IFAHS e.V.) for the German Society of Oncology Pharmacy (DGOP e.V.) as the result of the 11th North German Cytostatics Workshop (NZW), January 2003.

Richter, P., J. C. Calamera, M. C. Morgenfeld, et al. Effect of Chlorambucil on Spermatogenesis in the Human with Malignant Lymphoma. *Cancer.* 25 (1970): 1026–30.

Robbins, M. C. *OSHA's Wipe Sampling Policies and Procedures: Sampling and Analysis of Toxic Organics in the Atmosphere, STP 721*. West Conshohocken, PA: American Society for Testing Materials, 1980.

Rogers, B., and E. A. Emmett. Handling Antineoplastic Agents: Urine Mutagenicity in Nurses. *Image J. Nurs. Sch.* 19 (1987): 108–13.

Ros, J. J. W., K. A. Simons, J. M. Verzijl, G. A. de Bijl, and M. G. Pelders. Practical Applications of a Validated Method of Analysis for the Detection of Traces of Cyclophosphamide on Injection Bottles and at Oncological Outpatient Center. *Ziekenhuisfarmacie* 13 (1997): 168–71.

Rubino, F. M., L. Floridia, A. M. Pietropaolo, M. Tavazzani, and A. Colombi. Measurement of Surface Contamination by Certain Antineoplastic Drugs Using High-Performance Liquid Chromatography: Applications in Occupational Hygiene Investigations in Hospital Environments. *Med Lav.* 90 (1999): 572–83.

Schmaus, G., R. Schierl, and S. Funck. Monitoring Surface Contamination by Antineoplastic Drugs Using Gas Chromatography-Mass Spectrometry and Voltammetry. *Am. J. Health-Syst. Pharm.* 59 (2002): 956–61.

Scott, S. A. Antineoplastic Drug Information and Handling Guidelines for Office-Based Physicians *Am. J. Hosp. Pharm.* 41 (1984): 2402–403.

Selevan, S. G., M.-L. Lindbohm, R. W. Hornung, and K. Hemminki. A Study of Occupational Exposure to Antineoplastic Drugs and Fetal Loss in Nurses. *N. Eng. J. Med.* 313 (1985): 1173–78.

Selevan, S. H., M. L. Lindbohm, R. W. Hornung, et al. A Study of Occupational Exposure to Antineoplastic Drugs and Fetal Loss in Nurses. *N. Engl. J. Med.* 333 (1985): 1173–78.

Sessink, P. J. M., R. B. Anzion, P. H. H. Van den Broek, and R. P. Bos. Detection of Contamination with Antineoplastic Agents in a Hospital Pharmacy Department. *Pharm. Weekbl. (Sci)*. 14 (1992): 16–22.

Sessink, P. J., K. A. Boer, A. P. Scheefhals, et al. Occupational Exposure to Antineoplastic Agents at Several Departments in a Hospital: Environmental Contamination and Excretion of Cyclophosphamide and Ifosphamide in Urine of Exposed Workers. *Int Arch. Occup. Environ. Health.* 64 (1992): 105–12.

Sessink, P. J., and R. P. Bos. Drugs Hazardous to Healthcare Workers. *Drug Saf.* 20 (1999): 347–59.

Sessink, P. J., M. Cerna, P. Rossner, A. Pastorkova, H. Bavarova, K. Frankova, R. B. Anzion, and R. P. Bos. Urinary Cyclophosphamide Excretion and Chromosomal Aberrations in Peripheral Blood Lymphocytes after Occupational Exposure to Antineoplastic Agents. *Mutat Res.* 309, no. 2 (1994): 193–99.

Sessink, P. J. M., N. S. S. Friemèl, R. B. M. Anzion, and R. P. Bos. Biological and Environmental Monitoring of Occupational Exposure Caretakers of Pharmaceutical Plant Workers to Methotrexate. *Int. Arch. Occup. Environ. Health* 65 (1994): 401–3.

Sessink, P. J. M., H. C. Joost, F. H. Pierik, R. B. M. Anzion, and R. P. Bos. Occupational Exposure of Animal Caretakers to Cyclophosphamide. *J. Occup. Med.* 35 (1993): 47–52.

Sessink, P. J. M., E. D. Kroese, H. J. van Kranen, et al. Cancer Risk Assessment for Health Care Workers Occupationally Exposed to Cyclophosphamide. *Int. Arch. Occup. Environ. Health* 67 (1995): 317.

Sessink, P. J. M., M.-A. E. Rolf, and N. S. Ryden. Evaluation of the Phaseal Hazardous Drug Containment System. *Hosp. Pharm.* 34 (1999): 1311–17.

Sessink, P. J. M., B. C. J. Wittenhorst, R. B. M. Anzion, and R. P. Rob. Exposure of Pharmacy Technicians to Antineoplastic Agents: Reevaluation after Additional Protective Measures. *Arch. Environ. Health.* 52 (1997): 240–44.

Shahsavarani, S., R. J. Godefroid, and B. R. Harrison. Evaluation of Occupational Exposure to Tablet Trituration Dust. ASHP Midyear Clinical Meeting, 1993, P-59(E) abs.

Shortridge, L. A., G. K. Lemasters, B. Valanis, et al. Menstrual Cycles in Nurses Handling Antineoplastic Drugs. *Cancer Nurs.* 18 (1995): 439–44.

Smith, C. A. Managing Pharmaceutical Waste—What Pharmacists Should Know. *J. Pharm. Soc. Wisconsin,* Nov/Dec 2002, 17–22.

Sorsa, M., L. Pyy, S. Salomaa, L. Nyland, and J. W. Yager. Biological and Environmental Monitoring of Occupational Exposure to Cyclophosphamide in Industry and Hospitals. *Mutat. Res.* 204 (1988): 465–79.

Sotaniemi, E. A., S. Sutinen, A. J. Arranto, et al. Liver Damage in Nurses Handling Cytostatic Agents. *Acta. Med. Scand.* 214 (1983): 181–89.

Sottani, C., R. Turci, G. Micoli, M. L. Fiorention, and C. Minoia. Rapid and Sensitive Determination of Paclitaxel (Taxol) in Environmental Samples by High-Performance Liquid Chromatography Tandem Mass Spectrometry. *Rapid Comm. Mass. Spectrom.* 14 (2000): 930–35.

Spivey, S., and T. H. Connor. Determining Sources of Workplace Contamination with Antineoplastic Drugs and Comparing Conventional IV Drug Preparation with a Closed System. *Hosp. Pharm.* 38 (2003): 135–39.

Stein, G. C., and C. E. Myers. Limitations of the New OSHA Documents on Controlling Occupational Exposure to Hazardous Drugs. *Am. J. Health-Syst. Pharm.* 53 (1996): 1717–19.

Stephens, J. D., M. S. Golbus, T. R. Miller, et al. Multiple Congenital Abnormalities in a Fetus Exposed to 5-Fluorouracil During the First Trimester. *Am. J. Obstet. Gynecol.* 137 (1980): 747–49.

Stuart, A., A. D. Stephens, L. Welch, and P. H. Sugarbaker. Safety Monitoring of the Coliseum Technique for Heated Intra-operative Intraperitoneal Chemotherapy with Mitomycin C. *Ann. Surg. Oncol.* 9 (2002): 186–91.

Stucker, I., J. F. Caillard, R. Collin, M. Gout, D. Poyen, and D. Hemon. Risk Of Spontaneous Abortion among Nurses Handling Antineoplastic Drugs. *Scand. J. Work, Environ., Health* 16 (1990): 102–7.

Technical Bulletin, Medical (TB MED) 503. *Occupational and Environmental Health.* U.S. Army Army Industrial Hygiene Program.

Technical Bulletin, Medical (TB MED) 506. *Occupational Vision.* Aberdeen Proving Grounds, MD: U.S. Army Environmental Hygiene Agency, 1981.

TG No. 149. *Guidelines for Controlling Occupational Exposure to Hazardous Drugs.* USACHPPM.

TG No. 165. *Installation Industrial Hygiene Program Self-Assessment Guide.* USACHPPM.

Tuffnell, P. G., M. T. Gannon, A. Dong, et al. Limitations of Urinary Mutagen Assays for Monitoring Occupational Exposure to Antineoplastic Drugs. *Am. J. Hosp. Pharm.* 43 (1986): 344–48.

Turci, R., G. Micoli, and C. Minoia. Determination of Methotrexate in Environmental Samples by Solid Phase Extraction and High Performance Liquid Chromatorgraphy: Ultraviolet or Tandem Mass Spectrometry Detection. *Rapid Comm. Mass. Spectrom.* 14 (2000): 685–91.

Turci, R., C. Sottani, G. Spagnoli, and C. Minoia. Biological and Environmental Monitoring of Hospital Personnel Exposed to Antineoplastic Agents: A Review of Analytical Methods. *J. Chromatog. B.* 789 (2003): 169–209.

U.S. Army Regulation 11-34. *The Army Respiratory Protection Program.*

U.S. Army Regulation 40-5. *Preventive Medicine.*

U.S. Army Regulation 40-7. *Use of Investigational Drugs and Devices in Humans and the Use of Schedule I Controlled Drug Substances.*

U.S. Army Regulation 385-10. *The Army Safety Program.*

U.S. Army Regulation 385-30. *Safety Color Code Markings and Signs.*

U.S. Army Regulation 385-40. *Army Accident Reporting.*

U.S. Department of Labor, Occupational Safety and Health Administration (OSHA). *PL 91-596 Occupational Safety and Health Act of 1970.*

U.S. Department of Labor, Occupational Safety and Health Administration (OSHA). OSHA Standard, 29 CFR 1910.134. *Respiratory Protection.*

U.S. Department of Labor, Occupational Safety and Health Administration (OSHA). OSHA 29, CFR 1910.120. *Hazardous Waste Operations and Emergency Response.*

U.S. Department of Labor, Occupational Safety and Health Administration (OSHA). OSHA, 29 CFR1910 Subpart 1. *General Industry Standard for Personal Protective Equipment (PPE).*

U.S. Department of Labor, Occupational Safety and Health Administration (OSHA). OSHA instruction TED 1.15, Section II, Chapter 2. *Directorate of Technical Support: Controlling Occupational Exposure to Hazardous Drugs.* Washington, DC: Occupational Safety and Health Administration, 1999.

U.S. Department of Labor, Occupational Safety and Health Administration (OSHA). OSHA Technical Manual. Section II, Chapter 2. *Sampling for Surface Contamination*. Washington, DC: Occupational Safety and Health Administration, 1996.

U.S. Department of Labor, Occupational Safety and Health Administration (OSHA). OSHA Instruction CPL 2-2.20B CH-4. *Controlling Occupational Exposure to Hazardous Drugs*. Washington, DC: OSHA Office of Occupational Medicine, Directorate of Technical Support, 1995.

U.S. Department of Labor, Occupational Safety and Health Administration (OSHA). OSHA 29 CFR 1910.1200, as amended February 9, 1994. *Hazard Communication Standard*.

U.S. Department of Labor, Occupational Safety and Health Administration (OSHA). OSHA, 29 CFR 1910.1020. *Access to Employee and Medical Records Standard*.

U.S. Department of Labor, Occupational Safety and Health Administration (OSHA). OSHA, 29 CFR 1910.1030. *Occupational Exposure to Bloodborne Pathogens Standard*.

U.S. Department of Labor, Occupational Safety and Health Administration (OSHA). OSHA 3071 2002. *Job Hazard Analysis*.

USP 797—Barrier Isolators Summary. USP General Chapter 797, Pharmaceutical Compounding—Sterile Preparations. Rockville, MD: U.S. Pharmacopeia, 2004.

Vaccari, P. L., K. Tonat, R. DeChristoforo, J. F. Gallelli, and P. F. Zimmerman. Disposal of Antineoplastic Wastes at the National Institutes of Health. *Am. J. Hosp. Pharm.* 41, no. 1: 87–93.

Valanis, B. Environmental and Direct Measures of Exposure. *Occup. Med.* 1 (1986): 431–44.

Valanis, B., W. Vollmer, K. Labuhn, and A. Glass. Occupational Exposure to Antineoplastic Agents and Self-Reported Infertility among Nurses and Pharmacists. *J. Occup. Environ. Med.* 39 (1997): 574–80.

Valanis, B. G., W. M. Vollmer, K. T. Labuhn, et al. Association of Antineoplastic Drug Handling with Acute Adverse Effects in Pharmacy Personnel. *Am. J. Hosp. Pharm.* 50 (1993): 455–62.

Valanis, B., W. M. Vollmer, K. T. Labuhn, and A. G. Glass. Acute Symptoms Associated with Antineoplastic Drug Handling among Nurses. *Cancer Nurs.* 16, no. (1993): 288–95.

Valanis, B., W. M. Vollmer, and P. Steele. Occupational Exposure to Antineoplastic Agents: Self-Reported Miscarriages and Stillbirths among Nurses and Pharmacists. *J. Occ. Environ. Med.* 41 (1999): 632–638.

Van Raalte, J., C. Rice, and C. E. Moss. Visible Light System for Detecting Doxorubicin Contamination on Skin and Surfaces. *Am. J. Hosp. Pharm.* 47 (1990): 1067–74.

Venitt, S., C. Crofton-Sleigh, J. Hunt, et al. Monitoring Exposure of Nursing and Pharmacy Personnel to Cytotoxic Drugs: Urinary Mutation Assays and Urinary Platinum as Markers of Absorption. *Lancet.* 1 (1984): 74–76.

Volk, K. J., S. E. Hill, E. H. Kerns, et al. Profiling Degradants of Paclitaxel Using Liquid Chromatography-Mass Spectrometry and Liquid Chromatography-Tandem Mass Spectrometry Substructural Techniques. *J. Chromatogr. B. Biomed. Sci. Appl.* 696 (1997): 99–115.

Waksvik, H., O. Klepp, and A. Brogger. Chromosome Analyses of Nurses Handling Cytostatic Agents. *Cancer Treat. Rep.* 65 (1981): 607–10.

Wick, C., M. H. Slawson, J. A. Jorgenson, and L. S. Tyler. Using a Closed-System Protective Device to Reduce Personnel Exposure to Antineoplastic Agents. *Am. J. Health-Syst. Pharm.* 60 (2003): 2314–20.

Wilson, J. P., and D. A. Solimando. Aseptic Technique as a Safety Precaution in the Preparation of Antineoplastic Agents. *Hosp. Pharm.* 15 (1981): 575–81.

World Health Organization. *Breastfeeding and Maternal Medication, Recommendations for Drugs in the Eleventh WHO Model List of Essential Drugs*. Geneva: WHO, 2002.

World Health Organization. *Degradation of Antineoplastic Wastes*. Geneva: WHO.

Wren, A. E., C. D. Melia, S. T. Garner, and S. P. Denyer. Decontamination Methods for Cytotoxic Drugs. 1. Use of a Bioluminescent Technique to Monitor the Inactivation of Methotrexate with Chlorine-Based Agents. *J. Clin. Pharm. Therap.* 18 (1993): 133–37.

Yodaiken, R. *Safe Handling of Cytotoxic Drugs by Health Care Personnel*. Instructional Publication 8-1.1. Washington, DC: Occupational Safety and Health Administration, 1986.

Yodaiken, R., and D. Bennett. OSHA Work-Practice Guidelines for Personnel Dealing with Cytotoxic (Antineoplastic) Drugs. *Am. J. Hosp. Pharm.* 43 (1986): 1193–204.

Zeedijk, M., B. Greijdanus, F. B. Steenstra, and D. R. A. Uges. Monitoring Exposure of Cytotoxics on the Hospital Ward: Measuring Surface Contamination of Four Different Cytotoxic Drugs from One Wipe Sample. *Eur. J. Hosp. Pharm.* 1 (2005): 18–22.

Ziegler, E., H. J. Mason, and P. J. Baxter. *Occupational Exposure to Cytotoxic Drugs in Two UK Oncology Wards*.

LEUPRORELIN (*loo-PROH-lin*)
LEUPROLIDE
LEUPROLIDE ACETATE

Chemical Abstracts Service (CAS) Registry
  Numbers: 53714-56-0 74381-53-6
Registry of Toxic Effects of Chemical Substance
  (RTECS): OK6700000 OH6390000
National Cancer Institute: NSC 377526
C59-H84-N16-O12-C2-H4

Health & Safety Hazards/US Department of Transportation (DOT)/US Environmental Protection Agency (EPA)—Sources

Mutagen—Registry of Toxic Effects of Chemical Substance, Reproductive Effector—ToxReport, Pregnancy Category (X)—Food and Drug Administration, Toxic-Material Safety Data Sheet, Lactation Avoid Breastfeeding-US Navy Ref, Developmental Male & Female)—US California State Proposition 65, Hazardous Materials Identification System (R) and/or US Department of Defense System Health (1) Fire Hazard (0) Reactivity (0) Personal Protective Code (none stated)—Material Safety Data Sheet, Eye and Skin Irritant-Material Safety Data Sheet, Hazardous Materials Identification System (R) and/or US Department of Defense System Health (2) Fire Hazard (0) Reactivity (0) Personal Protective Code (X)—Material Safety Data Sheet, Developmental and Reproductive Effectors- US California Proposition 65.

LEUPROLIDE ACETATE is a white flocculent powder

LEUPROLIDE is available as injection (5 mg/m, 2.8 ml in a 6 ml vial) and implants

LEUPROLIDE ACTETATE for injection—is a clear, colorless, odorless liquid

First Aid/Medical Information/Occupational Exposure Limits

First Aid Measures to include: Use general first aid measures except for the following:

Ingestion: If LEUPROLIDE ACETATE is swallowed, call physician or poison control center for most current information. If professional advice is not available, DO NOT INDUCE Vomiting. Victim should drink milk, egg whites, or large quantities of water. Never induce vomiting or give diluents (milk or water) to someone who is unconscious, having convulsions, or who cannot swallow

Physician's note: No known antidote. Provide symptomatic and supportive care, monitoring hormone, or who cannot swallow.

Medical Information:

Caution and Warning Statements:

Caution: The chemical, physical, and toxicological properties have not been thoroughly investigated especially as it pertains to toxicological properties related to occupational exposure. LEUPROLIDE may impair fertility in males and females. Exposure may cause reproductive disorders.

Adverse effects following an injection may include fast or irregular heartbeat, hot flashes, blurred vision, decreased interest in sex, dizziness, swelling of feet or lower legs, headache, nausea or vomiting, swelling or tenderness of breasts, trouble sleeping, and weight gain. In males, adverse effects may also include constipation, decrease size of testicles, bone pain, and impotence. In females, adverse effects may also include stopping of menstrual periods; and light, irregular vaginal bleeding; pelvic pain; and burning, dryness, or itching of vagina. Possible allergic reaction to material if inhaled ingested or comes in contact with skin.

Caution: Avoid contact and inhalation. Exposure may cause reproductive disorders. Avoid inhalation. Avoid contact with eyes, skin, and clothing. Avoid prolonged or repeated exposure. May have actions similar to luteinizing hormone releasing hormone (LH-RH) and gonadotropin releasing hormone (GN-RH) which are the key mediators in the neuroregulation of the secreted of gonadotropins, luteinizing hormone (LH) and follicle stimulating hormone (FSH). LH-RH can modify sexual behavior by regulating plasma gonadotropin and sex steroid levels.

Therapeutic levels: There is a chance that LEUPROLIDE may cause birth defects if it is taken after becoming pregnant. It could also cause a miscarriage if taken or exposure occurs during pregnancy. It is not known whether LEUPROLIDE passes into breast milk.

Target organs/systems: Skin, eyes (anticipated at occupational exposure levels); reproductive systems, CNS, kidneys, cardiovascular system, fetus, and pituitary (therapeutic doses)

Medical conditions generally aggravated by exposure: The chemical, physical, and toxicological properties have not been thoroughly investigated.

LEUPROLIDE Patient Information: Any changes in vaginal bleeding form an unknown cause (for use for endometriosis or anemia due to tumors of the uterus) LEUPROLIDE may delay diagnosis or worsen condition.

Report health conditions to your occupational health staff that will increase the chances of developing thinning bones or osteoporosis, including your family history. Furthermore, report any medicine that you are taking that may increase broken bones. Some medicines, such as corticosteroids (cortisone-like medicines), can also cause thinning of the bones when used for long periods.

LEUPROLIDE ACETATE as administered in clinical use, this material reduces sex hormones in both men and women. It is a potent drug; target organs include the reproductive systems, fetus and pituitary. Report preexisting health conditions related to nervous, reproductive, and cardiovascular disorders.

Disorders involving the target organs of exposure to LEUPROLIDE ACETATE can be aggravated by exposures to this product (especially in doses/exposure approaching therapeutic levels for this product). Avoid exposure to LEUPROLIDE ACETATE during pregnancy and breastfeeding.

Specific medical surveillance information:

Reproductive and pregnancy counseling information: For men: leuprolide may cause sterility, which probably is only temporary. LEUPROLIDE ACETATE data suggest preexisting pituitary, ovarian, or testicular dysfunction; metastatic vertebral lesions and/or urinary tract obstruction.

Occupational Exposure Level/Limit (OEL) & Sampling Methods:

LEUPROLIDE ACETATE Innovators Exposure Limit: 20 ng/m3 TWA

Environmental Sentinel Contamination Action Level (ESCAL): Not otherwise specified (surface and air)

Supplemental Response Information

Extinguishing Media: Use extinguishing agent which is the most appropriate to extinguish surrounding fire (carbon dioxide, foam, dry chemical or water fog as extinguishing media).

Solubility: LEUPROLIDE ACETATE is water soluble with a pH range of 5.5 to 6.5.

Chemical Degradation/Neutralization Method: Not otherwise specified

Note: *If a specific degradation or neutralization method is not provided on this table and you do not have other specific information that will guide you on how to clean up the specific material spilled, and then follow the general spill procedure found in the introduction section of this handbook.*

Incompatibility: LEUPROLIDE ACETATE is incompatible with hypochlorite solutions and strong oxidizing agents.

ERGAMISOL®74 (*lee-VAM-i-sole*)
LEVAMISOLE
LEVAMISOLE HYDROCHLORIDE

Chemical Abstracts Service (CAS) Registry
    Numbers: 14769-73-4 16595-80-5 74381-53-6
Registry of Toxic Effects of Chemical Substance
    (RTECS): NJ5960000
National Cancer Institute:
($C_{11}H_{12}N_2$-S-HCL)

Health & Safety Hazards/US Department of Transportation (DOT)/US Environmental Protection Agency (EPA)—Sources

Mutagen—Registry of Toxic Effects of Chemical Substance, Mutagen—ToxReport, Reproductive Effector-ToxReport, FDA Pregnancy Category (X)—Food and Drug Administration and US Navy Reference, Teratogen—University of Maryland at College Park, Lactation: Avoid Breastfeeding—World Health Organization, Toxic-Material Safety Datasheet

First Aid/Medical Information/Occupational Exposure Limits

First aid measures to include: Use general first aid measures except for the following:

Physician's note: Levamisole-symptomatic treatment. After oral intake, Gastric lavage with aqueous potassium permanganate (20 mg/100 ml) may be performed afterwards, administer a purgative.

Caution and Warning Statements:

Exposure may cause skin and eye irritation. May be harmful if inhaled, material may be irritation to mucous membranes and upper respiratory tract. Toxic if swallowed. LEVAMISOLE HYDROCHLORIDE is hazardous in case of ingestion. This drug is slightly hazardous in case of skin contact (irritant) and of eye contact (irritant). Severe over-exposure can result in death. Exposure to dermis and eyes may cause irritation. Inhalation may cause respiratory tract and mucous membrane irritation. LEVAMISOLE HYDROCHLORIDE is classified as a possible female reproductive systems/toxin. Repeated or prolonged exposure to the drug can produce target organs damage. Repeated exposure to a highly toxic material may produce general deterioration of health by an accumulation in one or more human organs.

Adverse experiences reported in acute adult high dose trials (600 mg/day and higher) included: nausea, lethargy, cramps, diarrhea, headache, emesis, dizziness, and confusion. LEVAMISOLE (Ergamisol®74) is rapidly absorbed form the gastrointestinal tract.

Caution—Females and males planning to have a child, pregnant women, and nursing mothers should exercise caution regarding potential occupational exposure to this cytotoxic drug. No information or not enough information exists or was provided concerning occupational exposure that may potentially occur while handling this drug and its affects on reproductive systems, the fetus, and/or if it is secreted along with breast milk, which may harm nursing infants. Staff members should consult with the occupational health physician monitoring workers' health in your facility to be apprised of potential hazards and should be advised to avoid becoming pregnant and/or breast feeding or should be transferred in accordance with policy/procedures to other duties that do not involve preparation, handling, and administering this drug.

Therapeutic levels: there are no adequate and well-controlled studies in pregnant women and Ergamisol®74 should not be administered unless the potential benefits outweigh the risks. Women taking the combination of Ergamisol®74 and fluorouracil should be advised not to become pregnant. Nursing mothers: it is not known whether Ergamisol®74 is excreted in human milk; it is excreted in cows' milk. Because of the potential for serious adverse reactions in nursing infants from Ergamisol®74, a decision should be made whether to discontinue nursing or to discontinue the drug, taking into account the importance of the drug to the mother.

Target Organs/Systems:

LEVAMISOLE HYDROCHLORIDE may be toxic to immune system, blood, lungs, fetus, and central nervous system (CNS).

Medical Conditions Generally Aggravated by Exposure: Known hypersensitivity to this drug; reproductive and pregnancy issues

Specific Medical Surveillance Information: Reproductive and pregnancy counseling

Occupational Exposure Level/Limit (OEL) & Sampling Methods:

Environmental Sentinel Contamination Action Level (ESCAL): N.O.S.
LEUPROLIDE ACETATE OEL (ABBOTT LABORATORIES):
8 hr TWA   0.05 μ/m3 (ABBOTT LAB)
(Method Not Listed or Specified)

LEVAMISOLE OEL—JANSSEN PHARMACEUTICA:
0.15 mg/m3
(Method Not Listed or Specified)

LEVAMISOLE HCL (ACGIH TLV®):
2.5 mg/m3 TWA
5 mg/m3 STEL
(Method Not Listed or Specified)

Supplemental Response Information

Extinguishing Media: Use extinguishing agent most appropriate to extinguish surrounding fire (carbon dioxide, foam, dry chemical or water fog as extinguishing media)

Solubility: LEVAMISOLE (Ergamisol®74) is freely soluble in water (21g/100ml at 20 deg C). pH is reported to be 9.8 (at concentration: 6.5 g/l) LEVAMISOLE is soluble in alcohol, practically insoluble in ether, slightly soluble in dichloromethane.

Chemical Degradation/Neutralization Method: Not otherwise specified

Note: If a specific degradation or neutralization method is not provided on this table and you do not have other specific information that will guide you on how to clean-up the specific material spilled, then follow the general spill procedure found at the introduction section of this table.

Incompatibility: LEVAMISOLE HYDROCHLORIDE is incompatible with strong oxidizing agents.

LOMUSTINE (*lo-MUS-teen*)
CCNU
CEENU®75
CEENU

Chemical Abstracts Service (CAS) Registry
    Numbers: 13010-47-4
Registry of Toxic Effects of Chemical Substance
    (RTECS): YS4900000
National Cancer Institute:
$(C_9H_{16}C_1N_3O_2)$

Health & Safety Hazards/US Department of Transportation (DOT)/US Environmental Protection Agency (EPA)—Sources

Mutagen—Registry of Toxic Effects of Chemical Substance, Mutagen—ToxReport, Reproductive Effector—ToxReport, Pregnancy Category (D)—Food and Drug Administration, Cancer and Developmental Effector-US California State Proposition 65, Avoid Breastfeeding-US Navy Ref, Mutagen-University of Maryland at College Park, Carcinogen-University of Maryland at College Park, Carcinogen C2-US National Toxicology Program, Carcinogen G2A-International Agency For Research On Cancer, Carcinogen—US National Institute for Occupational Safety and Health,/ Material Safety Data Sheet, Teratogen—US National Institute for Occupational Safety and Health/Material Safety Data Sheet, Teratogen—University of Maryland at College Park, Embryotoxic—US National Institute for Occupational Safety and Health/Material Safety Data Sheet, Toxic—National Institute for Occupational Safety and Health/Material Safety Data Sheet
LOMUSTINE—Blue and clear capsules 40 mg
LOMUSTINE—A yellow crystalline powder

First Aid/Medical Information/Occupational Exposure Limits

First aid measures to include: Use general first aid measures
Medical information:
Dermal contact: Avoid rubbing of skin or increasing its temperature. Do not rinse with organic solvents.
Caution and Warning Statements:

LOMUSTINE is absorbed through the respiratory and intestinal tracts and transplacentally. RTECS lists LOMUSTINE as a suspected: cardiovascular or blood toxicant; as a gastrointestinal or as a liver toxicant; as a kidney toxicant and as a neurotoxicant. LOMUSTINE (1-(2-chloroethyl)-3-cyclo-hexyl-1-nitrosourea) can irritate the skin, eyes, nose and throat. Exposure may cause loss of appetite, nausea and vomiting. Liver and kidneys may sustain damage if exposure is high enough.

Caution: Females and males planning to have a child, pregnant women, and nursing mothers should exercise caution regarding potential occupational exposure to this cytotoxic drug. No information or not enough information exists or was provided concerning occupational exposure that may potentially occur while handling this drug and its affects on reproductive systems, the fetus and/or if it is secreted along with breast milk, which may harm nursing infants. Staff members should consult with the occupational health physician monitoring workers' health in your facility to be apprised of potential hazards and should be advised to avoid becoming pregnant and/or breast feeding or should be transferred in accordance with policy/procedures to other duties that do not involve preparation, handling, and administering this drug.

Therapeutic levels: LOMUSTINE is in the FD Pregnancy Category D. This means that LOMUSTINE is known to cause birth defects in an unborn baby. LOMUSTINE may also affect egg production in women and sperm production in men. Contraceptive measures are recommended during treatment with LOMUSTINE. It is not known whether LOMUSTINE passes into breast milk.

Target Organs/Systems: Bone marrow suppression, notably thrombocytopenia, leukopenia, liver, and kidneys (possibly reproductive and fetus)
Medical Conditions Generally Aggravated by Exposure: Reproductive and pregnancy issues.
Specific Medical Surveillance Information: Reproductive and Pregnancy Counseling. If symptoms develop and/or overexposure is suspected, it is recommended to perform liver and kidney functions tests.
Occupational Exposure Contamination Level/Limit (OEL) & Sampling Methods: Not otherwise specified
Environmental Sentinel Contamination Action Level (ESCAL): Not otherwise specified.

Supplemental Response Information

Extinguishing Media: Use extinguishing agent most appropriate to extinguish surrounding fire (carbon dioxide, foam, dry chemical or water fog as extinguishing media)

Solubility: LOMUSTINE is water insoluble (<0.05 mg/ml). Soluble in 10% ethanol (0.05 mg/ml) and in absolute alcohol (70 mg/ml), freely soluble in acetone and in dichloromethane

Chemical Degradation/Neutralization Method: Not otherwise specified

Note: If a specific degradation or neutralization method is not provided on this table and you do not have other specific information that will guide you on how to clean-up the specific material spilled, then follow the general spill procedure found at the introduction section of this table.

Incompatibility: Not otherwise specified

MEGESTROL ACETATE

(*me-HES-trole*)
MEGESTROL
MEGACE®77

Chemical Abstracts Service (CAS) Registry
  Numbers: 595-33-5 3562-63-8
Registry of Toxic Effects of Chemical Substance
  (RTECS): TU4075000
National Cancer Institute:
($C_{24}H_{32}O_4$)

Health & Safety Hazards/US Department of Transportation (DOT)/US Environmental Protection Agency (EPA)—Sources

Carcinogen G1-International Agency for Research on Cancer, Carcinogen—Material Safety Data Sheet, Reproductive—Material Safety Data Sheet, Teratogen—Material Safety Data Sheet, Developmental—US California State Proposition 65, Pregnancy Category (X)—Food and Drug Administration

MEGESTROL ACETATE is available as an oral suspension and in tablets (20 mg and 40 mg) form

MEGESTROL ACETATE is a white to creamy-white crystalline powder, essentially odorless

First Aid/Medical Information/Occupational Exposure Limits

First aid measures to include: Use general first aid measures except for:

Ingestion: Immediately notify medical personal and supervisor. Drink 2–3 glasses of water and seek medical assistance. Vomiting may be induced if directed by medical personnel.

Medical Information:
Caution and Warning Statements:

MEGESTROL ACETATE is a reproductive hazard and a carcinogen (limited evidence). Exposure may cause adverse reproductive effects in males and/or females. This material may cause cancer in animals and/or humans. Avoid exposure. Do not get on skin, eyes, on clothing. Do not breathe dust, vapor, mist or gas. Signs of overexposure are nausea, vomiting, and vaginal bleeding. Rare side effects are edema, deep vein thromobophlebitis, carpal tunnel syndrome and alopecia. Odor is a slight lemon-lime odor.

Caution: Females and males planning to have a child, pregnant women, and nursing mothers should exercise caution regarding potential occupational exposure to this cytotoxic drug. No information or not enough information exists or was provided concerning occupational exposure that may potentially occur while handling this drug and its affects on reproductive systems, the fetus and/or if it is secreted along with breast milk, which may harm nursing infants. Staff members should consult with the occupational health physician monitoring workers' health in your facility to be apprised of potential hazards and should be advised to avoid becoming pregnant and/or breast feeding or should be transferred in accordance with policy/procedures to other duties that do not involve preparation, handling, and administering this drug.

Therapeutic Levels: As the potential of teratogenic effects exists, pregnant women should avoid exposure (especially during the first four months of pregnancy).

Target Organs/Systems: (Female and male) reproductive, blood vessels, CNS, breast, and fetus congenital malformation.

Medical Conditions Generally Aggravated by Exposure: This compound is contraindicated in people with a known sensitivity to MEGESTROL ACETATE, a history or active case of thrombophlebitis, thromboembol disorders, cerebral apoplexy, carcinoma of the breast, asthma, and undiagnosed vaginal bleeding or pregnancy.

Specific Medical Surveillance Information: Reproductive and pregnancy counseling. Routine medical surveillance: a complete blood count differential should be taken to provide a baseline.

Occupational Exposure Level/Limit & Sampling Methods:

Environmental Sentinel Contamination Action Level (ESCAL):
PHARMACIA & UPJOHN /PHARMACIA & UPJOHN

40 µg/m3 TWA
(Method Not Listed or Specified)

ALAN(1) (*mel-fa-lan*)
PHENYLALANINE MUSTARD
ALKERAN®79

Chemical Abstracts Service (CAS) Registry
  Numbers: 8057-25-8 148-82-3
Registry of Toxic Effects of Chemical Substance
  (RTECS): AY3675000
National Cancer Institute: NSC 8806
$(C_{13}H_{18}Cl_2N_2O_2)$
(Two Degradation Methods)

Health & Safety Hazards/US Department of Transportation (DOT)/US Environmental Protection Agency (EPA)—Sources

Carcinogen C1-National toxicology Program/ Fact Sheet, Carcinogen G1-International Agency for Research on Cancer, Carcinogen—University of Maryland at College Park, Carcinogen-Berkeley University Hazardous Chemical List, Carcinogen—Material Data Sheet, Mutagen—ToxReport/Material Data Sheet, FDA Pregnancy Category (D)—Food and Drug Administration/Material Safety Data Sheet, Highly Toxic—Material Safety Data Sheet, Avoid Breastfeeding Ref., Reproductive Effector—ToxReport, reproductive Effector—Material Safety Data Sheet, Reproductive Effector—US National Institute of Environmental Health Sciences (NIEHS), Teratogen—Material Data Sheet, Cytotoxic—British Columbia Cancer Agency Canada/Material Safety Data Sheet, Vesicant—British Columbia Cancer Agency Canada, Skin Sensitizer—Material Safety Data Sheet, Developmental and Carcinogen—US California State Proposition 65

MELPHALAN—White tables 2 mg/or colorless fluid form powder

MELPHALAN—A white or almost white powder or off-white to buff powder with a faint odor

First Aid/Medical Information/Occupational Exposure Limits

First aid measures to include: Use general first aid measures except for the following:

Physician's note (A):

1. For recent ingestion, perform gastric lavage and administer activated charcoal.

2. Hematologic parameters should be closely followed for at least 3 to 6 weeks.
3. For bone marrow depression, transfusions of fresh blood may be required.
4. Individuals who develop leukopenia should be observed for signs of infection; antibiotic support may be required.
5. Treatment with colony stimulating factors may shorten the duration of pancytopenia. If mucositis prevents oral intake of nutrition, parenteral nutrition may be used.
6. General supportive measures should be employed; antibiotic therapy is advisable.

Physician's note (B): Medical treatment in cases of overexposure should be treated as an overdose of a cytotoxic agent. In allergic individuals, exposure to this material may require treatment for initial or delayed allergic symptoms and signs. This may include immediate and/or delayed treatment of anaphylactic reactions. Treat according to locally accepted protocols. For additional guidance, refer to the local poison control information center. Antidotes: no specific antidotes are recommended.

Medical Information:

Caution and Warning Statements:

MELPHALAN is a cytotoxic agent, which is highly toxic. Route of exposure: ingested, inhalation or through skin contact. MELPHALAN is known to react with DNA and as such may pose a carcinogenic, mutagenic and teratogenic risk. MELPHALAN may cause skin reactions and sensitization by contact. RTECS lists MELPHALAN as a suspected: cardiovascular or blood toxicant; and as a gastrointestinal or liver toxicant.

The immediate effects of overdose are severe nausea and vomiting. Decrease consciousness, convulsions, cholinomimetic effects and muscular paralysis are less frequently seen. Severe mucositis, stomatitis, colitis, diarrhea and hemorrhage of the gastrointestinal tract can occur at doses exceeding 100 mg/m2. The principle toxic effect in therapeutic use is bone marrow aplasia; resulting in pronounced decreased in numbers of formed elements (cells) of the blood (pancytopenia). No antidotes exist, but administration of autologous bone marrow or hematopoietic growth factors (gm-csf, g-csf) may shorten the period of pancytopenia.

Caution: Females and males planning to have a child, pregnant women, and nursing mothers should exercise caution regarding potential occupational exposure to this cytotoxic drug. No information or not enough information exists or was provided concerning occupational exposure that may potentially occur while handling this drug and its affects on reproductive systems, the fetus and/or if it is secreted along with breast milk, which may harm nursing infants. Staff members should consult with the occupational health physician monitoring workers' health in your facility to be apprised of potential hazards and should be advised to avoid becoming pregnant and/or breast feeding or should be transferred in accordance with policy/procedures to other duties that do not involve preparation, handling, and administering this drug.

Therapeutic Levels: there are no adequate and well-controlled studies in pregnant women. It is not known whether this drug is excreted in human milk.

Target Organs/Systems: Skin, liver and kidneys, dividing cells, GI tract, CNS, bone marrow, reproductive systems (adverse effects on fertility), fetus, and blood (may cause cancer).

Medical conditions generally aggravated by exposure: Hypersensitivity to material, blood disorders, a history or active case of thrombophlebitis, thromoboembolic disorders, cerebral apoplexy, carcinoma of the breast, asthma, undiagnosed vaginal bleeding, pregnancy, bone marrow depression, existing or recent chickenpox, herpes zoster, history of gout or urate renal stones, infection, impaired kidney function, and recent cytotoxic drug or radiation therapy. MELPHANAL—ocular symptoms may be indicative of allergic reaction. Reproductive and pregnancy issues

Specific Medical Surveillance Information: Reproductive and pregnancy counseling

If symptoms develop and/or overexposure is suspected, order a complete blood count should be performed along with liver and kidney functions tests.

Occupational Exposure Limits/Levels & Sampling Methods:

Environmental Sentinel Contamination Action Level:
   Not otherwise specified
OEL-GW
μ/m3 8-hr TWA (one MSDS)
1.0 μ/m3 8-hr TWA (one MSDS)
0.0025 mg/m3 (maximum exposure limit)
   (MSDS)(1996)
DOE: TEEL-3 23.0 mg/m3
(Method Not Listed or Specified)

Supplemental Response Information

Extinguishing Media: Use extinguishing agent most appropriate to extinguish surrounding fire (carbon di-oxide, foam, dry chemical or water fog as extinguishing media). **Warning**: Ignition of a dust cloud produces a weak explosion. Dust clouds are very sensitive to electrostatic ignition. Carbon dioxide extinguishers may not be effective.

Solubility: MELPHALAN is practically water insoluble; practically insoluble in chloroform and ether while being slightly soluble in ethanol, propylene glycol; dissolves in dilute mineral acids.

Chemical Degradation/Neutralization Method:

There are two or more recommended procedures for MELPHALAN. See below for optional method: The International Agency for Research on Cancer (IARC) recommended degradation method for MELPHALAN:

The IARC recommends treating spill surfaces with a 5.25% sodium hypochlorite (bleach) solution after absorbing liquids with inert absorbent pads or removing any powder present: allow solution to stand for up to one hour, and then thoroughly wash spilled surfaces with soap and water, sample to determine if surface contamination is still present (if sampling method is available). If it is still present repeat above steps, dispose of wastes in accordance with your local procedures, state, and federal regulations.

Incompatibility: Not otherwise specified
MELPHALAN: Conditions to avoid direct sunlight, conditions that might generate heat and dispersion of a dust cloud.

MELPHALAN(2) *(mel-fa-lan)*
PHENYLALANINE MUSTARD
ALKERAN®79

Chemical Abstracts Service (CAS) Registry
   Numbers: 8057-25-8 148-82-3
Registry of Toxic Effects of Chemical Substance
   (RTECS): AY3675000
National Cancer Institute: NSC 8806
($C_{13}H_{18}Cl_2N_2O_2$)
(Two Degradation Methods)

Health & Safety Hazards/US Department of Transportation (DOT)/US Environmental Protection Agency (EPA)—Sources

Carcinogen C1-National toxicology Program/ Fact Sheet, Carcinogen G1-International Agency for Research on Cancer, Carcinogen—University of Maryland at College Park, Carcinogen—Berkeley University Hazardous Chemical List, Carcinogen—Material Data Sheet, Mutagen—ToxReport/ Material Data Sheet, FDA Pregnancy Category (D)—

Food and Drug Administration/Material Safety Data Sheet, Highly Toxic—Material Safety Data Sheet, Avoid Breastfeeding Ref., Reproductive Effector—ToxReport, reproductive Effector—Material Safety Data Sheet, Reproductive Effector—US National Institute of Environmental Health Sciences (NIEHS), Teratogen-Material Data Sheet, Cytotoxic—British Columbia Cancer Agency Canada/Material Safety Data Sheet, Vesicant-British Columbia Cancer Agency Canada, Skin Sensitizer—Material Safety Data Sheet, Developmental and Carcinogen—US California State Proposition 65

MELPHALAN—White tables 2 mg/or colorless fluid form powder

MELPHALAN—A white or almost white powder or off-white to buff powder with a faint odor

First Aid/Medical Information/Occupational Exposure Limits

First Aid Measures to include: Use general first aid measures except for the following:

Physician's note (A):

1. For recent ingestion, perform gastric lavage and administer activated charcoal.
2. Hematologic parameters should be closely followed for at least 3 to 6 weeks.
3. For bone marrow depression, transfusions of fresh blood may be required.
4. Individuals who develop leukopenia should be observed for signs of infection; antibiotic support may be required.
5. Treatment with colony stimulating factors may shorten the duration of pancytopenia. If mucositis prevents oral intake of nutrition, parenteral nutrition may be use.
6. General supportive measures should be employed; antibiotic therapy is advisable.

Physician's note (B): Medical treatment in cases of overexposure should be treated as an overdose of a cytotoxic agent. In allergic individuals, exposure to this material may require treatment for initial or delayed allergic symptoms and signs. This may include immediate and/or delayed treatment of anaphylactic reactions. Treat according to locally accepted protocols. For additional guidance, refer to the local poison control information center. Antidotes: no specific antidotes are recommended.

Medical Information:

Caution and Warning Statements:

MELPHALAN is a cytotoxic agent, which is highly toxic. Route of exposure: ingested, inhalation or through skin contact. MELPHALAN is known to react with DNA and as such may pose a carcinogenic, mutagenic and teratogenic risk. MELPHALAN may cause skin reactions and sensitization by contact. RTECS lists MELPHALAN as a suspected: cardiovascular or blood toxicant; and as a gastrointestinal or liver toxicant.

The immediate effects of overdose are severe nausea and vomiting. Decrease consciousness, convulsions, cholinomimetic effects and muscular paralysis are less frequently seen. Severe mucositis, stomatitis, colitis, diarrhea and hemorrhage of the gastrointestinal tract can occur at doses exceeding 100 mg/m2. The principle toxic effect in therapeutic use is bone marrow aplasia; resulting in pronounced decreased in numbers of formed elements (cells) of the blood (pancytopenia). No antidotes exist, but administration of autologous bone marrow or hematopoietic growth factors (gm-csf, g-csf) may shorten the period of pancytopenia.

Caution: Females and males planning to have a child, pregnant women, and nursing mothers should exercise caution regarding potential occupational exposure to this cytotoxic drug. No information or not enough information exists or was provided concerning occupational exposure that may potentially occur while handling this drug and its affects on reproductive systems, the fetus and/or if it is secreted along with breast milk, which may harm nursing infants. Staff members should consult with the occupational health physician monitoring workers' health in your facility to be appraised of potential hazards and should be advised to avoid becoming pregnant and/or breast feeding or should be transferred in accordance with policy/procedures to other duties that do not involve preparation, handling, and administering this drug.

Therapeutic Levels: there are no adequate and well-controlled studies in pregnant women. It is not known whether this drug is excreted in human milk.

Target Organs/Systems: Skin, liver and kidneys, dividing cells, GI tract, CNS, bone marrow, reproductive systems (adverse effects on fertility), fetus, and blood (may cause cancer).

Medical Conditions Generally Aggravated by Exposure: Hypersensitivity to material, blood disorders, a history or active case of thrombophlebitis, thromoboembolic disorders, cerebral apoplexy, carcinoma of the breast, asthma, undiagnosed vaginal bleeding, pregnancy, bone marrow depression, existing or recent chickenpox, herpes zoster, history of gout or urate renal stones, infection, impaired kidney function, and recent cytotoxic drug or radiation therapy. MELPHALAN—ocular symptoms may be indicative of allergic reaction. Reproductive and pregnancy issues.

Specific Medical Surveillance Information: Reproductive and pregnancy counseling. If symptoms develop and/or overexposure is suspected, order a complete blood count should be performed along with liver and kidney functions tests.

Occupational Exposure Limits/Levels & Sampling Methods

Environmental Sentinel Contamination Action Level: OEL-GW
μ/m3 8-hr TWA (one MSDS)
1.0 μ/m3 8-hr TWA (one MSDS)
0.0025 mg/m3 (maximum exposure limit) (MSDS)(1996)
DOE: TEEL-3 23.0 mg/m3
(Method Not Listed or Specified)

Supplemental Response Information

Extinguishing Media: Use extinguishing agent most appropriate to extinguish surrounding fire (carbon dioxide, foam, dry chemical or water fog as extinguishing media).

Warning: Ignition of a dust cloud produces a weak explosion. Dust clouds are very sensitive to electrostatic ignition. Carbon dioxide extinguishers may not be effective.

Solubility: MELPHALAN is practically water insoluble; practically insoluble in chloroform and ether while being slightly soluble in ethanol, propylene glycol; dissolves in dilute mineral acids.

Chemical Degradation/Neutralization Method:
There are two or more recommended procedures for MELPHALAN. See below for optional method:

A manufacturer's MSDS recommends treating spill surfaces with a ~2 mol/liter (~8 g/100 ml), aqueous caustic soda (sodium hydroxide) solution after absorbing liquids with inert absorbent pads or removing any powder present: allow solution to stand for up to one hour, and then thoroughly wash spilled surfaces with soap and water, sample to determine if surface contamination is still present (if sampling method is available). If it is still present repeat above steps, dispose of wastes in accordance with your local procedures, state, and federal regulations.

While another MSDS states use a 5% solution of caustic soda. Then wash down with water.

Incompatibility: Not otherwise specified

MELPHALAN: Conditions to avoid direct sunlight, conditions that might generate heat and dispersion of a dust cloud.

MENOGARIL
7-O-METHYLNOGAROL

Chemical Abstracts Service (CAS) Registry
   Numbers: 71628-96-1 69256-91-3 74202-31-6
Registry of Toxic Effects of Chemical Substance
   (RTECS): KD1146400
National Cancer Institute: NSC 269148
C28-H31-NO10

Health & Safety Hazards/US Department of Transportation (DOT)/US Environmental Protection Agency (EPA)—Sources

Mutagen—Registry of Toxic Effects of Chemical Substance, Mutagen—ToxReport, Reproductive Effector—ToxReport, Pregnancy Category (None)—Food and Drug Administration.

First Aid/Medical Information/Occupational Exposure Limits

First aid measures to include: Use general first aid measures.

Ingestion: Have victim drink a suspension of flour/starch/beaten eggs/milk to dilute and slowly absorb (if conscious and alert). Induce vomiting. Give 1–2 cups of water. A cathartic given with 1 tbls of magnesium sulfate dissolved in a glass of water should be given by mouth. Seek medical attention.

Medical Information:

Caution and Warning Statements:

Primary routes of entry are inhalation and ingestion. MENOGARIL can cause skin irritation. Exposure to MENOGARIL may cause adverse reproductive effects and bone marrow depression. At high doses may damage the heart muscle.

Caution: Females and males planning to have a child, pregnant women, and nursing mothers should exercise caution regarding potential occupational exposure to this cytotoxic drug. No information or not enough information exists or was provided concerning occupational exposure that may potentially occur while handling this drug and its affects on reproductive systems, the fetus and/or if it is secreted along with breast milk, which may harm nursing infants. Staff members should consult with the occupational health physician monitoring workers' health in your facility to be appraised of potential hazards and should be advised to avoid becoming pregnant and/or breast feeding or should be transferred in accordance with policy/procedures to other duties that do not involve preparation, handling, and administering this drug.

Target Organs/Systems: Blood counts (white blood counts, platelet count, heart, immune system, and possible reproductive systems and fetus.

Medical Conditions Generally Aggravated by Exposure: Therapeutic levels: If you have any of the following medical problems: chickenpox or exposure to chickenpox, gout, heart disease, congestive heart failure, shingles, kidney stones, liver disease, or other forms of cancer. Reproductive and pregnancy issues.

Specific medical surveillance information: Reproductive and pregnancy counseling.

Occupational Exposure Limits/Levels & Sampling Methods: Not otherwise specified

Environmental Sentinel Contamination Action Level (ESCAL): Not otherwise specified

Supplemental Response Information

Extinguishing Media: Use extinguishing agent most appropriate to extinguish surrounding fire (carbon dioxide, foam, dry chemical or water fog as extinguishing media)

Solubility: MEMOGARIL is water insoluble.

Chemical Degradation/Neutralization Method:

A manufacturer's MSDS recommends treating spill surfaces with a 10% sodium hypochlorite (bleach) solution after absorbing liquids with inert absorbent pads or removing any powder present: allow solution to stand for up to one hour, and then thoroughly wash spilled surfaces with soap and water, sample to determine if surface contamination is still present (if sampling method is available). If it is still present repeat above steps, dispose of wastes in accordance with your local procedures, state, and federal regulations.

Incompatibility: Not otherwise specified

MERCAPTOPURINE®80 (*mer-cap-toe-pure-een*)

6-MERCAPTOPURIN
6-PMERCAPURIN
Purinethol®80

Chemical Abstracts Service (CAS) Registry
    Numbers: 6112-76-1 50-44-2
Registry of Toxic Effects of Chemical Substance
    (RTECS): U09800000 UP0400000
National Cancer Institute: NSC755

(C5H4N4S)
(C5-H4-N4-S-H20)

Health & Safety Hazards/US Department of Transportation (DOT)/US Environmental Protection Agency (EPA)—Sources

Carcinogen—Material Safety Data Sheet, Carcinogen Berkeley University Hazardous Chemical List, Reproductive Effector—Material Safety Data Sheet, Acutely Toxic—Material Safety Data Sheet, Teratogen—Material Safety Data Sheet, Teratogen—University of Maryland at College Park, Avoid Breastfeeding—US Navy Ref./World Health Organization, Mutagen—University of Maryland at College Park, Developmental—US California State Proposition 65, FDA Pregnancy Category (D)—Food and Drug Administration, Mutagen—Material Safety Data Sheet, Embryotoxic—Material Safety Data Sheet, Cytotoxic—Material Safety Data Sheet

MERCAPTOPURINE—50 mg yellow colored tablets or10 mg capsules

MERCAPTOPURINE is a light yellow-to-yellow, crystalline powder, odorless or practically odorless

First Aid Medical Information/Occupational Exposure Limits

First aid measures to include: Use general first aid measures except for the following:

Ingestion: If swallowed, rinse out mouth with water and drink 2–4 cups of milk or water provided person is conscious and alert. Do not induce vomiting.

Physician's note: Physicians treat symptomatically and supportively

Eye Exposure: Immediately check for contact lenses and remove any contact lenses. Irrigate immediately with sodium bicarbonate solution, followed by copious quantities of running water for at least 15 minutes occasionally lifting the upper and lower lids. Obtain ophthalmologic evaluation.

Dermal Contact: Avoid rinsing skin with organic solvents or scanned with UV light. Avoid rubbing of skin or increasing its temperature.

Medical Information:

Caution and Warning Statements: The chemical, physical, and toxicological properties have not been thoroughly investigated. May cause cancer if exposure occurs. May produce adverse effects on human fertility. May produce adverse effects on the development of human offspring.

Exposure to 6-MERCAPTOPURINE may cause skin, eye and respiratory tract irritation. Exposure to

6-MERCAPTOPURINE has caused adverse reproductive and fetal effects in animals. Mutagenic effects have occurred in experimental animals.

Caution: Females and males planning to have a child, pregnant women, and nursing mothers should exercise caution regarding potential occupational exposure to this cytotoxic drug. No information or not enough information exists or was provided concerning occupational exposure that may potentially occur while handling this drug and its affects on reproductive systems, the fetus and/or if it is secreted along with breast milk, which may harm nursing infants. Staff members should consult with the occupational health physician monitoring workers' health in your facility to be appraised of potential hazards and should be advised to avoid becoming pregnant and/or breast feeding or should be transferred in accordance with policy/procedures to other duties that do not involve preparation, handling, and administering this drug.

Therapeutic Levels: Females and males planning to have a child, pregnant women, and nursing mothers should exercise caution regarding potential exposure to this drug. Woman receiving MERCATOPURINE in the first trimester of pregnancy have an increased incidence of abortion; the risk of malformation in offspring surviving first trimester exposure is not accurately known. No information or not enough information was provided concerning if the drug and/or metabolites are potentially secreted into breast milk.

Target Organs/Systems: Bone marrow (blood), liver, skin, eyes, respiratory tract, dividing cells, GI tract, fetus, and immune and reproductive systems.

Medical Conditions Generally Aggravated by Exposure: 6-MERCAPTOPURINE is readily absorbed by various body tissues through the intestinal tract and transplacentally. Reproductive and pregnancy issues.

Specific Medical Surveillance Information: Reproductive and pregnancy counseling. Medical surveillance—determine baseline CBC and liver function tests.

Occupational Exposure Limits/levels & Sampling Methods:

OEL-GSK:
MERCAPTOPURINE MONHYDRATE (PURINETHOL®80 TABLETS)
10 μ/m3 (8-hr TWA)
(Reproductive Hazard, Carcinogen)

Environmental Sentinel Contamination Action Level (ESCAL): Not otherwise specified
(Method Not Listed or Specified)

Supplemental Response Information

Extinguishing Media: Use extinguishing agent most appropriate to extinguish surrounding fire (carbon dioxide, foam, dry chemical or water fog as extinguishing media). (Do not use water jet.)

Solubility: 6-MERCAPTOPURINE monohydrate is water insoluble. (Negligible) furthermore, slightly soluble in alcohol (hot); dissolves in solution of alkali hydroxides; dissolves in solution of 2 n sulfuric acid; insoluble in acetone and in ether.

Chemical Degradation/Neutralization Method:
The IARC recommends treating spill surfaces with a 5.25% sodium hypochlorite (bleach) solution after absorbing liquids with inert absorbent pads or removing any powder present: allow solution to stand for up to one hour, and then thoroughly wash spilled surfaces with soap and water, sample to determine if surface contamination is still present (if sampling method is available). If it is still present repeat above steps, dispose of wastes in accordance with your local procedures, state, and federal regulations.

Incompatibility: 6-MERCAPTOPURINE monohydrate is incompatible with strong oxidizing agents, strong acids and bases.

METHOTREXATE(1) *(m-tho-trex-ate)*
MTX
AMETHOPTERIN
METHOTREX
RHEUMATREX

Chemical Abstracts Service (CAS) Registry
    Numbers: 59-05-2
Registry of Toxic Effects of Chemical Substance
    (RTECS): MA1225000
National Cancer Institute: NSC740
C28-H22-N2-O5
(Two Degradation Methods)

Health & Safety Hazards/US Department of Transportation (DOT)/US Environmental Protection Agency (EPA)—Sources

Carcinogen G3—International Agency for Research on Carcinogen, Carcinogen—Berkeley University Hazardous Chemicals List, Acutely Toxic—Material Safety Data Sheet, Teratogen—University of Maryland at College Park, Avoid Breastfeeding—US Navy Ref./World Health Organization, Mutagen—Material Safety Data Sheet, Reproductive Effector—Material Safety Data Sheet, Cytotoxic—British Columbia

Cancer Agency Canada, Teratogen—US National Institutes of Health (NIH) and Material Safety Data Sheet, Developmental—US California State Proposition 65, Embryotoxic—US National Institutes of Health (NIH), Fetotoxic—Material Safety Data Sheet

First Aid Medical Information/Occupational Exposure Limits

First aid measures to include: Use general first aid measures except for the following:

Ingestion: If victim is conscious and alert, induce vomiting immediately and seek medical attention.

Dermal Contact: Readily absorbed through the skin, avoid rubbing of skin or increasing its temperature.

Physician's note (A): After following general first aid measure, an emollient (anti-bacterial cream) can be applied. Seek medical assistance.

Physician's note (B):
METHOTREXATE overdose treatment may include the following:

1. Administer LEUCOVORIN as soon as possible. The efficacy of LEUCOVORIN in reducing METHOTREXATE toxicity decreases with time.
2. Monitor serum METHOTREXATE concentration to determine required dose and treatment duration of LEUCOVORIN.
3. Initiate systemic hydration and urinary alkalinization to prevent precipitation of METHOTREXATE and metabolites in renal tubules.
4. Dialysis is of limited value.

Medical Information:
Caution and Warning Statements:
METHOTREXATE (MTX) is toxic if ingested. May cause harm to unborn child (fetus). Exposure to skin and eyes may cause irritation. May cause heritable genetic effects based on in vitro data. May impair fertility. May cause liver and kidney damage. May cause dermatitis. May cause blood abnormalities. May cause bone marrow depression.

Signs and symptoms of overexposure are irritation, nausea, vomiting, loss of appetite, diarrhea, coughing, anemia, coughing, and congestion of lungs.

RTECS lists METHOTREXATE as a suspected: cardiovascular or as a blood toxicant; as a gastrointestinal or liver toxicant; as a neurotoxicant; as a respiratory toxicant; and as a skin or sense organ toxicant (RTECS).

Caution: *The toxicological properties of most cytotoxic drugs have not been fully investigated, particularly as it pertains to occupational exposure. METHOTREXATE (MTX) is one of the drugs that have little occupational hazards information available. Therefore, therapeutic dose information was extrapolated below to assist in determining occupational toxicity, and signs and symptoms of overexposure. Therefore, it is prudent to minimize occupational exposure to METHOTREXATE (MTX).*

Possible side effects can include anemia, neutropenia, increased risk of bruising, and nausea. A small percentage of patients develop hepatitis, while there is an increased risk of pulmonary fibrosis. The higher doses of METHOTREXATE often used in cancer chemotherapy can cause toxic effects to the rapidly dividing cells of bone marrow and gastrointestinal mucosa. The resulting myelosuppression and mucositis are often prevented (termed METHOTREXATE "rescue") by using folinic acid supplements (not to be confused with folic acid).

Caution: Females and males planning to have a child, pregnant women, and nursing mothers should exercise caution regarding potential occupational exposure to this cytotoxic drug. No information or not enough information exists or was provided concerning occupational exposure that may potentially occur while handling this drug and its affects on reproductive systems, the fetus and/or if it is secreted along with breast milk, which may harm nursing infants. Staff members should consult with the occupational health physician monitoring workers' health in your facility to be appraised of potential hazards and should be advised to avoid becoming pregnant and/or breast feeding or should be transferred in accordance with policy/procedures to other duties that do not involve preparation, handling, and administering this drug.

Therapeutic Levels: METHOTREXATE is a highly teratogenic drug and categorized in pregnancy category X by the FDA. METHOTREXATE may pass through the placental barrier and may be excreted in maternal milk in human. May cause adverse reproductive effects (testicular and ovarian damage, sperm abnormalities, menstrual disorders, fetotoxicity, embryotoxicity, and post-implantation mortality). May affect genetic material (mutagenic).

Target Organs/Systems: Bone marrow, blood, immune system, liver and kidneys, GI tract, skin, lungs, fetus, and reproductive systems.

Medical Conditions Generally Aggravated by Exposure: Hypersensitivity to material, active alcoholism, ascites, pleural or peritoneal effusions, impaired liver or kidney function, bone marrow depression, immunodeficiency, infection, chickenpox (existing or recent), herpes zoster, oral mucositis, peptic ulcer or ulcerative colitis, and previous cytotoxic drug or radiation therapy.

Chronic therapeutic use of METHOTREXATE is reported to cause marked depression of bone marrow function (resulting in anemia [a decrease in the number of circulating red blood cells)], leukopenia [decrease in the number of white blood cells], and thrombocytopenia [decrease in platelets]), gastrointestinal bleeding, and liver damage. In addition, there are clinical reports of effects on fertility (male and female), menstrual dysfunction, liver function changes, hematologic (blood) changes, suppression of the immune system, induced lung disease (which may not be reversible), and chromosomal changes associated with the therapeutic use of this material. Eye irritation, possibly due to reduction in normal tear production, has been noted in approximately 25% of patients receiving METHOTREXATE therapeutically. Persons with pre-existing kidney function impairment may be more susceptible to the effects of METHOTREXATE due to elevated blood levels (a poorly-functioning kidney cannot get rid of the material in the urine, as normally occurs).

METHOTREXATE elimination is reduced in patients with impaired renal function, ascites, or pleural effusion.

Specific Medical Surveillance Information: Reproductive and pregnancy counseling. Complete homograms and liver/kidney function tests are recommended.

Occupational Exposure Limits/Levels & Sampling Methods:

Environmental Sentinel Contamination Action Level:
OEL: AMERICAN PHARMACEUTICAL
PARTNERS, INC.
OEL—METHOTREXATE: 0.5 µ/m3
OEL—AMERICAN CYANAMID
OEL—METHOTREXATE: 0.0007 mg/m3
OEL—AMERICAN CYANAMID
METHOTREXATE
Adult non-child bearing Potential:
5 consecutive days: 0.02 mg/m3
5 consecutive days: 0.01 mg/m3
Repeated at 7-to-9-day intervals
Daily exposure for 5 days or more: 0.001 mg/m3
Interrupted by not more than 2 days (e.g.,
   continuous repetition of a 5 day/week shift)
(Method Not Listed or Specified)

Supplemental Response Information

Extinguishing Media: Use extinguishing agent most appropriate to extinguish surrounding fire (carbon di-

oxide, foam, dry chemical or water fog as extinguishing media). (Do not use water jet.)

Solubility: METHOTREXATE is reported to be practically insoluble in (cold or hot) water. METHOTREXATE is insoluble in alcohol and chloroform. (pH = 8.5 to 8.7)

Chemical Degradation/Neutralization Method:

There are two recommended procedures for METHOTHREXATE. See below for methods:

A manufacturer's MSDS recommends treating spill surfaces with a ~2 mol/liter (~8 g/100 ml), aqueous caustic soda (sodium hydroxide) solution after absorbing liquids with inert absorbent pads or removing any powder present: allow solution to stand for up to one hour, and then thoroughly wash spilled surfaces with soap and water, sample to determine if surface contamination is still present (if sampling method is available). If it is still present repeat above steps, dispose of wastes in accordance with your local procedures, state, and federal regulations.

Incompatibility: METHOTREXATE (MTX) is incompatible with strong acid, strong alkaline solution and strong oxidizing agents. Furthermore, avoid storage near water reactive materials, light, heat and moisture.

METHOTREXATE(2) *(m-tho-trex-ate)*

MTX
AMETHOPTERIN
METHOTREX
RHEUMATREX

Chemical Abstracts Service (CAS) Registry
   Numbers: 59-05-2
Registry of Toxic Effects of Chemical Substance
   (RTECS): MA1225000
National Cancer Institute: NSC740
C28-H22-N2-O5
(Two Degradation Methods)

Health & Safety Hazards/US Department of Transportation (DOT)/US Environmental Protection Agency (EPA)—Sources

Carcinogen G3—International Agency for Research on Carcinogen, Carcinogen—Berkeley University Hazardous Chemicals List, Acutely Toxic—Material Safety Data Sheet, Teratogen—University of Maryland at College Park, Avoid Breastfeeding—US Navy Ref./World Health Organization, Mutagen-Material Safety Data Sheet, Reproductive Effector—Material Safety Data Sheet, Cytotoxic—British Columbia Cancer Agency Canada, Teratogen—US National Institutes of

Health (NIH) and Material Safety Data Sheet, Developmental—US California State Proposition 65, Embryotoxic—US National Institutes of Health (NIH), Fetotoxic—Material Safety Data Sheet

First Aid Medical Information/Occupational Exposure Limits

First aid measures to include: Use general first aid measures except for the following:

Ingestion: If victim is conscious and alert, induce vomiting immediately and seek medical attention.

Dermal Contact: Readily absorbed through the skin, avoid rubbing of skin or increasing its temperature.

Physician's note (A): After following general first aid measure, an emollient (anti-bacterial cream) can be applied. Seek medical assistance.

Physician's note (B):
METHOTREXATE overdose treatment may include the following:

1. Administer LEUCOVORIN as soon as possible. The efficacy of LEUCOVORIN in reducing METHOTREXATE toxicity decreases with time.
2. Monitor serum METHOTREXATE concentration to determine required dose and treatment duration of LEUCOVORIN.
3. Initiate systemic hydration and urinary alkalinization to prevent precipitation of METHOTREXATE and metabolites in renal tubules.
4. Dialysis is of limited value.

Medical Information:
Caution and Warning Statements:
METHOTREXATE (MTX) is toxic if ingested. May cause harm to unborn child (fetus). Exposure to skin and eyes may cause irritation. May cause heritable genetic effects based on in vitro data. May impair fertility. May cause liver and kidney damage. May cause dermatitis. May cause blood abnormalities. May cause bone marrow depression.

Signs and symptoms of overexposure are irritation, nausea, vomiting, loss of appetite, diarrhea, coughing, anemia, coughing, and congestion of lungs.

RTECS lists METHOTREXATE as a suspected: cardiovascular or as a blood toxicant; as a gastrointestinal or liver toxicant; as a neurotoxicant; as a respiratory toxicant; and as a skin or sense organ toxicant (RTECS).

Caution: *The toxicological properties of most cytotoxic drugs have not been fully investigated, particularly as it pertains to occupational exposure. METHOTREXATE (MTX) is one of the drugs that have little occupational hazards information available. Therefore, therapeutic dose information was extrapolated below to assist in determining occupational toxicity, and signs and symptoms of overexposure. Therefore, it is prudent to minimize occupational exposure to METHOTREXATE (MTX).*

Possible side effects can include anemia, neutropenia, increased risk of bruising, and nausea. A small percentage of patients develop hepatitis, while there is an increased risk of pulmonary fibrosis. The higher doses of METHOTREXATE often used in cancer chemotherapy can cause toxic effects to the rapidly dividing cells of bone marrow and gastrointestinal mucosa. The resulting myelosuppression and mucositis are often prevented (termed METHOTREXATE "rescue") by using folinic acid supplements (not to be confused with folic acid).

Caution: Females and males planning to have a child, pregnant women, and nursing mothers should exercise caution regarding potential occupational exposure to this cytotoxic drug. No information or not enough information exists or was provided concerning occupational exposure that may potentially occur while handling this drug and its affects on reproductive systems, the fetus and/or if it is secreted along with breast milk, which may harm nursing infants. Staff members should consult with the occupational health physician monitoring workers' health in your facility to be appraised of potential hazards and should be advised to avoid becoming pregnant and/or breast feeding or should be transferred in accordance with policy/procedures to other duties that do not involve preparation, handling, and administering this drug.

Therapeutic levels: METHOTREXATE is a highly teratogenic drug and categorized in pregnancy category X by the FDA. METHOTREXATE may pass through the placental barrier and may be excreted in maternal milk in human. May cause adverse reproductive effects (testicular and ovarian damage, sperm abnormalities, menstrual disorders, fetotoxicity, embryotoxicity, and post-implantation mortality). May affect genetic material (mutagenic).

Target Organs/Systems: Bone marrow, blood, immune system, liver and kidneys, GI tract, skin, lungs, fetus and reproductive systems.

Medical Conditions Generally Aggravated by Exposure: Hypersensitivity to material, active alcoholism, ascites, pleural or peritoneal effusions, impaired liver or kidney function, bone marrow depression, immunodeficiency, infection, chickenpox (existing or recent), herpes zoster, oral mucositis, peptic ulcer or ulcerative colitis, and previous cytotoxic drug or radiation therapy.

Chronic therapeutic use of METHOTREXATE is reported to cause marked depression of bone marrow function (resulting in anemia [a decrease in the number of circulating red blood cells], leukopenia [decrease in the number of white blood cells], and thrombocytopenia [decrease in platelets]), gastrointestinal bleeding, and liver damage. In addition, there are clinical reports of effects on fertility (male and female), menstrual dysfunction, liver function changes, hematologic (blood) changes, suppression of the immune system, induced lung disease (which may not be reversible), and chromosomal changes associated with the therapeutic use of this material. Eye irritation, possibly due to reduction in normal tear production, has been noted in approximately 25% of patients receiving METHOTREXATE therapeutically. Persons with preexisting kidney function impairment may be more susceptible to the effects of METHOTREXATE due to elevated blood levels (a poorly functioning kidney cannot get rid of the material in the urine, as normally occurs).

METHOTREXATE elimination is reduced in patients with impaired renal function, ascites, or pleural effusion.

Specific Medical Surveillance Information: Reproductive and pregnancy counseling. Complete homograms and liver/kidney function tests are recommended.

Occupational Exposure Limits/Levels & Sampling Methods:

Environmental Sentinel Contamination Action Level:
OEL: AMERICAN PHARMACEUTICAL
    PARTNERS, INC.
OEL—METHOTREXATE: 0.5 μ/m3
OEL—AMERICAN CYANAMID
OEL—METHOTREXATE: 0.0007 mg/m3
OEL—AMERICAN CYANAMID

METHOTREXATE
Adult non-child bearing Potential:
5 consecutive days: 0.02 mg/m3
5 consecutive days: 0.01 mg/m3
Repeated at 7-to-9-day intervals
Daily exposure for 5 days or more: 0.001 mg/m3
Interrupted by not more than 2 days (e.g.,
    continuous repetition of a 5 day/week shift)
(Method Not Listed or Specified)

Supplemental Response Information

Extinguishing Media: Use extinguishing agent most appropriate to extinguish surrounding fire (carbon dioxide, foam, dry chemical or water fog as extinguishing media). (Do not use water jet.)

Solubility: METHOTREXATE is reported to be practically insoluble in (cold or hot) water. METHOTREXATE is insoluble in alcohol and chloroform. (pH = 8.5 to 8.7)

Chemical Degradation/Neutralization Method:

There are two recommended procedures for METHOTHREXATE. See below for methods:

A manufacturer's MSDS recommends treating spill surfaces with 5% ammonium hydroxide solution after absorbing liquids with inert absorbent pads or removing any powder present: allow solution to stand for up to one hour, and then thoroughly wash spilled surfaces with soap and water, sample to determine if surface contamination is still present (if sampling method is available). If it is still present repeat above steps, dispose of wastes in accordance with your local procedures, state, and federal regulations.

Incompatibility: METHOTREXATE (MTX) is incompatible with strong acid, strong alkaline solution and strong oxidizing agents. Furthermore, avoid storage near water reactive materials, light, heat and moisture.

INDEXES 4

General Index

CAS Number	Drug Name (Nomenclature)	Page	Page
N.O.S.	Abatacept	15	15
57576-44-0	Acarubicin	15	17
75443-99-1	Aclarubicin	15	17
25316-40-9	Adriamycin	17	18
32214-92-8	Adriamycin	17	18
110942-02-4	Aldesleukin, Proleukin	18	20
216503-57-0	Alemtuzumab, Campath	20	21
150399-23-8	Altimta, Pemetrexed	21	22
645-05-6	Altretamine, Hexalen, Hemel	22	24
125-84-8	Aminoglutethimide, Cytadren	24	24
54301-15-4	Amsacrine	25	26
51264-14-3	Amsacrine, Amsacrine HCL	25	26
120511-73-1	Anastrozole, Arimidex	26	27
1327-53-3	Arsenic trioxide, Trisenox	27	30
9015-68-3	Asparaginase, l-Asparaginase	30	33
216974-75-3	Avastin, Bevacizumab	33	34
320-67-2	Azacytidine,	34	35
446-86-6	Azathioprine, Imuran	35	38
153559-49-0	Bexarotenum, Bexarotene	38	39
90357-06-5	Bicalutamide, Cascodex	39	40
71439-68-4	Bisantrene Hydrochloride	40	41
78186-34-2	Bisantrene Hydrochloride	40	41
9041-93-4	Bleomycin, Blenoxane	41	43
11056-06-7	Bleomycin, Blenoxane	41	43
67763-87-5	Bleomycin, Blenoxane	41	43
55-98-1	Busulfan, Myleran	43	44
136572-09-3	Camptosar, CPT	44	46
7689-03-4	Camptosar, CPT-11	44	46
97682-44-5	Camptosar, Irinotecan HCL, Camptothecin	44	46
100286-90-6	Camptosar, Irinotecan HCL, Camptothecin	44	46
111348-33-5	Camptosar, Irinotecan HCL, Camptothecin	44	46
154361-50-6	Capecitabine, Xeloda	46	47
158798-73-3	Capecitabine, Xeloda	46	47
41575-94-4	Carbonplatin, Diammine	47	51
7440-06-4	Carboplatin, Paraplatin	47	51

CAS Number	Drug Name (Nomenclature)	Page	Page
154-93-8	Carmustine, BCNU	51	52
305-03-3	Chlorambucil, CCNU, Leukeran	52	54
51-75-2	Chlormethine, Nitrogen Mustard	54	57
54749-90-5	Chlorozotocin, DCNU	57	58
113852-37-2	Cidofovir, Vistide	58	59
149394-66-1	Cidofovir, Vistide	58	59
15663-27-1	Cisplatin, Platinol AQ	59	61
4291-63-8	Cladribine, Leustatin	61	62
147-94-4	Cytarabine, Cytosar-u, Udicil	62	64
69-74-9	Cytosine Arabinoside, Alexan	66	67
6007-96-7	Cytoxan Anhydrous, Cycolophospamide	62	64
6007-95-6	Cytoxan Anhydrous, Cycolophospamide	62	64
6055-19-2	Cytoxan Anhydrous, Cycolophospamide	62	64
50-18-0	Cytoxan Anhydrous, Cycolophospamide, Neosar	62	64
60030-72-0	Cytoxan Anhydrous, Cycolophosphamide	62	64
4342-03-4	Dacarbazine, DTIC-DOME	69	70
37626-23-6	Dacarbazine, DTIC-DOME	69	70
55390-090-10	Dacarbazine, DTIC-DOME	69	70
50-76-0	Dacinomycin , Actinomycin D, Cosmegen	70	72
20830-81-3	Daunorubicin HCL, Cerubidine, Daunoxome	72	79
23541-50-6	Daunorubicin HCL, Cerubidine, Daunoxome	72	79
61825-94-3	Diaminocyclohexane Oxalatoplatinum, Elocatin	79	80
21436-03-3	Diaminocyclohexane Oxalatoplatinum, Eloxatin	79	80
23261-20-3	Dianhydrogalactitol (DAD), DAG	80	80
57998-68-2	Diaziquone, AZQ	80	81
528-74-5	Dichloromethotrexate	81	82
88442-77-7	Dichloromethotrexate	81	82
66395-18-4	Diethylstilbestrol Tozocin, Zanosar, Streptozocin	82	83
66395-17-3	Diethylstilbestrol Tozocin, Zanosar, Streptozocin	82	83
18883-66-4	Diethylstilbestrol Tozocin, Zanosar, Strptozocin	82	83
56420-45-2	Epirubicin, Ellen	84	86
56390-90-1	Epirubicin, Ellence	84	86
205923-56-4	Erbitux, Cetuximab	86	87
63521-85-7	Esorubicin	87	88
63950-06-1	Esorubicin	87	88
2998-57-4	Estramustine phosphate, Emcyt	88	89
33419-42-9	Etoposide, Vespesid	89	97
33419-42-0	Etoposide, Vespesid	89	97
98319-26-7	Finasteride, Proscar, Propecia	97	98
50-91-9	Floxuridine	98	99
51-21-8	Fluorouracil, 5-Fu	99	103
76-43-7	Fluoxymesterone, Halotestin	103	105
13311-84-7	Flutamide, Eulexin	105	106
84245-13-6	Ganciclovir, Cytovene	106	109
82410-32-0	Ganciclovir, Cytovene, Valcyte	106	109
220578-59-6	Gemtuzumab, Mylotarg	109	112
12211-03-9	Gemzar, Gemcitabine	112	113
95058-81-4	Gemzar, Gemcitabine HCL	112	113
65807-02-5	Goserelin Acetate, Zoladex	113	114

CAS Number	Drug Name (Nomenclature)	Page	Page
127-07-1	Hydroxyurea, Droxia	114	115
206181-63-7	Ibritumomab tiuxetan, Zevalin	115	116
57852-57-0	Idarubicin	116	118
58957-92-9	Idarubicin , Idamycin	116	118
3778-73-2	Ifosfamide, Ifex	118	120
66849-34-1	Ifosfamide, Ifex	118	120
66849-33-0	Ifosfamide, Ifex	118	120
84711-20-6	Ifosfamide, Ifex	118	120
19767-45-4	Ifosfamide, Ifex, Iphospamide	118	120
152459-95-5	Imatinib Mesylate, Gleevec	120	121
220127-57-1	Imatinibmesylate, Gleevec	120	121
9015-68-3	L-Asparaginase, Elspar. Leunase	30	33
53714-56-0	Leuprorelin, Leuprolide, Leuprolide Acetate	327	328
14769-73-4	Levamisole, Ergamiso	328	330
16595-80-5	Levamisole, Ergamisol	328	330
13010-47-4	Lomustine, CCNU, CEENU, CEECENU	330	331
55-86-7	Mechlorethamine HCL, Nitrogen Mustard	54	57
595-33-5	Megestrol acetate, Megace	331	332
3562-63-8	Megestrol acetate, Megace	331	332
8057-25-8	Melphalan, Alkeran	332	333
148-82-3	Melphalan, BCNU	333	335
69256-91-3	Menogaril	335	336
71628-96-1	Menogaril	335	336
74202-31-6	Menogaril	335	336
50-44-2	Mercaptopurine, Mercapurin	336	337
6112-76-1	Mercaptopurine, Mercapurin	336	337
59-05-2	Methotrexate, Amethopterin	337	341
75020-13-2	Methyl-gag, Mitogauazone	121	122
459-86-9	Methyl-gag, Mitoguazone	121	122
7059-23-6	Methyl-gag, Mitoguazone	121	122
50-07-7	Mitomycin C, Mutamycin	122	126
53-19-0	Mitotane, Lysodren	126	127
65271-80-9	Mitoxantrone HCL, Novantrone, DHAD	127	130
70476-82-3	Mitoxantrone HCL, Novantrone, DHAD	127	130
63612-50-0	Nilutamide, Anandron	130	131
61825-94-3	Oxaliplatin, Eloxatin	130	131
13909-02-9	PCNU	133	133
130167-69-0	Peg-Aspar, Oncaspar	133	134
150399-23-8	Pemetrexed, Alimta	21	22
140-64-7	Pentamidine, Ebupent	134	135
53910-25-1	Pentostatin, Nipent	135	136
18378-89-7	Plicamycin, Mithracin	137	138
53-03-2	Prednisone	138	139
366-70-1	Procarbazine, Matulane	139	141
24584-09-6	Razoxane, Zinecard	141	142
21416-67-1	Razoxane, Zinecard, Dexrazoxane	141	142
170277-31-3	Remicade, Inflixnab	142	143
331731-18-1	Remicade, Inflixnab	142	143
174722-31-7	Rituxan, Mobthera, Rituximab	143	144

CAS Number	Drug Name (Nomenclature)	Page	Page
13909-09-6	Semustine, Me-CCNU	144	145
33073-59-5	Semustine, ME-CCNU	144	145
33185-87-4	Semustine, ME-CCNU	144	145
56748-54-0	Semustine, ME-CCNU	144	145
56605-16-4	Spiromustine	145	146
10540-29-1	Tamoxifen Citrate, Nolvadex	146	147
54965-24-1	Tamoxifen Citrate, Nolvadex	146	147
33069-62-4	Taxol, Paclitaxel	147	151
114977-28-5	Taxotere, Docetaxel	151	152
17902-23-7	Tegafur, Ftorafur	152	153
37076-68-9	Tegafur, Ftorafur	153	153
85622-93-1	Temozolomide, Methazolastone	153	154
29767-20-2	Teniposide	154	155
154-42-7	Thioguanine	155	157
52-24-4	Thiotepa, Thioplex	157	160
123948-87-8	Topotecan, Hycamtin	160	162
192391-48-3	Tositumomab, Bexxar	162	163
208921-02-2	Tositumomab, Bexxar	162	163
31368-48-6	Triazinate	163	163
41191-04-2	Triazinate	163	163
82952-64-5	Trimetrexate, Neutrexin	163	165
66-75-1	Uramustine, Uracil Mustard	165	166
56124-62-0	Valrubicin, Valsar	166	167
179324-69-7	Velcase, Bortexomib	168	173
865-21-4	Vinblastine	168	173
143-67-9	Vinblastine, Velsar	166	167
57-22-7	Vincristine, Leurocristine	168	173
2068-78-2	Vincristine, Leurocristine	168	173
5364-48-4	Vindesine, Eldisine	175	176
71486-22-2	Vinorelbine tartrate, Navelbine	176	178
125317-39-7	Vinorelbine Tartrate, Navelbine	176	178

Index of CAS Number for Cytotoxic Drugs from Section 2.1

4.3

CAS Number	Drug Name (Nomenclature)	Page	Page
N.O.S.	Abatacept	15	15
50-91-9	Floxuridine	98	99
55-98-1	Busulfan, Myleran	43	44
55-86-7	Mechlorethamine HCL, Nitrogen Mustard	54	57
51-75-2	Chlormethine, Nitrogen Mustard	54	57
50-76-0	Dacinomycin , Actinomycin D, Cosmegen	70	72
69-74-9	Cytosine Arabinoside, Alexan	66	67
66-75-1	Uramustine, Uracil Mustard	165	166
50-44-2	Mercaptopurine, Mercapurin	336	337
51-21-8	Fluorouracil, 5-Fu	99	103
52-24-4	Thiotepa, Thioplex	157	160
76-43-7	Fluoxymesterone, Halotestin	103	105
57-22-7	Vincristine, Leurocristine	168	173
50-18-0	Cytoxan Anhydrous, Cycolophospamide, Neosar	62	64
125-84-8	Aminoglutethimide, Cytadren	24	24
53-19-0	Mitotane, Lysodren	126	127
50-07-7	Mitomycin C, Mutamycin	122	126
53-03-2	Prednisone	138	139
147-94-4	Cytarabinc, Cytosar-u, Udicil	62	64
59-05-2	Methotrexate, Amethopterin	337	341
154-93-8	Carmustine, BCNU	51	52
148-82-3	Melphalan, BCNU	337	341
143-67-9	Vinblastine, Velsar	166	167
140-64-7	Pentamidine, Ebupent	134	135
154-42-7	Thioguanine	155	157
127-07-1	Hydroxyurea, Droxia	114	115
320-67-2	Azacytidine,	34	35
366-70-1	Procarbazine, Matulane	139	141
305-03-3	Chlorambucil, CCNU, Leukeran	52	54
446-86-6	Azathioprine, Imuran	35	38
459-86-9	Methyl-gag, Mitoguazone	121	122
528-74-5	Dichloromethotrexate	81	82
595-33-5	Megestrol acetate, Megace	331	332
645-05-6	Altretamine, Hexalen, Hemel	22	24
865-21-4	Vinblastine	168	173
1327-53-3	Arsenic trioxide, Trisenox	27	30
2068-78-2	Vincristine, Leurocristine	168	173

CAS Number	Drug Name (Nomenclature)	Page	Page
2998-57-4	Estramustine phosphate, Emcyt	88	89
3562-63-8	Megestrol acetate, Megace	331	332
3778-73-2	Ifosfamide, Ifex	118	120
4291-63-8	Cladribine, Leustatin	61	62
4342-03-4	Dacarbazine, DTIC-DOME	69	70
5364-48-4	Vindesine, Eldisine	175	176
6007-96-7	Cytoxan Anhydrous, Cycolophospamide	62	64
6007-95-6	Cytoxan Anhydrous, Cycolophospamide	62	64
6055-19-2	Cytoxan Anhydrous, Cycolophospamide	62	64
6112-76-1	Mercaptopurine, Mercapurin	336	337
7059-23-6	Methyl-gag, Mitoguazone	121	122
7440-06-4	Carboplatin, Paraplatin	47	51
7689-03-4	Camptosar, CPT-11	44	46
8057-25-8	Melphalan, Alkeran	332	333
9015-68-3	Asparaginase, L-Asparaginase	30	33
9041-93-4	Bleomycin, Blenoxane	41	43
9015-68-3	L-Asparaginase, Elspar. Leunase	30	33
10540-29-1	Tamoxifen Citrate, Nolvadex	146	147
11056-06-7	Bleomycin, Blenoxane	41	43
12211-03-9	Gemzar, Gemcitabine	112	113
13010-47-4	Lomustine, CCNU, CEENU, CEECENU	330	331
13311-84-7	Flutamide, Eulexin	105	106
13909-09-6	Semustine, Me-CCNU	144	145
13909-02-9	PCNU	133	133
14769-73-4	Levamisole, Ergamiso	328	330
15663-27-1	Cisplatin, Platinol AQ	59	61
16595-80-5	Levamisole, Ergamisol	328	330
17902-23-7	Tegafur, Ftorafur	152	153
18378-89-7	Plicamycin, Mithracin	137	138
18883-66-4	Diethylstilbestrol Tozocin, Zanosar, Strptozocin	82	83
19767-45-4	Ifosfamide, Ifex, Iphospamide	118	120
20830-81-3	Daunorubicin HCL, Cerubidine, Daunoxome	72	79
21416-67-1	Razoxane, Zinecard, Dexrazoxane	141	142
21436-03-3	Diaminocyclohexane Oxalatoplatinum, Eloxatin	79	80
23261-20-3	Dianhydrogalactitol (DAD), DAG	80	80
23541-50-6	Daunorubicin HCL, Cerubidine, Daunoxome	72	79
24584-09-6	Razoxane, Zinecard	141	142
25316-40-9	Adriamycin	17	18
29767-20-2	Teniposide	154	155
31368-48-6	Triazinate	163	163
32214-92-8	Adriamycin	17	18
33069-62-4	Taxol, Paclitaxel	147	151
33073-59-5	Semustine, ME-CCNU	144	145
33185-87-4	Semustine, ME-CCNU	144	145
33419-42-9	Etoposide, Vespesid	89	97
33419-42-0	Etoposide, Vespesid	89	97
37076-68-9	Tegafur, Ftorafur	153	153
37626-23-6	Dacarbazine, DTIC-DOME	69	70
41191-04-2	Triazinate	163	163
41575-94-4	Carbonplatin, Diammine	47	51
51264-14-3	Amsacrine, Amsacrine HCL	25	26
53714-56-0	Leuprorelin, Leuprolide, Leuprolide Acetate	327	328

CAS Number	Drug Name (Nomenclature)	Page	Page
53910-25-1	Pentostatin, Nipent	135	136
54301-15-4	Amsacrine	25	26
54749-90-5	Chlorozotocin, DCNU	57	58
54965-24-1	Tamoxifen Citrate, Nolvadex	146	147
55390-090-10	Dacarbazine, DTIC-DOME	69	70
56124-62-0	Valrubicin, Valsar	166	167
56390-90-1	Epirubicin, Ellence	84	86
56420-45-2	Epirubicin, Ellen	84	86
56605-16-4	Spiromustine	145	146
56748-54-0	Semustine, ME-CCNU	144	145
57576-44-0	Acarubicin	15	17
57852-57-0	Idarubicin	116	118
57998-68-2	Diaziquone, AZQ	80	81
58957-92-9	Idarubicin , Idamycin	116	118
60030-72-0	Cytoxan Anhydrous, Cycolophosphamide	62	64
61825-94-3	Diaminocyclohexane Oxalatoplatinum, Elocatin	79	80
61825-94-3	Oxaliplatin, Eloxatin	130	131
63521-85-7	Esorubicin	87	88
63612-50-0	Nilutamide, Anandron	130	131
63950-06-1	Esorubicin	87	88
65271-80-9	Mitoxantrone HCL, Novantrone, DHAD	127	130
65807-02-5	Goserelin Acetate, Zoladex	113	114
66395-18-4	Diethylstilbestrol Tozocin, Zanosar, Streptozocin	82	83
66395-17-3	Diethylstilbestrol Tozocin, Zanosar, Streptozocin	82	83
66849-34-1	Ifosfamide, Ifex	118	120
66849-33-0	Ifosfamide, Ifcx	118	120
67763-87-5	Bleomycin, Blenoxane	41	43
69256-91-3	Menogaril	335	336
70476-82-3	Mitoxantrone HCL, Novantrone, DHAD	127	130
71439-68-4	Bisantrene Hydrochloride	40	41
71486-22-2	Vinorelbine tartrate, Navelbine	176	178
71628-96-1	Menogaril	335	336
74202-31-6	Menogaril	335	336
75020-13-2	Methyl-gag, Mitogauazone	121	122
75443-99-1	Aclarubicin	15	17
78186-34-2	Bisantrene Hydrochloride	40	41
82410-32-0	Ganciclovir, Cytovene, Valcyte	106	109
82952-64-5	Trimetrexate, Neutrexin	163	165
84245-13-6	Ganciclovir, Cytovene	106	109
84711-20-6	Ifosfamide, Ifex	118	120
85622-93-1	Temozolomide, Methazolastone	153	154
88442-77-7	Dichloromethotrexate	81	82
90357-06-5	Bicalutamide, Cascodex	39	40
95058-81-4	Gemzar, Gemcitabine HCL	112	113
97682-44-5	Camptosar, Irinotecan HCL, Camptothecin	44	46
98319-26-7	Finasteride, Proscar, Propecia	97	98
100286-90-6	Camptosar, Irinotecan HCL, Camptothecin	44	46
110942-02-4	Aldesleukin, Proleukin	18	20
111348-33-5	Camptosar, Irinotecan HCL, Camptothecin	44	46
113852-37-2	Cidofovir, Vistide	58	59
114977-28-5	Taxotere, Docetaxel	151	152
120511-73-1	Anastrozole, Arimidex	26	27

CAS Number	Drug Name (Nomenclature)	Page	Page
123948-87-8	Topotecan, Hycamtin	160	162
125317-39-7	Vinorelbine Tartrate, Navelbine	176	178
130167-69-0	Peg-Aspar, Oncaspar	133	134
136572-09-3	Camptosar, CPT	44	46
149394-66-1	Cidofovir, Vistide	58	59
150399-23-8	Altimta, Pemetrexed	21	22
150399-23-8	Pemetrexed, Alimta	21	22
152459-95-5	Imatinib Mesylate, Gleevec	120	121
153559-49-0	Bexarotenum, Bexarotene	38	39
154361-50-6	Capecitabine, Xeloda	46	47
158798-73-3	Capecitabine, Xeloda	46	47
170277-31-3	Remicade, Inflixnab	142	143
174722-31-7	Rituxan, Mobthera, Rituximab	143	144
179324-69-7	Velcase, Bortexomib	168	173
192391-48-3	Tositumomab, Bexxar	162	163
205923-56-4	Erbitux, Cetuximab	86	87
206181-63-7	Ibritumomab tiuxetan, Zevalin	115	116
208921-02-2	Tositumomab, Bexxar	162	163
216503-57-0	Alemtuzumab, Campath	20	21
216974-75-3	Avastin, Bevacizumab	33	34
220127-57-1	Imatinibmesylate, Gleevec	120	121
220578-59-6	Gemtuzumab, Mylotarg	109	112
331731-18-1	Remicade, Inflixnab	142	143

About the Author

Samuel J. Murff is currently a civilian Department of Defense contractor. Previously, he served as senior industrial hygienist with the US Army Center for Health Promotion and Preventive Medicine, providing cytotoxic drug consulting services.